Research and Innovation on the Road to Modern Child Psychiatry

Volume 2

Classic papers by

Professor Sir Michael Rutter

Research and Innovation on the Road to Modern Child Psychiatry

Volume 2

Classic papers by
Professor Sir Michael Rutter

Edited by Eric Taylor and Jonathan Green

GASKELL

© The Royal College of Psychiatrists 2001

Cover images:
Front: photographers Anita and John O'Grady, © The British Council 1989
Back: © The Wellcome Trust Medical Library 1996

Gaskell is an imprint of the Royal College of Psychiatrists
17 Belgrave Square, London SW1X 8PG
http://www.rcpsych.ac.uk

British Library Cataloguing-in-Publication Data
A catalogue record for this book is available from the British Library.
Volume 1: ISBN 1-901242-62-5
Volume 2: ISBN 1-901242-63-3

Distributed in North America by American Psychiatric Press, Inc.

The views presented in this book do not necessarily reflect those of the Royal College of Psychiatrists, and the publishers are not responsible for any error of omission or fact.

Gaskell is a registered trademark of the Royal College of Psychiatrists.
The Royal College of Psychiatrists is a registered charity (no. 228636).

Printed by Bell & Bain Limited, Glasgow, UK.

Contents

The development of developmental psychiatry:
a collection of writings 1965–1999
by Professor Sir Michael Rutter FRS

The scientific contribution of Michael Rutter

An appreciation

Eric Taylor

To look back over the past 40 years of child psychiatry is to witness an intellectual transformation. Forty years ago the subject was a marginal branch of medicine, seen with some puzzlement by the rest of the profession, treating small numbers of patients and isolated from the intellectual currents of the time. Now, it is an established medical speciality in many European countries, it often provides an advanced form of service delivery and organisation, and its scientific basis is growing. Many of the key current scientific concepts in medicine – developmental approaches to pathology, childhood contributions to adult disorders, the continuities and discontinuities between normality and pathology, and the interaction of genetic and environmental factors – draw on child psychiatric investigations and contribute to them. There is, of course, much to be done: many causes for regret at failures of the subject to develop, many challenges for the future. Nevertheless, the change in the subject has been remarkable.

Nobody has contributed more to this development than Michael Rutter. He not only provided classic studies that lie at the heart of the discipline: he also showed that they could be done. This volume provides a selection of his (and his collaborators') papers that have had a high impact on the development of the field. It is accompanied by another volume (Green & Yule, 2001), in which some of his colleagues and students describe the current state of topics that he illuminated. Together, they emphasise how much his contributions have been pervasive and have drawn upon a wide range of different scientific techniques and traditions. At one extreme, these have involved hard biological science, such as the sophisticated DNA neuroimaging technology involved in his autism work (this volume, pp. 85–102). At another extreme have been the methods of social science, quasi-experimental designs and analysis of nationally gathered indicator figures. Examples here include the studies of change in the mental health of pupils in schools when a new head teacher arrives (Rutter *et al*, 1979) and of the reasons for secular changes in adolescent psychopathology (Rutter & Smith, 1995). At the centre of the enterprise have been the methods and concepts of epidemiological medicine (this volume, pp. 32–41) and developmental psychology (this volume, pp. 3–31).

Eclecticism on this scale is not a weakness, but an essential part of the early development of a medical specialism. Clinical science sets out to investigate disorders where it is uncertain which scientific discipline will have most to contribute. The clinical scientist must collaborate with those basic disciplines in a leading and guiding way. It can be all too easy for a clinician trained in a basic discipline to develop exclusively down pathways that are of fundamental importance to the basic science and to neglect the applications that are most likely to illuminate pathology. The management and focusing of scientific approaches onto clinical questions is a key challenge that faces the clinical scientist.

I will not try here to enumerate the twists and turns of Michael Rutter's uniquely productive career. In the space of a chapter this would reduce to a listing of titles of studies. It would do scant justice to the contribution of someone who has been rightly critical of enumerative history – the listing of events and dates rather than the concentration on issues and themes. Rather, I shall try to select some themes from his work that are pervasive throughout his career and characteristic of his contribution.

Application of scientific method to new subjects

Forty years ago, child psychiatry was in the grip of certainties. There was a dominant ideology, built upon psychoanalysis, Piagetian psychology and social learning theory. Clinical services were organised around a 'Holy Trinity' of psychiatrists interviewing children, social workers interviewing parents and psychologists assessing cognitive and educational function. There was a clear view of pathogenesis. Juvenile delinquency was thought to result essentially from the long-standing sequelae of early failures of the attachment relationship; autism to result from an even more profound and earlier failure of the mother–child bond. Children were believed not to show the main disorders of adult life such as depression. When they did show such disorders it was supposed to be in a different form – 'masked depression' or 'childhood schizophrenia' presenting as autism. The main treatments were play-based psychotherapy and casework. As late as the 1960s in the UK, women were still being referred and accepted for psychotherapy because they had a child with autism whose disability testified to their supposed inability to love. There were disputes between psychiatrists on the developmental significance of an individual symptom that could only be resolved, and in practice were resolved, by which psychiatrist commanded the highest status. There was much that was insightful and humane in the profession, and we must take care that that is not lost in oversimple considerations of cost and price of treatment. Nevertheless, the intellectual basis needed a spring-clean. The tools that were needed, and Rutter brought, were scepticism and rigorous inquiry. The successive editions of the textbook *Child and Adolescent Psychiatry: Modern Approaches*, of which he has been senior editor for some 20 years, had as an epigraph a quotation from Al-Ghazari: "He who does not doubt, does not investigate, and he who does not investigate does not perceive, and he who does not perceive remains in blindness and error."

An example can be drawn from one of his most influential early reviews, on the role played by 'maternal deprivation' in the genesis of child psychiatric disorders (Rutter, 1972). This review was critical of some formulations of types of child psychopathology as specific manifestations of disruption of early attachment relationships. This criticism in its turn was attacked and misunderstood as an assertion of the opposite – that disruptions of attachment had no consequences whatever for psychopathology. The conclusion that should have been drawn was that empirical science could illuminate the area. This has proved to be the case. Social science was indeed able to replace the unexamined certainties of clinicians with empirical knowledge of the effects of early childhood experience (this volume, pp. 249–271). Longitudinal investigations have used reliable objective measures to identify different attachment problems in young children and to follow them forward to clarify the problems to which they are the antecedents. It is clear both that there are links and that these links are complex. Early adversity exerts strong effects through transactional influences, in which the adversity persists and brings about other forms of problems.

The true picture is both more worrying and more optimistic than that from the early formulations. More worrying, because the chain of adverse circumstances in young people's lives can have progressively more deleterious effects on personality and cognitive development as they grow. More optimistic, because the findings also emphasise resilience and plasticity in children and the extent to which it is possible to recover from dreadful adversity, provided – and the proviso is a difficult one – that the adversity is reversed. Michael Rutter's current investigations include work that has returned to just this issue of the consequences of early deprivation of maternal care. An experiment of nature – the adoption into British homes of children who had undergone devastating early privation in the orphanages of Romania – has allowed a longitudinal investigation of the consequences of that privation, the course of recovery, the limitations and constraints on recovery and the factors promoting resilience (Rutter & English Romanian Adoptees Study Team, 1998).

Many other examples could be adduced. Rutter's critique of so-called dyslexia (Rutter *et al*, 1970) was interpreted as an attack on the concept of reading disorders by neurologists who were firmly wedded to a simple neuromythology of a specific neurological deficit underlying disabilities in written language. Again, his position was not the assertion that there was no brain basis to reading problems, but an objection to the acceptance of that view without evidence and a concern that empirical science should guide the debate. Findings since then have emphasised the heterogeneity and complexity of the determinants of reading problems, as well as their association with some forms of neuropsychological deviation. Recent research by Rutter and his collaborators includes studies that take a longitudinal approach to explaining the course of people who have shown reading disability. It has, for instance, demonstrated that the development of psychiatric problems is not a fixed pathway and that, although reading problems persist, they need not be in themselves a risk for other forms of psychopathology (Maughan *et al*, 1996). This is in contrast to the findings of strong links in childhood between reading disability and psychopathology, and it emphasises how risks may work in different ways at different ages.

The ability to pose clinical issues in a way that makes them amenable to scientific investigations has done much to accelerate the quantity of scientific study. Rutter has achieved much in this by scientific administration as well as by direct example. One result has been the fall of grand theories. The great overarching systems developed by Freud, Piaget and the architects of social learning theory no longer have a major role in generating clinical and scientific hypotheses. What has taken their place has been, first, a growth in microtheories applied to particular areas (such as the reasons for the relationships between genetic constitution and environmental stresses in children's lives); and second, an approach that unifies a wide range of microtheories into a type of enquiry – developmental psychopathology. This approach, which is still being worked out, owes much to Rutter's formulations (e.g. this vol., pp. 3–31 & 32–41). It is categorised by a set of principles that will recur in this chapter: the interaction of biological and social factors in aetiology, and an emphasis on protective and risk factors rather than on taxons of psychopathology, and on the continuity and discontinuity between normal and pathological development. This approach is reviewed and taken further by Cicchetti in Volume 1 (Green & Yule, 2001: pp. 93–103).

Development and application of theory

■ ix

Recognition of biological factors

A major recent trend in child psychopathology has been the rise in biological explanations of disorder. The clearest example is perhaps that of autism (this vol., pp. 85–102 & 103–124); see also Volkmar's review in Volume 1 (Green & Yule, 2001: pp. 37–53). Rutter's early researches focused on delineating the necessary and sufficient clinical features for the recognition of this severe handicap and on describing the natural course of the disorder. Among other things this showed strong evidence for neurological dysfunction, rather than psychosocial stress, in the aetiology of the disorder. For example, the development of epilepsy in the subsequent course of children who had been diagnosed with autism was a frequent event and a strong pointer to the significance of brain dysfunction.

At that time, many very confident speculations were advanced by others, and brain damage mythologies were taking over from psychological mythologies in the guidance of clinical practice. We now know the major importance of genetic causes, but this was not at all apparent at the time. It is quite rare for a person with autism to have a sibling with the disorder and virtually unknown for autism to be handed down from parent to child. All these aspects had diverted the thinking of clinicians away from the possible role of genetic factors, and it is only when research with strongly informative genetic designs could be mounted that the truth became clear.

The development of an informative twin study of autism was a major step forward in investigation. It required several things – notably, a clear and accurate scheme of case-finding, which had been developed by the previous clinical investigations; and the identification of a national sample of twins with this rare disorder, which required not only the necessary administration but also the collaboration of an educated population of scientifically minded clinicians in the UK. Finally, of course, it needed the input of technically strong genetics. The result was very influential, because the ascertainment of the series had avoided the biases towards over-identifying concordant cases that come in self-selected series. The results were straightforward – the genetic contribution to autism is very strong, stronger indeed than that to any other psychiatrically defined syndrome.

This finding in turn led to further genetically informative studies on the mode of inheritance, with the strong suggestion that a relatively small number of genes is involved in the disorder. This step made feasible a current study, involving Europe-wide collaboration, applying DNA techniques to identify the actual genes involved, which has already reported replicated linkage sites (International Molecular Genetic Study of Autism Consortium, 1998).

Interaction of biological and psychosocial factors

The discovery of biological roots of disorder has been of great importance, but it is only the beginning of understanding. Current ideology in biological psychiatry sometimes seems to suggest that the physical disturbance of brain dysfunction is a sufficient means of understanding the expression of a disorder. There is no particular basis in science for this – it could be that all forms of psychopathology have associated brain dysfunctions, yet that their causes are psychosocial rather than physical; or, of course, it could be that the exact details of DNA variation and neurophysiological deviation will explain everything about a disorder, unlikely though this sounds. Rutter's work has consistently emphasised the complexity of factors that determine the expression of a biological risk (see also Taylor's review in Volume 1 (Green & Yule, 2001: pp. 81–92). For instance, some of his studies have focused on the reasons for the appearance of psychopathology in children with brain disorder. This has been a strong interest since the beginning of his investigative career. The epidemiological surveys in the Isle of Wight (see below) were designed in part to identify, without selection and referral bias, a group of children with known organic neurological dysfunction. The detailed investigation of these children made several things clear. Brain damage was a very strong risk, especially when there was evidence of pathological brain function (such as epilepsy) rather than simply loss of function of a region of brain. The risk was not for any one syndrome of brain damage: most children showed the same kinds of disorder that were shown by those with neurologically intact brains, albeit at increased rate. The lessons from this were continued in surveys of children with localised head injury, children recovering from severe head injury and the outcome of children with specific disorders of learning. The conclusions were plain and different from the conventional clinical wisdom that held sway before. The idea that there is a characteristic psychiatric syndrome of 'minimal brain damage' did not survive this combination of clear questioning and epidemiological evidence (this vol., pp. 199–211). While brain dysfunction is a very strong factor, it is also a diffuse one, and one whose manifestations depend critically upon interaction with the psychological environment.

Emphasis on social factors

The demonstration of the role of social factors in disorder has been one of the characteristic contributions of British psychiatry. It can be seen, for instance, in the Social Psychiatry Unit set up by Aubrey Lewis at the Maudsley Hospital in London, where Rutter worked in the 1960s. A recurring motif in Rutter's work has been the identification of the effects of social stress. For example, epidemiological comparisons of geographical areas have uncovered the impact of social stresses that differ between areas (this vol., pp. 314–318). Twin and adoptive studies (this vol., pp. 45–55) have given good evidence for the presence of both environmental and genetic contribution to common disorders and have emphasised the non-shared environment. The influence of parent–child relationships is strong (this vol., pp. 272–293, 294–313). There are other important programmes of investigation, for instance, into the effect of school qualities on the educational outcome of children and into the course of children who have spent part of their childhood in institutional care (see Maughan in Green & Yule, 2001: pp. 1–19). The importance of this work is not just to identify risk factors. It is not surprising to find that social adversity can be linked to adverse outcome. The interest of the studies lies much more in their approach to identifying the mechanisms involved in the operation of risk.

Longitudinal and epidemiological approaches to studying interactions

The mapping of the human genome and the clarification of genetic influences add new urgency to Rutter's emphasis that they act through interactions with environmental factors. The interplay between nature and nurture, rather than the polar opposition of their influences, becomes the focus of investigation. It makes very little sense to ask "Nature or nurture?" A whole family of questions must be considered, such as "How does nature restrict or expand the range of nurturing experience?" "How do nurturing influences modify the expression of nature?" and "Which precise aspects of nature and nurture are necessary, sufficient and contributory for individual forms of psychopathology?" It seems likely that the clarification of these will be the major preoccupation of child psychiatric investigators for some years to come.

Risk and protective factors must interact over periods of time to produce disorder. Simply to study their cross-sectional associations is unlikely to make it possible to say what is cause and what is effect. But to examine the risks in prospective longitudinal design has offered Rutter a powerful way of moving from the finding of an association to the demonstration of a pathogenetic mechanism. Several examples of this could be offered. Let us take the question of the associations between risk factors in children's upbringing and the development of behaviour disorders. The risks are strong, but what accounts for them?

One study focused on children reared by parents with mental illness, based on epidemiological samples and requiring both longitudinal study and comparisons with a general population sample (Rutter & Maughan, 1997). The expectation was that parental mental disorder would be a major risk factor in its own right. In the event, comparison between the sample of families with parental mental illness and a general population community sample showed that the two groups differed greatly in marital discord and in adverse parent–child relationships. Children in families with parental mental illness were much more likely to be exposed to hostile parenting than were those in the general population. In fact, the main effect on the children derived from hostile parenting, rather than from parental personality disorder.

At the time that this study was undertaken, the main focus in the research literature was on family-wide marital discord. The distinctive and unusual feature of this investigation was obtaining measures on the family environment as it impinged on each child at an individual level. It made it possible to show that the risk for the children derived mostly from child-specific risk experience within the family rather than overall family circumstances. Children with difficult temperaments tended to attract the hostility of parents with mental illness.

Another example can be drawn from the association between behaviour in childhood and adult experiences. One particularly important aspect of that effect concerns the choice of spouse or partner. A follow-up of children who had spent much of their upbringing in group foster homes showed that, compared with the general population sample, they were much more likely to have a partner with deviant behaviour involving antisocial activities, drug taking or alcohol problems. When women from high-risk backgrounds did happen to have a 'non-deviant' supportive partner, their adult functioning was very much better. The key question was whether that was simply because these women had been less antisocial themselves in childhood. The institutional sample was therefore combined with a general population sample also followed into adult life. It proved that there was a true turning-point effect by which the presence of support from a non-deviant partner was associated with a much better adult outcome among girls who had shown conduct disturbance in childhood. In the absence of such support, antisocial behaviour showed a strong likelihood of leading to pervasive social malfunction in adult life. By sharp contrast, women who were antisocial as children, but received support from a non-deviant partner, went on to good adult social functioning.

To understand how this protective effect came about, the intervening years were studied in greater detail. The question was why some young people with antisocial behaviour succeeded in making a harmonious relationship with a non-deviant partner whereas many did not. Both the age at which the women married and had their first child and (for any given age) the likelihood of the partner being antisocial were important.

Girls showing antisocial behaviour in childhood were much more likely to become a teenage parent and to have a 'deviant' partner. A range of possible influences were examined. Being part of a deviant peer group and having had an institutional rearing were associated with an increased risk of cohabitation with a deviant partner by age 20. A tendency to plan (to make deliberate decisions about key life choices) and the presence of a harmonious family environment were associated with a decreased risk. Early cohabitation with a deviant partner was associated with a markedly decreased likelihood of the young women being with a current non-deviant supportive partner at the time of follow-up in their mid-twenties.

These two examples could be multiplied, but they exemplify an important point. Both childhood and adult experiences are very influential on whether young people who have had behaviour problems in childhood will go on to an antisocial adjustment. The course of development is not a trajectory set in childhood, but a continuing interaction with circumstances. Much of the reason for an adverse outcome is a cumulative set of disadvantages. These can be set in motion by the child's own problems; but they then have a strong effect on continuity. There is a chain of transactions, in which a person with disorder evokes the risks from the environment that will in their turn come to be the major determinants of disorder.

Developmental psychologists have long drawn attention to the extent to which dysfunction in childhood can represent the extreme of a continuum rather than categorically separate disorder. Ideologies have developed about this as well, often crystallised around disciplinary positions. For the clinical psychiatrist, binary categories – of disorder or no disorder, treatment

Continuities and discontinuities between normality and pathology

xi

or no treatment – are a natural way of thinking. For the educational psychologist, and to some extent the psychodynamic psychotherapist, it is equally natural to focus upon the operation of factors that influence the normal range of variation within the whole population. Neither of these can possibly represent the whole truth.

The approach towards developmental psychopathology that Rutter has been developing certainly addresses the question of the extent to which continuities or discontinuities from normality are the best description of psychopathology; but it does so in a way that allows for both possibilities.

Some disorders, such as autism, probably present qualitative differences from normal development and others, probably including conduct disorder, represent quantitative variation. The latter show strong effects of factors such as family discord and stress that, in milder degrees, influence normal variations in personality development. We need to clarify the extent to which these different models apply and the mechanisms that apply in both. The more that one deals with multiple influences, each of small effect, the more need there is for a developmental approach that stresses the interplay between factors and the details of their mutual interaction.

Links between research and practice

Rutter's role as a clinican has also been distinguished. Many of his key contributions have been in clinical nosology – for example, in dispelling the myth that 'adolescent turmoil' is a distinct disorder (this vol., pp. 224–245). His development of assessment schemes for children with autism, trial evaluation of educational approaches, and evidence-based recommendations for treatment are still the foundation for therapeutic approaches (this vol., pp. 103–124). His papers with Tony Cox and others on the psychiatric interview were pioneering applications of experimental method to the understanding of the ways in which clinically important information should be elicited (this vol., pp. 72–81). Clinical progress has been built on good communication between researcher and clinicians, and sound classification systems are indispensable for this type of communication. Shaffer's chapter in Volume 1 (Green & Yule, 2001: pp. 109–114) expands on them; they are the basis of our discourse. The major contribution to classification has come from Michael Rutter. From the clarity of his early formulation of the key issues (this vol., pp. 59–71) to his key role in developing the World Health Organization's multi-axial scheme (now ICD–10) and encouraging compatibility between that and the American Psychiatric Association's manual (DSM–IV), he has been effective in refinining the dialectic of the tribe.

Conclusion

This outline of Michael Rutter's wide investigative interests – and indeed this whole volume – can only sample some of the aspects that seem most distinctive. I hope that it has given an idea of his determination that research should tackle big and pressing questions, focus on the mechanisms of development of disorder and ask new questions about how it arises; and that research and clinical practice should illuminate one another. The selection of papers in this volume has been guided by illustrating these major themes. The final advice to the reader can therefore be to go directly to his writings.

References

Green, J. & Yule, W. (eds) (2001) *Research and Innovation on the Road to Modern Child Psychiatry. Vol. 1: Festschrift for Professor Sir Michael Rutter*. London: Gaskell.

International Molecular Genetic Study of Autism Consortium (1998) A full genome screen for autism with evidence for linkage to a region on chromosome 7q. *Human Molecular Genetics*, **119**, 571–578.

Maughan, B., Pickles, A., Hagell, A., *et al* (1996) Reading problems and antisocial behaviour: developmental trends in comorbidity. *Journal of Child Psychology and Psychiatry*, **37**, 405–418.

Rutter, M. (1972) *Maternal Deprivation Reassessed*. Harmondsworth: Penguin.

—— & English and Romanian Adoptees (ERA) Study Team (1998) Developmental catch-up, and deficit, following adoption after severe global early privation. *Journal of Child Psychology and Psychiatry*, **39**, 465–476.

—— & Maughan, B. (1997) Psychosocial adversities in childhood and adult psychopathology. *Journal of Personality Disorders*, **11**, 4–18.

—— & Smith, D. (1995) *Psychosocial Disorders in Young People: Time Trends and Their Causes*. Chichester: John Wiley & Sons.

——, Tizard, J. & Whitmore, K. (eds) (1970) *Education, Health and Behaviour*. London: Longman & Green.

——, Maughan, B., Mortimore, P., *et al* (1979) *Fifteen Thousand Hours*. London: Open Books.

Part I
Developmental psychopathology

Journal of Child Psychology and Psychiatry, 1989, vol. 30, pp. 23–51

Pathways from Childhood to Adult Life*

Michael Rutter†

Abstract—Principles and concepts of development are reviewed in relation to life-span issues noting the need to consider: development in its social context; timing of experiences; intrinsic and experiential factors; continuities and discontinuities; parallels and differences between normal and abnormal development; heterotypic and homotypic continuities; key life transitions; risk and protective factors; indirect chain affects; mediating mechanisms; age as an index of maturational and experiential factors. Developmental findings from childhood to adult longitudinal studies are reviewed for possible mediating factors. These include: genetic mechanisms; the (non-genetic) biological substrate; shaping of the environment; cognitive and social skills; self-esteem and self-efficacy; habits, cognitive sets and coping styles; links between experiences.

Keywords: Life-span development, developmental continuities/discontinuities, turning points in development, personality development

■3

Introduction

Throughout his highly productive life, Jack Tizard was strongly committed to the application of research methods in psychology to issues of relevance for social policy and practice (see Clarke & Tizard, 1983). However, he was equally committed to the need for basic research that is focused on the elucidation of the processes and mechanisms underlying normal and abnormal development. In his letter to the Chief Scientist outlining the philosophy of the Thomas Coram Research Unit, he was forthright in arguing that it was essential to combine both approaches. Research must bring forth new ideas and fresh knowledge so that patterns of practice may be improved in the future; it is not enough simply to assess the best of what is being done today.

My own debt to Jack is enormous; not only in gaining an appreciation of how research and policy interact but, more particularly, in learning how epidemiological and longitudinal research methods may be used in this connection. Our collaboration in the Isle of Wight studies (Rutter, Tizard & Whitmore, 1970; Rutter, Tizard, Yule, Graham & Whitmore, 1976) was an exciting learning experience for me. Jack was an extremely generous as well as immensely stimulating teacher, whose combination of unwavering methodological rigour and intellectual openness provided a model that

Accepted manuscript received 12 *August* 1988

*Jack Tizard Memorial Lecture. Delivered on 1 July 1988 at the Association for Child Psychology and Psychiatry Annual Conference, London.
†Honorary Director, MRC Child Psychiatry Unit, Institute of Psychiatry, University of London, U.K.
Requests for reprints to: Professor M. Rutter, Department of Child and Adolescent Psychiatry, Institute of Psychiatry, De Crespigny Park, Denmark Hill, London SE5 8AF, U.K.

Journal of Child Psychology and Psychiatry, 1989, vol. 30, pp. 23–51

all of us who worked with him strove to follow. The longitudinal element in the Isle of Wight studies, four years, was relatively short, but it served to alert me to the importance of understanding how developmental processes served to bring about both stability and change. This elucidation of the mechanisms underlying continuities and discontinuities of development over the life-span is crucial if we are to devise improved means of intervening to bring about long term gains for children suffering intrinsic or extrinsic hazards during their growing years.

It has to be said that Jack was always sceptical of claims that short term experiences could have long term effects and that permanent change should be the goal of treatment. In his presidential address to the British Psychological Society (Tizard, 1976), he argued for the importance of the immediate environment as the main influence on a person's behaviour, and he urged that we should abandon notions about the long term value of preventive interventions such as Headstart, and that instead we should examine the characteristics of the environment that contribute to immediate happiness and well being. Those cautions remain apposite today, and both of the first two Jack Tizard lectures—by Alan Clarke (Clarke & Clarke, 1984) and by Ron Clarke (1985)—developed these themes well and showed their importance.

On the other hand, Jack was well aware that, in some circumstances, adverse experiences could have long term sequelae, as he demonstrated in his own collaborative research on the development of children who suffered the combination of malnutrition and psychosocial privation (Hertzig, Birch, Richardson & Tizard, 1972; see also Tizard, 1975). His point was *not* that continuities did not occur, but rather that simplistic concepts of immutable effects needed to be put aside and replaced by more dynamic notions of the continuing interplay over time between intrinsic and extrinsic influences on individual development. This is the theme that I seek to explore in this paper.

Over the last three decades there have been major changes in the ways in which the developmental process has been conceptualized. During the 1950s beliefs in the consistency of personality and in the lack of major changes after the first few years of life held sway (see Kelly, 1955). Longitudinal studies sought to chart this early stabilization of personality (see Moss & Susman, 1980), and it was urged that maternal deprivation in infancy led to permanent, irreversible damage (Bowlby, 1951). However, longitudinal studies failed to show high temporal stability and the claims on maternal deprivation were subjected to severe academic criticism (e.g. O'Connor, 1956; Orlansky, 1949; Yarrow, 1961). It became clear that people changed a good deal over the course of development and that the outcome following early adversities was quite diverse, with long-term effects heavily dependent on the nature of subsequent life experiences (Clarke & Clarke, 1976). Even markedly adverse experiences in infancy carry few risks for later development if the subsequent rearing environment is a good one (Rutter, 1981).

The pendulum swung and it came to be argued that there was little continuity in psychological development, such continuity as there was being dependent on people's interpretation of their experiences (Kagan, 1984). Mischel (1968, 1969) challenged the very notion of personality traits and argued that much behaviour was highly situation-specific. These claims gave rise to equally vigorous dispute on both the concepts and the empirical findings (Block, 1979; Epstein, 1979; Epstein & O'Brien,

1985; Hinde, 1987; Hinde & Bateson, 1984; McCall 1977; Magnusson, 1988; Nesselroade, 1988; Olweus, 1979).

In recent years there has been a limited swinging back of the pendulum, as investigators have been faced with evidence demonstrating a rather complex mix of both continuities and discontinuities (Rutter, 1987a). That mix applies to all phases in the developmental process, but my focus today is on the longer time span of connections between childhood and adult life.

Principles and concepts of development

∎5

Before proceeding to consider some of the key findings from several major longitudinal studies, it may be useful first to outline some of the principles and concepts of development that derive from research findings both on normal development (Rutter, 1987a) and on psychopathology (Rutter, 1984a,b; Rutter, 1988).

The first point is that a life-span perspective is necessary (Rutter, 1984b). That is because *Homo sapiens* is a social animal and because social development occurs in relation to a person's interactions and transactions with his or her social environment (Erikson, 1963; Bronfenbrenner, 1979; Hinde, 1987; Hinde & Stevenson-Hinde, 1988). Because key social experiences such as marriage or childbearing tend not to occur during the childhood years, social development needs to be extended into adult life. A related point is that development includes the *content* of emotions and social relationships as well as *capacities* in these areas of functioning. Maccoby (1984) made the point that, although there are important universals in development, social development follows more than one pathway and has more than one endpoint— hence the plural of pathways in the title of this paper.

A related issue is that the *timing,* as well as the nature, of experiences is likely to influence their impact. The importance of timing arises for several different reasons. First, the effects on neural structure and functioning will be affected by what is happening at the time in neural development. This is illustrated by the effects of prenatal androgens on both brain organization and sexually dimorphic behaviours in later life (Mayer-Bahlburg, Ehrhardt & Feldman, 1986), by the varying effects of brain damage at different ages (Goodman, 1987; Rutter, 1982) and by the effects on binocular vision of uncorrected strabismus in infancy. Secondly, the effects will also be influenced by sensitivities and vulnerabilities deriving from the psychological processes that are emerging at the time. Thus, very young infants are protected from separation experiences because they have yet to develop strong attachments; older children are protected because they have learned to maintain relationships over time and space; but toddlers are most at risk because attachments are first becoming established at that age and because they lack the cognitive skills required to maintain relationships during an absence (Rutter, 1981, 1987a). Thirdly, timing may be important because experiences may be felt differently, or give rise to different societal responses, if they arise at non-normative times. For example, this may apply to the links between teenage pregnancy and difficulties in parenting (Hayes, 1987), to those between early marriage and an increased risk of divorce (Otto, 1979), to the differences in effects between redundancy in middle life and retirement in old age (Warr, 1987)

Journal of Child Psychology and Psychiatry, 1989, vol. 30, pp. 23–51

and to the psychological consequences of unusually early puberty (Graham & Rutter, 1985).

A biological perspective, of course, requires an emphasis on both intrinsic and experiential influences on development. Genetic factors will play a part in shaping not only individual differences in psychological characteristics but also their developmental course (Plomin, 1986; Plomin & Thompson, 1988). In addition, it is likely that physiological transitions such as puberty, which involve major changes in hormonal output and in bodily configuration, will have a psychosocial impact (Petersen, 1988; Rutter, in press a). However, development is also affected by environmental factors that are not accompanied by somatic alteration. Experiences within and outside the home have been shown to make an impact on intellectual (Rutter, 1985a) and behavioural development (Rutter, 1985b).

A fourth consideration, also stemming from a biological perspective, is that both continuities and discontinuities are to be expected (Hinde, 1988; Hinde & Bateson, 1984; Rutter, 1987a). The process of development is concerned with change and it is not reasonable to suppose that the pattern will be set in early life. Physiological alterations, as at puberty, and new experiences will both serve to shape psychological functioning. However, continuities will occur because children carry with them the results of earlier learning and of earlier structural and functional change. This does not necessarily mean that a person's characteristics at one age will predict the degree or type of *change* over a later time period, but it does mean that it is likely to predict later *levels* of functioning, because they will incorporate earlier levels. The importance of this distinction is well shown in the excellent recent study of primary school effectiveness undertaken by Mortimore, Sammons, Stoll, Lewis and Etab (1988). Final attainment level was strongly correlated with family background and with the child's level of skills at school entry, but *progress* between 7 and 11 yrs was most strongly associated with school characteristics. The importance of differentiating between progress and final attainment level is also shown in Tizard, Blatchford, Burk, Farquahar and Plewis' (1988) important longitudinal study of children attending inner city infant schools.

The next issue is that there can be no presupposition that normal and abnormal development do, or do not, involve the same mechanisms or do, or do not, share the same qualities; rather there must be a concern empirically to test for similarities and dissimilarities (Rutter & Sandberg, 1985; Rutter, 1988). It is clear that both occur. Thus, it may well be that the features associated with the development of a pattern of heavy drinking in the general population parallel those that play a role in the emergence of alcoholism; by contrast it is possible that the pathways leading to schizophrenia or bipolar affective disorder include elements that do not constitute any part of normal development.

A sixth consideration is that there must be a search for heterotypic as well as homotypic continuities. In other words, we must recognize that behaviours may change in *form* whilst still reflecting the same basic *process*. There are, however, methodological hazards that must be avoided in any consideration of heterotypic continuity. The mere finding that behaviour X at one age is correlated with behaviour Y at a later age provides no basis for assuming continuity. In any complex statistical analysis, many such correlations are bound to arise by chance. To infer continuity it is important either to show that both behaviours, although different in form, function similarly in their association with risk factors and/or consequences, or to replicate the longitudinal correlation in another sample (or preferably both). Nevertheless, it is clear that there are heterotypic continuities that have withstood these tests. For example, there is continuity between social isolation, peer rejection, odd unpredictable behaviour and attention deficits in childhood and schizophrenic psychosis in adult life (Nuechterlein, 1986; Rutter, 1984a). It has also been found that conduct disorder in childhood leads not only to antisocial personality disorders in adult life, but also to a broader range of social malfunctions associated with an increased risk of depressive disorder—the former pathway being more common in males and the latter in females (Robins, 1986; Quinton, Rutter & Gulliver, in press; Zeitlin, 1986).

■7

A life-span perspective requires attention to the variety of transitions that occur during the course of development, such as leaving the parental home, starting work, getting married and becoming a parent. However, it also brings a further consideration—the need to focus on the process of *negotiation* of life transitions, and not just their occurrence or the behavioural outcome that follows. Thus, the fact of getting married at a particular age is one thing, but it is equally important to consider why and how the decision was taken when it was, as well as the social context of the decision and the characteristics of the spouse.

An eighth consideration is the need to take into account individual differences in the meaning of, and response to, such transitions. Thus, parenthood that arises unwanted at the age of 15 yrs will not be the same as a wanted child being born to a young adult in the context of a happy marriage, and both will differ from the experience of having a first child after a decade's unsuccessful attempts to conceive associated with multiple treatments for infertility. All three will differ yet again from parenthood as a result of artificial insemination by donor or adoption or fostering.

A ninth issue is that an emphasis is needed on both risk *and* protective factors, together with interactions between them (Rutter, 1983; in press a). Both good and bad experiences influence development. However, it is also crucial that some experiences that seem negative at the time may nevertheless be protective. Just as a resistance to infection stems from "successful" encounters with the infective agent in a modified or attentuated form (the basis of immunization), perhaps too resistance to psychosocial adversity is fostered by successful copying with earlier stressful experiences. Elder's (1974, 1979) example of the strengthening effect of older children having to take on family responsibilities during the great economic depression is a case in point.

A related issue is the need to recognize the importance of indirect chain and strand effects in the developmental process (Brown, 1988), as well as direct influences. In other words, the impact of some factor in childhood may lie less in the immediate behavioural change it brings about than in the fact that it sets in motion a chain reaction in which one "bad" thing leads to another or, conversely, that a good experience makes it more likely that another one will be encountered. For example, academic success at school is likely to increase the chance of a well-paid job in adult life and better living conditions—not because passing exams alters personality but simply because academic credentials open the doors to career advancement which in turn is associated with a range of social advantages in adult life.

Journal of Child Psychology and Psychiatry, 1989, vol. 30, pp. 23–51

The penultimate principle is that there must be a concern to elucidate the processes and mechanisms involved in such indirect and direct effects. It is, of course, important to determine the various factors associated with an adaptive psychosocial outcome. Thus, it has been useful that research has shown that these are more likely if the child has positive characteristics such as high self-esteem and a positive social orientation; if the family shows warmth, harmony and cohesion; and if adequate social supports are available (Masten & Garmezy, 1985). However, if we are to use this information to develop effective means of fostering normal development and of preventing mental disorder, we must go on to ask *how* self-esteem develops, which experiences or biological qualities are likely to foster it, and by which mechanisms does it operate.

Finally, in studying these processes and mechanisms, it is necessary to appreciate that age is an ambiguous variable; the finding that some psychological function increases as children grow older does not, in itself, provide an answer as to why or how this happens (Rutter, in press b). It may occur as a result of physiological maturation (but, if so, there is the further question of which aspect of maturity is crucial; thus, cognitive and endocrinological maturity do not necessarily proceed hand in hand). Equally, however, the psychological advance may derive from the cumulative effect of certain sorts of experiences or from the occurrence of particular types of experiences that usually arise only later in childhood or adolescence.

In short, the investigation of pathways from childhood to adult life requires an analysis of a quite complicated set of linkages over time. It is not simply a matter of determining the level of correlation for particular behaviours from one age to some later age.

Some childhood to adult life longitudinal studies

With these considerations as a background, let me turn to the empirical evidence on pathways from childhood to adult life. I will not dwell on the findings on correlations over time for particular psychological characteristics, as these have been extensively reviewed previously (see e.g. Moss & Sussman, 1980; Rutter, 1987a). Suffice it to say that the correlations between early or middle childhood and adult life for most psychological features are general positive, but quite low. There is some tendency for children's behaviour to predict adult behaviour, but the correlations are too weak for much useful prediction at the individual level.

Psychopathological continuities

That conclusion, however, applies to normally distributed characteristics as assessed in the general population. The situation with respect to psychopathological features is somewhat different in that some types of disorder, especially conduct disturbances, do exhibit substantial continuity between childhood and adult life. Robins (1978) showed that antisocial personality disorder in adulthood was almost always preceded by conduct disturbance in childhood, so that continuity looking backwards is very strong indeed. However, because conduct disturbance in the childhood years is very common, and because only about a third persist into adulthood, continuity looking forwards is less impressive. This finding raises several important issues. First, there is the question of whether the apparent reduction in conduct problems is real or whether, rather, the form of disturbance has changed but the disorder nevertheless continues—the issue of heterotypic continuity. As already noted, conduct problems do indeed lead on to a broader range of adult disorders. Using the ECA retrospective data, Robins (1986) reported that when women had had three or more conduct problems in childhood, 85% had some form of psychiatric disorder in adult life compared with 41% of the remainder. The relative risk (a four-fold increase) was greatest for drugs, alcohol and antisocial problems, but there was also a two-fold increase for emotional disorders.

■9

The second issue is what features differentiate the individuals who are most likely to show persistence of disorder into adult life. The Stockholm longitudinal study (Magnusson, 1988) showed that the risk was particularly great for boys who exhibited the combination of aggression, hyperactivity and poor peer relationships. Compared with well-adjusted boys, the risk of having adult criminality *and* alcohol abuse *and* psychiatric disorder was 20 times higher and, compared with the total population rate, it was still more than seven times higher! The children with multiproblem patterns were few in number but they accounted for much of the persistence.

The findings from the Cambridge longitudinal study of working class London boys confirm the markedly increased risk for persistent adult criminality associated with both hyperactivity and conduct disturbance in childhood. In that longitudinal study of 411 boys, only 24 had as many as six convictions by their 26th birthday. Twenty of these 24 men had shown hyperactivity and/or conduct disturbance at 8–10 yrs; a ten-fold increase in risk that accounted for 83% of chronic adult offenders (Farrington, Loeber & Van Kammen, in press).

Parker and Asher's (1987) excellent recent review of the association between poor peer relationships in childhood and adult disorder emphasizes the importance of both low peer acceptance and aggressiveness as predictors of school dropout, adult criminality and probably also other types of adult problems. Shyness/withdrawal does not seem to carry the same risks. As Parker and Asher point out, many issues remain to be resolved. Thus, it is not clear whether the risk stems from lack of social skills, lack of social ties or negative socially disapproved behaviour. Moreover, it remains uncertain whether low peer acceptance is merely an incidental correlate of persisting psychopathological disturbance or whether it plays a causal role in continuities over time because it predisposes to deviant socialization experiences and opportunities. Nevertheless, the evidence from longitudinal studies that have examined hyperactivity, conduct disturbance and poor peer relationships is that when present in marked pervasive form they carry a markedly increased risk for adult disorder of one kind or another.

This does not necessarily mean that the continuities stem from intrinsic psychological processes. It could be that the persistence of disorder simply reflects the continuation of the psychosocial risk factors that gave rise to the children's problems in the first place. This is a very real possibility because conduct disorders are particularly associated with types of family discord and disorganization and of parental deviance that tend to be very persistent (Rutter, 1985b). We need to focus on circumstances where children's environments have changed markedly for the better in order to see if this

Journal of Child Psychology and Psychiatry, 1989, vol. 30, pp. 23–51

is accompanied by parellel improvements in the children's conduct disturbance. Richman, Stevenson and Graham (1982), in their longitudinal study from age 3–8 yrs, found that a reduction in marital disharmony made no difference to the likelihood that children's problems would remit; however, improved parent–child relationships (as reflected in increased parental warmth and reduced criticisms) were associated with benefits for the children. It seems that the specifics of children's interpersonal interactions may be more important in continuity than the overall family circumstances.

A more dramatic change in children's circumstances was investigated by Hodges and Tizard (1989 a,b) in their follow-up to age 16 yrs of children reared in residential nurseries until at least age 2 yrs and then adopted or restored to their biological parents at some time between 2 and 7 yrs (Tizard & Hodges, 1978). The restored group, whose families tended to be disturbed and disadvantaged, showed a high rate of antisocial behaviour, with almost all having had contact with the police and/or psychiatric services. The adoptees, most of whom were in stable harmonious homes, were much less likely to show this pattern, but tended to be more worried, unhappy and fearful than the comparison group children. These differences would seem to reflect their current circumstances more than their early institutional experiences. However, both the adoptees and restored children were very similar to each other, and different from controls, in being more oriented towards adult attention and in having more difficulties with peers and fewer close peer relationships. As the experiences of the adoptees and of the restored children were so different over the decade preceding the 16 yr follow-up, it must be inferred that the institutional upbringing for the first few years of life had left some social sequelae that were somewhat resistant to later influences, at least up to the age of 16 yrs. Nevertheless, it is notable that this persistence in terms of subtle qualities of peer relationships stands out as different from the pattern exhibited by other behaviours.

A further possibility that has to be considered is that the children's behaviour, as a result of its impact on other people, makes later stressful environments more likely. It is clear that both conduct disturbance and poor peer relationships, the two types of psychopathology most likely to persist, carry that potential. Thus, Robins (1986) reported that the ECA data showed that women aged 30–49 yrs who showed three or more conduct problems in childhood had a two-fold increased risk of job loss during the 6 mths before interview, a two-fold increased risk of break-up with a spouse or lover and a four-fold increased risk of break-up with a best friend during the same time period. These retrospective data require confirmation from longitudinal studies, but the strong implication is that behavioural disturbance predisposes to an increased likelihood of adverse psychosocial experiences or life events in adult life. Kandel and Davies (1986), using longitudinal questionnaire data, similarly showed that adolescent depression was associated with an increased risk of certain kinds of social stress situations in early adult life.

Psychosocial pathways

With that possibility in mind, let me turn to a few of the long term longitudinal studies that have attempted to chart the various steps that might be involved in

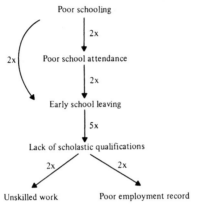

Fig. 1. **Simplified pathway from poor schooling to poor job success (Gray**
et al., **1980).**

pathways from childhood to adult life. The first investigation to mention is our follow-up of inner London children from age 10 yrs to one year after leaving school (Gray, Smith & Rutter, 1980). Figure 1 summarizes the pathways leading from poor schooling to poor job success. We found no effect of schooling that was independent of later circumstances, but the indirect continuities were quite strong. The children who went to less effective schools were twice as likely as other children to show poor school attendance; poor attenders were twice as likely to leave school early without sitting national examinations—necessarily this meant that all left without scholastic qualifications, compared with only a fifth of other pupils; those without qualifications were in turn twice as likely to go into unskilled work and were twice as likely to have a poor employment record as shown by their getting dismissed from jobs. These continuities were still evident after controlling for other variables such as the individual's measured intelligence and social circumstances.

Of course, the chain of adversity was far from inevitable, in that each link was open to other influences that could break (or strengthen) the chain. For example, black girls were particularly likely to have a good attendance record and to stay on at school beyond the period of compulsory education (Maughan, Dunn & Rutter, 1985a; Maughan & Rutter, 1986). As a result of their unusual educational persistence they left school with exam qualifications that were substantially better than might have been expected on the basis of their reading skills on entering secondary school or the quality of the schools they attended. Conversely, boys with poor reading skills tended to leave school without exam qualifications, not so much because their academic limitations meant that they failed exams, but rather because their conduct problems tended to be associated with leaving school early without sitting any exams (Maughan, Gray & Rutter, 1985b).

The second study to mention is the follow-up of institution-reared children undertaken by David Quinton and myself, together with colleagues (Quinton & Rutter, 1988). The young people were interviewed in depth in their mid 20s and comparable data were obtained for a general population sample, reared at home by their biological parents, and followed up over a comparable time period. The findings showed a chain by which parenting breakdown in one generation *sometimes* led to parenting breakdown

Journal of Child Psychology and Psychiatry, 1989, vol. 30, pp. 23–51

12 ▪

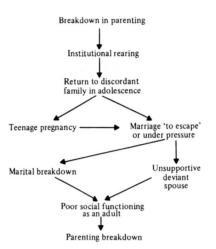

Fig. 2. Simplified model of intergenerational transmission of parenting breakdown (Quinton & Rutter, 1988).

in the next. Not surprisingly, perhaps, the adult outcome of the institution-reared girls was significantly worse than that of the comparison group, and overt parenting breakdown was found only in the institutional sample, occuring in a third of cases. Numerous statistical analyses were undertaken to determine the possible mechanisms underlying the heterogeneity in outcome.

Figure 2 presents a selection of the findings in terms of the intervening steps leading to eventual parenting breakdown. The story begins with a variety of psychosocial problems in the girls' parents; these problems were associated with parenting difficulties and with lack of social support, which in turn led to the girls' admission to residential nurseries or Group Homes where they remained off and on, or continuously, until adolescence. On leaving the institutions, many of the girls either had no family to which to go or they returned to the same discordant families from which they had been 'rescued' when young. Faced with these stressful circumstances, many married hastily to 'escape' or under pressure as a result of a teenage pregnancy. An institutional upbringing led many of the girls to feel that they could not control their lives and they tended not to plan ahead with either work or marriage. As one might have expected, these impulsive marriages undertaken for negative reasons were often to deviant men from similarly disadvantaged backgrounds and many of the marriages broke down. Alternatively, the women were left unsupported in a conflictful, unrewarding marital relationship. These adult circumstances were then associated with a markedly increased risk of poor social functioning in adult life which, in turn, was accompanied by an increased risk of parenting breakdown.

It will be appreciated that this chain of adversities is made up of a series of contingencies which, if not met, are likely to result in different consequences. Figure 3 provides one example of how a more adaptive chain of circumstances could arise. The girls who were admitted to the institution after the age of 2 yrs, not having experienced early disruptions of parenting, were much more likely to return to a harmonious family on leaving the Children's Home in adolescence. The presence

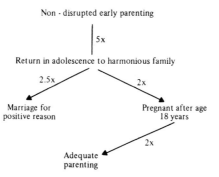

Non - disrupted early parenting

5x

Return in adolescence to harmonious family

2.5x   2x

Marriage for   Pregnant after age
positive reason   18 years

2x

Adequate
parenting

**Fig. 3. Simplified adaptive chain of circumstances in institution-reared
women (1) (Quinton & Rutter, 1988).**

of such a harmonious home at that time made it more than twice as likely that the
girls would marry for positive reasons (i.e. not under pressure or to escape) and that
they would not become pregnant until age 19 or later. Both these circumstances
increased the likelihood of adequate or good parenting.

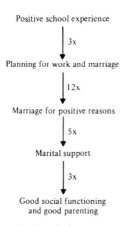

Positive school experience

3x

Planning for work and marriage

12x

Marriage for positive reasons

5x

Marital support

3x

Good social functioning
and good parenting

**Fig. 4. Simplified adaptive chain of circumstances in institution-reared
women (2) (Quinton & Rutter, 1988).**

In a sense, that chain involved a series of partially interconnected social
circumstances. However, some risk pathways were turned into more adaptive routes
as a result of adventitious happenings. Thus, for example, it was a policy of the
Children's Homes to distribute the children among many different schools in order
to avoid an undue weighting of institutional children in any one school, which could
lead to adverse labelling. As a consequence, some children had much more positive
school experiences than others. Those who had good experiences were three times
as likely to show planning in their choice of careers and of marriage partner. This
meant that they were much more likely to marry for positive reasons which, in turn,
much increased the likelihood that they would marry a non-deviant man with whom
they developed a warm confiding relationship. The presence of such marital support

Journal of Child Psychology and Psychiatry, 1989, vol. 30, pp. 23–51

greatly increased the likelihood that they would show good social functioning and good parenting as a young adult. This chain of connections remained after controlling for other variables, such as the girls' non-deviant behaviour in childhood and adolescence.

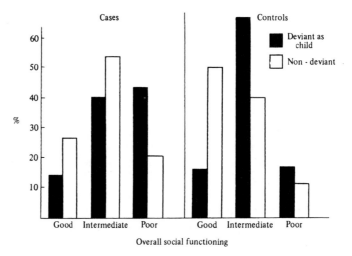

Fig. 5. Childhood deviance and adult outcome (males) (based on Rutter, Quinton & Hill, in press).

Nevertheless, deviant behaviour was itself associated with outcome, and this statistical relationship was substantially stronger in males than in females (Rutter, Quinton & Hill, in press). The findings for males showed that childhood deviance was significantly associated with poor overall social functioning in adult life, there being a two-fold increase in risk. However, among those showing childhood deviance, an institutional rearing was still associated with a two-fold increase in poor social functioning. In other words, there was a pathway involving childhood deviance, but also one or more that involved other features.

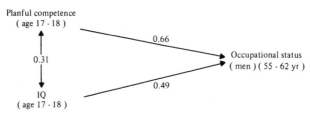

Fig. 6. Berkeley longitudinal studies: the role of planful competence (Clausen, 1986).

Our data suggested the important role of planning as a factor associated with good adult outcomes. However, we had to measure planning retrospectively, with all the uncertainties that retrospective measurement involves. The Berkeley longitudinal studies (Clausen, 1986) provided the opportunity to assess the same effect prospectively. What was termed 'planful competence' was measured at age 17–18 yrs, when there was also an assessment of IQ. The two measures intercorrelated only modestly at the 0.31 level. Strikingly, planful competence correlated 0.66 with occupational status in late middle life, at age 55–62 yrs, a stronger correlation than that found with IQ.

Table 1. Number of marriages according to Senior High School level of planful competence (percentage distribution) (men)

| | Planful competence | | |
	High	Inter.	Low
Total	100	100	100
None	—	5	—
One	82	75	55
Two	18	15	32
Three or more	—	5	14
Number of subjects	28	20	22

(Data from Clausen, 1986)

As in our institution-reared sample, a lack of planful competence was also associated with an increased risk of marital breakdown. Nearly half (46%) of those who lacked such planning had two or more marriages, compared with 18% of those with high planning. The comparable figures for females (based on a slightly different measure) were 46% versus 6%. It is evident that characteristics shown in adolescence were quite strongly predictive of marital and occupational circumstances in middle life, some 40 yrs later. Note, however, that what is evident is *not* unchanging behaviour over time, but rather a style of dealing with life circumstances that increased the chances of things turning out less well.

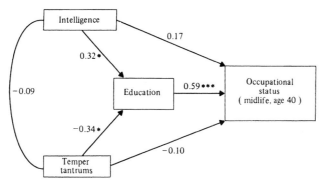

Fig. 7. Temper tantrums in childhood and occupational status in adult life (based on Caspi, Elder & Herbener, in press).

The Berkeley and Oakland studies were also used as a data-base by Caspi, Elder and Herbener (in press). Once again, a variety of chain reactions are to be seen. Figure 7 summarizes the consequences of a pattern of frequent temper tantrums in childhood. This type of 'explosive' behaviour made it significantly more likely that there would be an early exit from school and hence less likely that the person would

Journal of Child Psychology and Psychiatry, 1989, vol. 30, pp. 23–51

end up with good educational attainments in early adult life. Poor attainments were, in turn, associated with lower occupational status in mid life. The childhood behaviour had no direct effect on occupational level, but it had an important indirect effect via its impact on scholastic attainment.

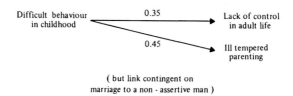

Fig. 8. Longitudinal study of Berkeley women: adult sequelae of difficult behaviour in childhood (Caspi & Elder, 1988).

Difficult behaviour in childhood was also associated with an increased risk of ill-tempered parenting and of poor social control in adult life in women (Caspi & Elder, 1988). Interestingly, however, this outcome was contingent on marriage to a non-assertive man. Difficult behaviour made it significantly more likely that the women *would* marry men with these characteristics and, if they did, they were more likely to show poor social control in mid life. If they did not, however, there was *no* such tendency.

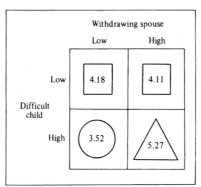

Fig. 9. The behavioural consequences of difficult girls' mate-selection patterns. Dependent variable: women's undercontrolled behaviour at midlife (1 = low, 9 = high) (Caspi & Elder, 1988).

The findings are summarized in Fig. 9. The score in the triangle in the bottom right hand corner shows the lack of adult control score when there was the combination of difficult childhood behaviour in the women and unassertive withdrawal in the spouse. The rate of poor control is significantly higher than that in all other cells. Caspi and Elder (1988) concluded that the continuities reside in interactional styles that operate in two ways: firstly, through selection of environments and relationships (as shown by the effect on choice of spouse); secondly, through elicitation of interactions that bring out maladaptive behaviours (the interactive effect shown in Fig. 9).

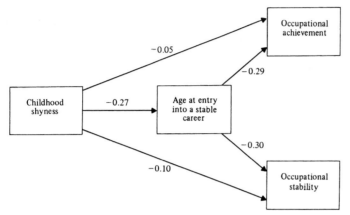

Fig. 10. Adult sequelae of childhood shyness (based on Caspi, Edler & Herbener, in press).

Childhood shyness, another early manifest characteristic, showed a rather different causal chain. It was accompanied by an increased likelihood of late entry into a stable occupational career; late entry was then associated with a lower level of occupational achievement and greater occupational instability. It seemed as if career entry at an atypically late point meant a lesser investment in career skills and benefits and hence an increased career vulnerability.

However, it should not be assumed that people who undergo key life transitions unusually late are always thereby disadvantaged. Elder (1986) showed that, in some circumstances, it could be protective if the late transitions opened up new opportunities. In the Berkeley Guidance Study, low achieving youths from a deprived background who, in adolescence, scored low on measures of social competence tended to join the Armed Forces unusually early, often dropping out from high school to do so (this was in the late 1940s during a period of conscription). Military service was associated with a prolongation of education (the great majority took up schooling again in the Army) and with a delay in both marriage and the starting of careers. For these deprived youths, military service proved to be an important turning point that enabled them to acquire scholastic and occupational skills that they would not have had otherwise; also their later marriage meant that they were marrying at a time when they were more self-sufficient and part of a better functioning social group. Follow-up into middle life showed that this was accompanied by a beneficial change in life trajectory; their outcome was significantly better than expected on the basis of their background and their functioning in adolescence. Of course, in the population as a whole, military service was not likely to have this beneficial effect and it is not argued that it should be recommended as a solution to deprivation. Rather, the point is that even experiences with many negative aspects can be helpful if they serve to provide adaptive opportunities that would not otherwise have been available.

The importance of timing is evident in another longitudinal project, the Stockholm study reported by Magnusson (1988). Unusually early puberty in girls, a menarché under the age of 11 yrs, was associated with a marked increase in drunkenness and in other forms of norm-breaking in mid adolescence. It was found that this increase was a function of a greater tendency to be part of an older peer group. The early

■17

Journal of Child Psychology and Psychiatry, 1989, vol. 30, pp. 23–51

maturing girls who did not mix with older teenagers did not exhibit any increase in norm-breaking. It seemed that the stimulus was physiological but the mechanism was psychosocial (Magnusson, Stattin & Allen, 1986). However, later follow-up in the mid 20s showed that early maturity was no longer associated with an increase in norm-breaking. It was inferred that the early maturing girls had adopted an older adolescent style of behaviour that was evanescent, because as peer groups changed so the influences on behaviour altered; hence there was no long term persistence.

The early maturing girls were also more likely to drop out of school, again following the pattern of older girls. However, unlike the school leaving of older girls who had completed their education, the premature drop-out of the early maturers meant that they left with lower educational attainments. This outcome was persistent; probably because to reverse it would have required a return to education at a later age. Although this was possible, it required a major step that few took. The continuity stemmed from a closing down of opportunities rather than from any intrinsic personality change as such. Similarly, leaving school meant that many turned to marriage and home making. As a consequence, the early maturers had significantly more children at age 26 yrs than the remainder of the sample. Again, this was a continuity that lay in the consequences of early behaviour rather than in internal change in the women themselves.

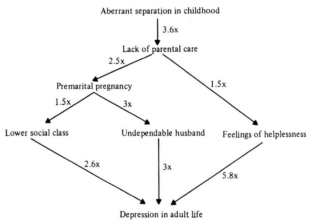

Fig. 11. Simplified model of the links between aberrant separation in childhood and depression in adult life (based on data from Brown *et al.*, 1986).

Several of the studies that have been discussed have drawn attention to pregnancy, marriage and choice of occupation as important turning points in people's lives. The importance of these life transitions is shown again in the study of adult women by Brown and his colleagues (Brown, Harris & Bifulco, 1986; Harris, Brown & Bifulco, 1986, 1987). Figure 11 summarizes some of the main findings. The pathway starts with aberrant separations from parents in childhood (sometimes leading to institutional admission). This was associated with an increased risk (3.6 ×) that parental care would be poor. Poor parental care was then associated with a 2.5 times increase in the likelihood of a premarital pregnancy. Such a pregnancy increased the risk that the girl would land up with an undependable husband and also it made it more likely that the girl would not rise in social class. Lack of parental care separately increased the probability of the woman showing feelings of helplessness. Each of these three strands (i.e. to a lower social class, to a poor marriage and to feelings of helplessness) was associated with an increased vulnerability to depression in adult life. It was notable, as in the other studies, that each link in the chain was contingent on how the life transitions were negotiated. Thus, parental separation carried no risk if it did not lead to poor parental care. Similarly, if the premarital pregnancy was coped with well it did not have the ill-effects noted in Fig. 11.

■19

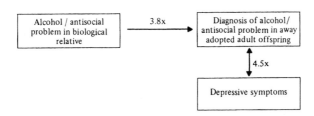

Fig. 12. Simplified model of links between genetic risk factor for alcohol/antisocial problems and occurrence of depression (Cadoret *et al.*, in press).

Another pathway that requires mention is that through genetic influences. In their investigation of children who were adopted in early life and therefore not reared by their biological parents, Cadoret, Troughton, Morens and Whitters (in press) found both direct and indirect genetic effects. They found that alcohol or antisocial problems in biological relatives were associated with a 3.8 times risk of similar problems in the away-adopted adult offspring—a direct genetic effect. These problems in the biological family were not associated with any direct effect on depression in the offspring. On the other hand, individuals with alcohol or antisocial problems were over four times as likely to show depressive symptoms—a substantial indirect genetic effect. It remains uncertain just why antisocial disorder is associated with an increased risk of depression, but many studies have shown that it is. One explanation is probably that the deviant behaviour leads to both stressful interpersonal interactions and social disadvantage (cf. Robins, 1986), both of which in turn predispose to depression.

My account of long-term longitudinal studies has been deliberately incomplete. The pattern of findings in the studies cited is more complex than I have been able to indicate and, of course, there are many other studies that could have been considered. Nevertheless, the overall patterns that I have presented are, I think, reasonably representative of those reported in the literature and, as I have shown, many of the key patterns have been replicated across studies. These patterns fall far short of anything approaching a complete explanation of developmental connections. Nevertheless, they do point to some of the ways in which chain effects may arise. It remains to bring the findings together in a consideration of the various processes and mechanisms that might underlie these continuities (and discontinuities) between childhood and adult life (see Maughan & Champion, in press; Rutter, 1984c).

Journal of Child Psychology and Psychiatry, 1989, vol. 30, pp. 23–51

20 ▪

Possible mediating factors for continuities and discontinuities

Genetic mechanisms

The first possibility is that both continuities and change may be mediated genetically. This may occur in several different ways. Thus, the persistence of a disorder from childhood to adult life may be a function of the intrinsic qualities of a genetically determined condition; this may apply to autism where there seems to be a strong genetic component (Folstein & Rutter, 1987; Smalley, Asarnow & Spence, 1988). Less obviously, however, genetic factors need to be considered in relation to the continuity between conduct disorder in childhood and personality disorder in adult life. Although the broad run of conduct problems and of delinquent behaviour in childhood seems to have only a weak genetic component, the evidence suggests that genetic factors may well be more important in the subgroup that persist into adult life (Rutter, MacDonald, Le Couteur, Harrington, Bolton & Bailey, submitted). Equally, however, genetic mechanisms may play a part in the continuities between two different forms of behaviour. Thus, this may apply to the connections between social oddities and attentional deficits in childhood and schizophrenic psychoses in adult life (Nuechterlein, 1986; Gottesman & Shields, 1976) and to depression in early adult life as a precursor of Huntington's disease in middle age (Folstein, Franz, Jensen, Chase & Folstein, 1983).

In addition, however, genetic factors may also operate indirectly in leading to types of psychopathology that then are associated with an increased vulnerability to other forms of psychiatric disorder. Thus, the study of Cadoret *et al.* (in press) showed that this probably occurred with genetic mechanisms in relation to antisocial disorders which were, in turn, associated with an increased risk of depressive symptomatology.

Biological substrate

Secondly, mediation may lie in aspects of the biological substrate that are not genetically determined. For example, several investigations have shown statistical associations between pregnancy and birth complications and schizophrenia in adult life (Lewis & Murray, 1987; Murray *et al.,* in press; Parnas, Schulsinger, Teasdale, Schulsinger, Feldman & Mednick, 1982). The mechanisms involved in this association remain uncertain but it may be that the later maturation of brain systems linked with schizophrenia, possibly dopaminergic neural systems, activates the mental disorder because the relevant brain structures were damaged at birth (Weinberger, 1987). The brain pathology as such is not progressive, but the effects are not manifest until much later because the brain systems associated with schizophrenia have yet to develop. The suggestion remains speculative so far as schizophrenia is concerned but there are well-established medical examples of similar late effects or of changing manifestations with age. Thus, there is the link between encephalitis lethargica (or brain damage from boxing) in early adult life and the later development of Parkinsonism. Similarly, there are the well established associations between viral infections and the development of various forms of cancer some decades later. The association between high alcohol exposure *in utero* and attentional deficits in childhood provides an example of a prenatal effect (Porter, O'Conner & Whelan, 1984); the adult sequelae are as yet unknown.

However, the mediation does not necessarily have to involve organic brain damage. For example, the animal experiments of Levine and others (Hennessy & Levine, 1979; Hunt, 1979) showed that physical stress in infancy led to both enlarged adrenal glands and increased resistance to later stressors. Also, the administration of prenatal adrenogens is associated with an increased tendency for females to show tomboyish behaviour (Mayer-Bahlberg *et al.,* 1986). Adequate sensory experiences are necessary for the development of the related neural systems. This has been well demonstrated for vision, but the sensory deprivation of non-visual stimuli has also been shown to have effects on brain structure and function (Greenough, Black & Wallace, 1987; Rosenzweig & Bennett, 1977).

■21

Shaping of environment

A third mediating mechanism is to be found in the ways in which a person's behaviour or experiences in childhood serve to shape the environment experienced in adult life. This is seen most obviously in the connections between eduational achievement and later occupational status, as shown in several of the longitudinal studies discussed. It is important to emphasize that the link is *not* just a secondary consequence of individual qualities such as IQ. The Stockholm Study (Magnusson, 1988; Magnusson *et al.,* 1986) showed how early puberty in girls could lead to drop-out from education; our own longitudinal studies (Maughan *et al.,* 1985b) showed a similar effect from conduct disturbances, as did the Berkeley studies (Caspi *et al.,* in press); the latter also showed how joining the Armed Forces could lead to a prolongation of education (Elder, 1986); and our studies of black school children showed how their greater persistence in education had benefits in the form of higher scholastic achievement (Maughan & Rutter, 1986). In these instances, drop-out from, or persistence in, education closed down or opened up career opportunities that were likely to affect social circumstances in adult life. It is important to appreciate that people's living conditions are in part a consequence of steps that they themselves have taken, steps that serve to shape their later experiences (cf. Scarr & McCartney, 1983).

An equally important factor in shaping the adult environment is the choice of marriage partner. Our study of institution-reared girls (Quinton & Rutter, 1988) showed the strong tendency for them to marry in haste at an early age to escape from what they felt to be an intolerable family situation—a tendency that much increased the likelihood that they would land up with an unsatisfactory marriage that would break down. The same investigation, and the Berkeley study (Clausen, 1986), demonstrated the protective effect of planning, an effect that was associated with a significant increase in marital stability. The studies of Brown *et al.* (1986) have also shown the key role of a premarital pregnancy, and numerous investigations have indicated the greater likelihood of divorce for teenage marriages.

A more continuing shaping of environments stems from the effects of people's behaviour on other people's responses to them. There is much evidence to show that this occurs. For example, experimental investigations have shown how oppositional children elicit different types of adult behaviour than do passive compliant children (Brunk & Henggeler, 1984). Observational studies, too, have demonstrated that aggressive boys tend to elicit negative behaviour from their peers (Dodge, 1980). I

Journal of Child Psychology and Psychiatry, 1989, vol. 30, pp. 23–51

mentioned earlier the ECA finding that conduct disturbance in childhood was associated with an increased risk of social rebuffs and job loss in adult life (Robins, 1986).

It should be added that antisocial behaviour also will influence later environments through the societal responses that it induces—such as custodial or correctional actions that may serve both to 'label' and to strengthen antisocial peer group influences, as well as potentially to create more adaptive environments.

On the beneficial side, the available evidence suggests that, insofar as the gains associated with good early educational experiences persist, they do so because they make it more likely that the children will develop a positive approach to schooling that makes them rewarding to teach and *not* because there is a lasting effect on cognitive capacity (Pedersen, Faucher & Eaton, 1978; Berreuta-Clement, Schweinart, Barnett, Epstein & Weikart, 1984).

Of course, too, the fact that a person has children means that they will be exposed to the influence of those children on themselves as adults. The stresses and rewards of parenthood derive from their own behaviour in becoming parents. The circumstances in which they do so (e.g. as a single teenager or a happily married adult) and the number and timing of children are likely to help determine whether the effects are mainly positive or negative.

Cognitive and social skills

The enhancement or reduction of cognitive and/or social skills constitutes a fourth possible mediating mechanism. A variety of studies of children reared in high risk environments have shown that those of higher IQ or better scholastic attainments are less likely to develop later psychiatric disorders (Cohler, 1987; Garmezy, 1983; Rutter, 1979). The reasons why greater cognitive skills are protective remain obscure. Doubtless part of the explanation is that such skills bring their own rewards in terms of enhanced self-esteem and are associated with environmental advantages. But perhaps, too, the skills are protective because they mean that the individuals have a greater repertoire of adaptive strategies to deal with later life challenges and hazards.

However, it is likely that social skills are as important as those in the strictly cognitive domain. Thus, Dodge's work (Dodge, 1983; Dodge, Pettit, McClaskey & Brown, 1986) has shown that aggressive boys lack interpersonal skills and deal ineptly with social interactions. This lack of social skills is likely to play a role in the further perpetuation of their conduct problems. As already noted, social incompetence and poor peer relationships are predictive of later psychopathology (Parker & Asher, 1987).

A major tenet of attachment theory is that early parent–child relationships constitute the basis for all later relationships and that a failure to develop secure attachments in the first few years leads to a relatively lasting impairment in the ability to form close confiding relationships as an adult (Bowlby, 1969, 1988; Bretherton & Waters, 1985; Waters, Hay & Richters, 1986). Early writings, heavily influenced by psychoanalysis, postulated a rather fixed effect on personality organization (Bowlby, 1951). Influences from ethology led to suggestions that parent–child attachment was equivalent to imprinting of the following response seen in certain species of birds (Bowlby, 1969). However, Bowlby's (1988) current views hypothesize a much more fluid process involving developmental pathways that remain open to change throughout life. What remains distinctive, nevertheless, is the notion that the key thread underlying continuities derives from the effect of early relationships as shaping influences on later ones. There is a lack of good data on the extent to which such an association does in fact exist and, insofar as it does, on the mechanisms involved. Nevertheless, the data from Hodges and Tizard's (1989 a,b) follow-up of children who spent their first few years in a residential nursery suggests that there may be something in the proposition. The effects are not as extreme as once suggested but, nevertheless, an early institutional rearing was associated with less intense and less selective relationships in adolescence. It remains to be seen whether this feature will persist into adult life.

■ 23

Our own follow-up of institution-reared girls also showed that, compared with girls reared in ordinary families, they were more likely to develop disorder when faced with social adversity in adult life (Quinton & Rutter, 1988). Given good social circumstances, their outcome was fairly comparable with controls but they were more likely to succumb when faced with social difficulties. Whether or not this was because they lacked coping skills is not known, but that may have been part of the explanation. Similarly, in the Kauai longitudinal study (Werner & Smith, 1982; Werner, 1985) it was noted that resilience was associated with superior problem-solving skills.

It is often argued that vulnerability of this kind is a consequence of not 'working through', or otherwise coming to terms with, earlier stressful experiences. For example, this is particularly emphasized in relation to grief following bereavement, where it is suggested that there is an increased risk of later psychiatric disorder when grief has not been manifest at the time. It is certainly possible that the ways in which the grieving processes are dealt with psychologically at the time are associated with increased or decreased vulnerabilities to later disorder. However, such evidence as there is shows that an absence of depression following bereavement is not a risk factor; rather the reverse (Wortman & Silver, in press). Similarly, Vaillant's follow-up of the Glueck's inner city sample of deprived children showed that good functioning in adult life tended to have been preceded by the same in childhood—an absence of disturbance is *not* a risk factor (Felsman & Vaillant, 1987). Nevertheless, it could still be the case that the way someone conceptualizes earlier adverse experiences is important in determining later sequelae (Main, Kaplan & Cassidy, 1985; Bowlby, 1988).

Self-esteem and self-efficacy

A related notion is that childhood adversities may create a vulnerability to later psychiatric disorder because they lead to a diminished self-esteem and sense of self-efficacy. For example, this has been postulated as one of the mechanisms mediating the link between lack of affectionate care in childhood and a vulnerability to depression in adult life (Brown *et al.,* 1986). There are findings that are consistent with the hypothesis, but direct longitudinal evidence is so far lacking. However, there is evidence that successful coping and/or positive experiences tend to be protective, and it is plausible that the protection lies in the enhanced self-confidence that derives from the experiences (Rutter, 1987a, in press a). Thus, in the follow-up of institution-reared girls, it was found that positive school experiences were associated with an

Journal of Child Psychology and Psychiatry, 1989, vol. 30, pp. 23–51

increased tendency to exert 'planning' in relation to both marriage and careers (Quinton & Rutter, 1988; Rutter *et al.*, in press). It was suggested that this was because the successful coping in one situation—school—increased the likelihood that the girls would feel in control of other aspects of their lives and able to do something about their situation. Similarly, Elder (1974, 1979) found that older children who took on family responsibilities successfully in the Great Depression tended to have better outcomes.

Habits, cognitive sets and coping styles

24 ▪   A sixth mediating mechanism concerns established habits, cognitive sets and coping styles. In a sense, this is the main way that continuities have been conceptualized in the past. The general notion is that through repetition we develop habitual ways of behaving that become both self-reinforcing and reinforced by others. Moreover, these traits become internally organized through the development of cognitive sets about ourselves, our relationships and our environment (Rutter, 1987a, b, c). The notion that this is one way by which personality functions develop and become stabilized is plausible, but we lack knowledge on the processes involved. Research that focused on the associations between cognitions and manifest behaviour, and on the circumstances in which each altered in relation to circumstances, would be helpful. Examples of personality functions conceptualized in this way are provided by 'working models of relationships' (Bretherton & Waters, 1985), styles of coping with stress situations (Moos, 1986; Snyder & Ford, 1987) and the variety of routines and patterns that most people develop in organizing their lives. It is relevant to note that these habits, cognitive sets and coping styles may be important not just—perhaps not even mainly—in the perpetuation of the same behaviours, but also through their effects in leading to other consequences. For example, the use of drugs (such as nicotine, alcohol, opioids or tranquillizers) as a way of dealing with either stress or boredom is likely to predispose to problems from the drugs themselves if their usage increases when stressors increase in later life. Involvement in a satisfying job may be protective in many circumstances but increase vulnerability if the job is lost through redundancy. As with the other mechanisms, it is necessary to consider the ways in which their operation may lead to changes in, as well as stabilization of, behaviour, as both occur.

Links between experiences

    The last possible mediating mechanism to mention is the link between experiences. There are many examples of circumstances in which there is a major change of environment, yet nevertheless one bad environment tends to make it likely that another different bad environment will be experienced or, conversely, that one set of advantages predisposes to other advantages. That was evident in our follow-up of institution-reared children (Quinton & Rutter, 1988), as I have indicated. There was a chain of events by which parental mental disorder led to family discord, which was associated with parenting breakdown, which led to institutional admission. On discharge from the institution in adolescence, early parenting breakdown often meant that there was no family home to which the young people could go so that they were largely left to their own resources at a time of vulnerability. In comparable fashion, marital discord may lead to divorce which, in turn, may be followed by disputes over custody and access and then by the additional change brought about by the entry of a step-parent into the family (Hetherington, 1988; Hetherington, Cox & Cox, 1982, 1985). All of this entails several changes of environment, but there is an essential continuity of potentially stressful circumstances. Advantages frequently involve similar mutually reinforcing chains. Children from privileged homes are more likely to go to better quality schools, the experience of good education will make it more likely that the person will go on to higher education, which in turn may open the way to social advantages as well as career success.

■ 25

Conclusions

In conclusion, it is evident that the limited empirical evidence available on the connections between childhood and adult life emphasizes the need to account for both continuities and discontinuities, and to recognize the multiplicity of pathways across the life-span and the diversity of end points. Life-span transitions have a crucial role in the processes involved, both in strengthening emerging patterns of behaviour and in providing a means by which life trajectories may change direction. Traditionally, such transitions have been thought of in terms of a ladder-like progression through predictable stages, each of which has its own set of tasks—as evident in both Erikson's (1963) and Levinson's (1976) concepts. However, that seems a rather misleadingly rigid way of viewing transitions. Most transitions are not universals—not everyone has a career, not everyone marries, not everyone has children, not everyone outlives their parents and so experiences parental death, some people never retire from work. Moreover, there are hugely important transitions that may be purely individual— as brought about, for example, by migration or by late adoption or by leaving an institutional environment. Transitions need to be considered in personal terms.

Also, however, there is immense individual variability in the number, type and timing of transitions, as is obvious when considering people's experiences of marriage or divorce, retirement, bereavement and physical illness. Equally, there is marked individual variability in the meaning of transitions. There is a world of difference between a much-wanted retirement from a stressful job and involuntary retirement from a rewarding one.

The point that comes over most strongly from longitudinal studies, however, is that the outcome of transitions, and the ways in which they are dealt with, is partially determined by people's past behaviour and experiences. People act in ways that serve to shape their experiences, and there are equally important links between different types of environment. Of course, too, the transitions will be influenced by societal factors. Career progression will be affected by job opportunities; the experience of marriage and childrearing by housing conditions; the choice of jobs and housing by racial or other forms of discrimination. Finally, the negotiation of transitions will similarly be influenced by the past and by societal factors.

The implication, I suggest, is that just as we have learned not to polarize nature and nurture as if they were mutually exclusive alternative explanations, so also we need to get away from the unduly simplified question of whether a person's behaviour

Journal of Child Psychology and Psychiatry, 1989, vol. 30, pp. 23–51

is the result of past or present experiences. Not only will behaviour be shaped by the biological substrate, genetically and non-genetically determined, as well as by psychosocial influences, but equally both the past and present are likely to have effects. Most crucially, however, they are not independent of one another. To an important extent the past helps to determine the present environment through a variety of different mechanisms. Chain effects are common and, if we are to understand the developmental process, we need to analyse each of the links in the chain, to determine how the links interconnect and to study how changes in life trajectory come about. In this way, life transitions have to be considered both as end products of past processes and as instigators of future ones—in data analysis terms as both independent and dependent variables. It is important to search for unifying principles in the mechanisms underlying the diversity of pathways from childhood to adult life, but in so doing we must consider the pathways in personal terms and in the context of possible person–environment interactions. The elucidation of the processes giving rise to these varied pathways should provide useful leads for both prevention and treatment through improved knowledge on how changes take place, for that is what development is all about.

References

Berreuta-Clement, J. R., Schweinart, L. J., Barnett, W. S., Epstein, A. S. & Weikart, D. P. (1984). *Changed lifes: The effects of the Perry Pre-School Program on youths through age 19.* Ypsilanti: High Scope.

Block, J. (1979). Advancing the science of personality: Paradigmatic shift or improving the quality of research? In D. Magnusson and M. S. Endler (Eds), *Psychology at the crossroads: Current issues and interactional psychology.* Hillsdale, NJ: Erlbaum.

Bowlby, J. (1951). *Maternal care and mental health.* Geneva: World Health Organization.

Bowlby, J. (1969/82). *Attachment and loss:* Vol. 1: *Attachment.* London: Hogarth.

Bowlby, J. (1988). *A secure base: Clinical applications of attachment theory.* London: Routledge.

Bretherton, I. & Waters, E. (Eds) (1985). Growing points of attachment theory and research. *Monographs of the Society for Research in Child Development,* Serial No. 209, 50, Nos 1–2.

Bronfenbrenner, U. (1979). *The ecology of human development: Experiments by nature and design.* Cambridge, MA: Harvard University Press.

Brown, G. W. (1988). Causal paths, chains and strands. In M. Rutter (Ed.), *Studies of psychosocial risk: The power of longitudinal data.* Cambridge: Cambridge University Press.

Brown, G. W., Harris, T. O. & Bifulco, A. (1986). The long term effects of early loss of parent. In M. Rutter, C. E. Izard & P. B. Read (Eds), *Depression in young people: Clinical and developmental perspectives* (pp. 251–296). New York: Guilford.

Brunk, M. A. & Henggeler, S. W. (1984). Child influences on adult controls. An experimental investigation. *Developmental Psychology,* **20,** 1074–1081.

Cadoret, R. J., Troughton, E., Moreno, L. & Whitters, A. (in press). Early life psychosocial events and adult affective symptoms. In L. N. Robins & M. Rutter (Eds), *Straight and devious pathways from childhood to adult life.* Cambridge: Cambridge University Press.

Caspi, A. & Elder, G. H. (1988). Emergent family patterns: The intergenerational construction of problem behaviors and relationships. In R. A. Hinde & J. Stevenson-Hinde (Eds), *Relationships within families: Mutual influences.* Oxford: Clarendon Press.

Caspi, A., Elder, G. H. & Herbener, E. S. (in press), Childhood personality and the prediction of life-course patterns. In L. N. Robins & M. Rutter (Eds), *Straight and devious pathways from childhood to adult life.* Cambridge: Cambridge University Press.

Clarke, A. D. B. & Clarke, A. M. (1984). Consistency and change in the growth of human characteristics. *Journal of Child Psychology and Psychiatry,* **25,** 191–210.

Clarke, A. D. B. & Tizard, B. (Eds) (1983). *Child development and social policy: The life and work of Jack Tizard.* Leicester: British Psychological Society.

26

Clarke, A. M. & Clarke, A. D. B. (1976). *Early experience: Myth and evidence.* London: Open Books.

Clarke, R. B. G. (1985). Delinquency, environment and intervention. *Journal of Child Psychology and Psychiatry,* **26,** 505–523.

Clausen, J. A. (1986). Early adult choices and the life course. *Zeitschrift fur Sozialisations Forschung und Erzielungsozioligie,* **6,** 313–320.

Cohler, B. J. (1987). Adversity, resiliance and the study of lives. In E. J. Anthony & B. J. Cohler (Eds), *The invulnerable child* (pp. 363–424). New York: Guilford.

Dodge, K. A. (1980). Social cognition and children's aggressive behavior. *Child Development,* **51,** 162–172.

Dodge, K. A. (1983). Behavioral antecedents of peer social status. *Child Development,* **54,** 1386–1399.

Dodge, K. A., Pettit, G. S., McClaskey, C. L. & Brown, M. M. (1986). Social competence in children. *Monographs of the Society for Research in Child Development,* Serial No. 213.

Elder, G. H. (1974). *Children of the great depression.* Chicago: University of Chicago Press.

Elder, G. H. (1979). Historical change in life patterns and personality. In P. Baltes & O. G. Brim (Eds), *Life span development and behavior,* Vol. 2. New York: Academic Press.

Elder, G. H. (1986). Military times and turning points in men's lives. *Developmental Psychology,* **22,** 233–245.

Epstein, S. (1979). The stability of behavior: I: On predicting most of the people much of the time. *Journal of Personality and Social Psychology,* **37,** 1097–1126.

Epstein, S. & O'Brien, E. J. (1985). The person-situation debate in historical and current perspectives. *Psychological Bulletin,* **98,** 513–537.

Erikson, E. H. (1963). *Childhood and society* (2nd edn). New York: W. W. Norton.

Farrington, D. P., Loeber, R. & van Kammen, W. B. (in press). Long-term criminal outcomes of hyperactivity–impulsivity–attention deficit and conduct problems in childhood. In L. N. Robins & M. Rutter (Eds), *Straight and devious pathways from childhood to adult life.* Cambridge: Cambridge University Press.

Felsman, J. K. & Vaillant, G. E. (1987). Resiliant children as adults: A 40-year study. In E. J. Anthony & B. J. Cohler (Eds), *The invulnerable child.* (pp. 289–374). New York: Guilford.

Folstein, S. & Rutter, M. (1987). Family aggregation and genetic implications. In E. Schopler & G. Mesibov (Eds), *Neurobiological issues in autism* (pp. 83–105). New York: Plenum.

Folstein, S. E., Franz, M. L., Jensen, B. A., Chase, G. A. & Folstein, M. F. (1983). Conduct disorder and affective disorder among the offspring of patients with Huntington's disease. *Psychological Medicine,* **13,** 45–52.

Garmezy, N. (1983). Stressors of childhood. In N. Garmezy & M. Rutter (Eds), *Stress, coping and development in children* (pp. 43–84). New York: McGraw-Hill.

Goodman, R. (1987). The developmental neurobiology of language. In W. Yule & M. Rutter (Eds), *Language development and disorders: Clinics in developmental medicine, No. 101/102.* London: MacKeith/Blackwell.

Gottesman, I. I. & Shields, J. (1976). A critical review of recent adoption, twin and family studies of schizophrenia: Behavioral genetics perspective. *Schizophrenia Bulletin,* **2,** 360–400.

Graham, P. & Rutter, M. (1985). Adolescent disorders. In M. Rutter & L. Hersov (Eds), *Child and adolescent psychiatry: Modern Approaches* (2nd edn) (pp. 351–367). Oxford: Blackwell Scientific.

Gray, G., Smith, A. & Rutter, M. (1980). School attendance and the first year of employment. In L. Hersov & I. Berg (Eds), *Out of school: Modern perspectives in truancy and school refusal* (pp. 343–370). Chichester: Wiley.

Greenough, W. T., Black, J. E. & Wallace, C. S. (1987). Experience and brain development. *Child Development,* **58,** 539–559.

Harris, T., Brown, G. W. & Bifulco, A. (1986). Loss of parent in childhood and adult psychiatric disorder: The role of lack of adequate parental care. *Psychological Medicine,* **16,** 641–659.

Harris, T., Brown, G. W. & Bifulco, A. (1987). Loss of parent in childhood and adult psychiatric disorder: The role of social class position and premarital pregnancy. *Psychological Medicine,* **17,** 163–183.

Hayes, C. D. (Ed.) (1987). *Preventing adolescent pregnancy: An agenda for America.* Washington DC: National Academy Press.

Hennessy, J. & Levine, S. (1979). Stress, arousal and the pituitary–adrenal system: A psychoendocrine hypothesis. In J. M. Sprague & A. N. Epstein (Eds), *Progress in psychobiology and physiological psychology* (pp. 133–178). New York: Academic Press.

■27

Journal of Child Psychology and Psychiatry, 1989, vol. 30, pp. 23–51

Hertzig, M. E., Birch, H. G., Richardson, S. A. & Tizard, J. (1972). Intellectual levels of school children severely malnurished during the first two years of life. *Pediatrics,* **49,** 814–824.

Hetherington, E. M. (1988). Parents, children and siblings: 6 years after divorce. In R. A. Hinde & J. Stevenson-Hinde (Eds), *Relationships within families: Mutual influences.* Oxford: Clarendon Press.

Hetherington, E. M., Cox, M. & Cox, A. (1982). Effects of divorce on parents and Children. In M. E. Lamb (Ed.), *Nontraditional families* (pp. 223–288). Hillsdale, NJ: Erlbaum.

Hetherington, E. M., Cox, M. & Cox, A. (1985). Long-term effects of divorce and remarriage on the adjustment of children. *Journal of the American Academy of Child Psychiatry,* **24,** 518–530.

Hinde, R. A. (1987). *Individuals, relationships and culture: Links between ethology and the social sciences.* Cambridge: Cambridge University Press.

Hinde, R. A. (1988). Continuities and discontinuities: Conceptual issues and methodological considerations. In M. Rutter (Ed.), *Studies of psychosocial risk: The power of longitudinal data.* Cambridge: Cambridge University Press.

Hinde, R. A. & Bateson, P. A. (1984). Discontinuities versus continuities in behavioural development and the neglect of process. *International Journal of Behavioural Development,* **7,** 129–143.

Hinde, R. A. & Stevenson-Hinde, J. (Eds) (1988). *Relationships within families: Mutual influences.* Oxford: Clarendon Press.

Hodges, J. & Tizard, B. (1989 a). IQ and behavioural adjustment of ex-institutional adolescents. *Journal of Child Psychology and Psychiatry,* **30,** 53–75.

Hodges, J. & Tizard, B. (1989 b). Social and family relationships of ex-institutional adolescents. *Journal of Child Psychology and Psychiatry,* **30,** 77–97.

Hunt, J. McV. (1979). Psychological development: Early experience. *Annual Review of Psychology,* **30,** 103–143.

Kagan, J. (1984). *The nature of the child.* New York: Basic Books.

Kandel, D. B. & Davies, M. (1986). Adult sequelae of adolescent depressive symptoms. *Archives of General Psychiatry,* **43,** 255–262.

Kelly, E. L. (1955). Consistency of the adult personality. *American Psychologist,* **10,** 659–681.

Levinson, D., with Darrow, D. N., Klein, E. B., Levinson, M. H. & McKee, D. (1976). *The seasons of a man's life.* New York: Alfred Knopf.

Lewis, S. W. & Murray, R. M. (1987). Obstetric complications, neurodevelopmental deviance and risk of schizophrenia. *Journal of Psychiatric Research,* **21,** 413–421.

Maccoby, E. E. (1984). Socialization and developmental change. *Child Development,* **55,** 317–328.

Magnusson, D. (1988). *Individual development from an interactional perspective: A longitudinal study.* Hillsdale, NJ: Erlbaum.

Magnusson, D., Stattin, H. & Allen, V. L. (1986). Differential maturation amongst girls and its relation to social adjustment: A longitudinal perspective. In D. Featherman & R. M. Lerner (Eds), *Life span development,* Vol. 7. New York: Academic Press.

Main, M., Kaplan, N. & Cassidy, J. (1985). Security in infancy, childhood, and adulthood: A move to the level of representation. In I. Bretherton & E. Waters, (Eds), Growing points of attachment theory and research. *Monographs of the Society for Research in Child Development,* Serial No. 209, 50, Nos 1–2. (pp. 66–106).

Masten, A. S. & Garmezy, M. (1985). Risk, vulnerability, and protective factors in developmental psychopathology. In B. B. Lahey & A. E. Kazdin (Eds), *Advances in clinical child psychology,* Vol. 8 (pp. 1–52). New York: Plenum.

Maughan, B. & Rutter, M. (1986). Black pupils' progress in secondary schools: II: Examination attainments. *British Journal of Developmental Psychology,* **4,** 19–29.

Maughan, B. M. & Champion, L. (in press). Risk and protective factors in the transition of young adults. In P. B. Baltes & M. M. Baltes (Eds), *Successful aging: Research and theory.* New York: Cambridge University Press.

Maughan, D., Dunn, G. & Rutter, M. (1985a), Black pupils' progress in secondary schools: I: Reading attainment between 10 and 14. *British Journal of Developmental Psychology,* **3,** 113–121.

Maughan, B., Gray, G. & Rutter, M. (1985b). Reading retardation and antisocial behaviour: A follow-up into employment. *Journal of Child Psychology and Psychiatry,* **26,** 741–758.

Mayer-Bahlberg, H. F. L., Ehrhardt, A. A. & Feldman, J. F. (1986). Long-term implications of the prenatal endocrine milieu for sex-dimorphic behavior. In L. Erlenmeyer-Kimling & N. E. Miller (Eds), *Life-span research on the prediction of psychopathology* (pp. 17–30). Hillsdale, NJ: Erlbaum.

28 ▪

McCall, R. B. (1977). Challenges to a science of developmental psychology. *Child Development,* **48,** 333–344.

Mischel, W. (1968). *Personality and assessment.* New York: Wiley.

Mischel, W. (1969). Continuities and change in personality. *American Psychologist,* **24,** 1012–1018.

Moos, R. H. (Ed.) (1986). *Coping with life crises: An integrated approach.* New York: Plenum.

Mortimore, P., Sammons, P., Stoll, L., Lewis, D. & Etob, R. (1988). *School matters: The junior years.* Wells, Somerset: Open Books.

Moss, H. A. & Susman, E. J. (1980). Longitudinal study of personality development. In O. G. Brim & J. Kagan (Eds), *Constancy and change in human development* (pp. 530–595). Cambridge, MA: Harvard University Press.

Murray, R. M., Lewis, S. W., Owen, M. J. & Foerster, A. (in press). The neurodevelopmental origins of demenia precox. In P. McGuffin & P. Bebbington (Eds), *Schizophrenia: The major issues.* London: Heinemann.

Nesselroade, J. (1988). Some implications of the trait–state distinction for the study of development over the life-span: Case of personality. In P. B. Baltes, D. L. Featherman & R. M. Lerner (Eds), *Life span development and behaviour,* Vol. 8 (pp. 163–189). Hillsdale, NJ: Erlbaum.

Nuechterlein, K. H. (1986). Childhood precursors of adult schizophrenia. *Journal of Child Psychology and Psychiatry,* **27,** 133–144.

O'Connor, N. (1956). The evidence for the permanently disturbing effects of mother–child separation. *Acta Psychologica,* **12,** 174–191.

Olweus, D. (1979). Stability of aggressive reaction patterns in males: a review. *Psychological Bulletin,* **86,** 852–875.

Orlansky, H. (1949). Infant care and personality. *Psychological Bulletin,* **46,** 1–48.

Otto, L. B. (1979). Antecedents and consequences of marital timing. In W. R. Burr, R. Hill, F. I. Nye & I. L. Reiss (Eds), *Contemporary theories about the family,* Vol. 1. (pp. 101–126). New York: Free Press.

Parker, J. G. & Asher, S. R. (1987). Peer relations and later personal adjustment: Are low-accepted children at risk? *Psychological Bulletin,* **102,** 357–389.

Parnas, J., Schulsinger, R., Teasdale, T. W., Schulsinger, H., Feldman, P. M. & Mednick, S. A. (1982). Perinatal complications and clinical outcome within the schizophrenia spectrum. *British Journal of Psychiatry,* **140,** 416–420.

Pedersen, E., Faucher, T. A. & Eaton, W. W. (1978). A new perspective on the effects of first grade teachers on children's subsequent adult status. *Harvard Educational Review,* **48,** 1–31.

Petersen, A. C. (1988). Adolescent development. *Annual Review of Psychology,* **39,** 583–607.

Plomin, R. (1986). *Development, genetics and psychology.* Hillsdale, NJ: Erlbaum.

Plomin, R. & Thompson, L. (1988). Life-span developmental behavioral genetics. In P. B. Baltes, D. L. Featherman & R. M. Lerner (Eds), *Life-span development and behavior,* Vol. 8 (pp. 1–31). Hillsdale, NJ: Erlbaum.

Porter, R., O'Conner, M. & Whelan, J. (Eds) (1984). *Alcohol damage in utero.* Ciba Foundation Symposium No. 105. London: Pitman.

Quinton, D. & Rutter, M. (1988). *Parental breakdown: The making and breaking of intergenerational links.* Aldershot: Gower.

Quinton, D., Rutter, M. & Gulliver, L. (in press). Continuities in psychiatric disorders from childhood to adulthood, in the children of psychiatric patients. In L. N. Robins & M. Rutter (Eds), *Straight and devious pathways from childhood to adult life.* Cambridge: Cambridge University Press.

Richman, N., Stevenson, J. & Graham, P. (1982). *Preschool to school: A behavioural study.* London: Academic Press.

Robins, L. (1978). Sturdy childhood predictors of adult antisocial behaviour: Replications from longitudinal studies. *Psychological Medicine,* **8,** 611–622.

Robins, L. N. (1986). The consequences of conduct disorder in girls. In D. Olweus, J. Block & M. Radke-Yarrow (Eds), *Development of antisocial and prosocial behaviour: Research, theories and issues* (pp. 385–408). New York: Academic Press.

Rosenzweig, M. R. & Bennett, E. L. (1977). Effects of environmental enrichment or impoverishment on learning and on brain values in rodents. In A. Oliviero (Ed.), *Genetics, environment and intelligence* (pp. 163–196). Amsterdam: North Holland.

Journal of Child Psychology and Psychiatry, 1989, vol. 30, pp. 23–51

Rutter, M. (1979). Protective factors in children's responses to stress and disadvantage. In M. W. Kent & J. E. Rolf (Eds), *Primary prevention of psychopathology*, Vol. 3: *Social competence in children* (pp. 49–74). Hanover, NH: University Press of New England.

Rutter, M. (1981). *Maternal deprivation reassessed* (2nd edn). Harmondsworth: Penguin.

Rutter, M. (1982). Developmental neuropsychiatry: Concepts, issues and prospects. *Journal of Clinical Neuropsychiatry*, **4**, 91–115.

Rutter, M. (1983). Statistical and personal interactions: Facets and perspectives. In D. Magnusson & V. Allen (Eds), *Human development: An interactional perspective* (pp. 295–319). New York: Academic Press.

Rutter, M. (1984a). Psychopathology and development. I: Childhood antecedents of adult psychiatric disorder. *Australian and New Zealand Journal of Psychiatry*, **18**, 225–234.

Rutter, M. (1984b). Psychopathology and development. II: Childhood experiences and personality development. *Australian and New Zealand Journal of Psychiatry*, **18**, 314–327.

Rutter, M. (1984c). Continuities and discontinuities in socioemotional development: Empirical and conceptual perspectives. In R. Emde & R. Harmon (Eds), *Continuities and discontinuities in development* (pp. 41–68). New York: Plenum.

Rutter, M. (1985a). Family and school influences on cognitive development. *Journal of Child Psychology and Psychiatry*, **26**, 683–704.

Rutter, M. (1985b). Family and school influences on behavioural development. *Journal of Child Psychology and Psychiatry*, **26**, 349–368.

Rutter, M. (1987a). Continuities and discontinuities from infancy. In J. Osofsky (Ed.), *Handbook of infant development* (2nd edn) (pp. 1256–1298). New York: Wiley.

Rutter, M. (1987b). Temperament, personality and personality development. *British Journal of Psychiatry*, **150**, 443–458.

Rutter, M. (1987c). The role of cognition in child development and disorder. *British Journal of Medical Psychology*, **60**, 1–16.

Rutter, M. (1988). Epidemiological approaches to developmental psychopathology. *Archives of General Psychiatry*, **45**, 486–495.

Rutter, M. (in press a). Psychosocial resilience and protective mechanisms. In J. E. Rolf, A. S. Masten, D. Cicchetti, K. Nuechterlein & S. Weintraub (Eds), *Risk and protective factors in the development of psychopathology*. New York: Cambridge University Press.

Rutter, M. (in press b). Age as an ambiguous variable in developmental research. *International Journal of Behavioural Development*.

Rutter, M., Macdonald, H., Le Couteur, A., Harrington, R., Bolton, P. & Bailey, A. (submitted). Genetic factors in child psychiatric disorders: H: Empirical findings.

Rutter, M., Quinton, D. & Hill, J. (in press). Adult outcome of institution-reared children: Males and females compared. In L. N. Robins & M. Rutter (Eds), *Straight and devious pathways from childhood to adult life*. Cambridge: Cambridge University Press.

Rutter, M. & Sandberg, S. (1985). Epidemiology of child psychiatric disorder: Methodological issues and some substantive findings. *Child Psychiatry and Human Development*, **15**, 209–233.

Rutter, M., Tizard, J. & Whitmore, K. (1970). *Education, health and behaviour*. London: Longman.

Rutter, M., Tizard, J., Yule, W., Graham, P. & Whitmore, K. (1976). Isle of Wight Studies 1964–1974. *Psychological Medicine*, **6**, 313–332.

Scarr, S. & MacCartney, K. (1983). How people make their own environments: A theory of genotype-environment effects. *Child Development*, **54**, 424–435.

Smalley, S. L., Asarnow, R. F. & Spence, M. A. (1988). Autism and genetics: A decade of research. *Archives of General Psychiatry*, **45**, 953–961.

Snyder, C. R. & Ford, C. E. (Eds) (1987). *Coping with negative life events: clinical and social psychological perspectives*. New York: Plenum.

Tizard, B. & Hodges, J. (1978). The effect of early institutional rearing on the development of eight-year old children. *Journal of Child Psychology and Psychiatry*, **19**, 99–118.

Tizard, B., Blatchford, D., Burk, J., Farquahar, C. & Plewis, I. (1988). *Young children at school in the inner city*. London: Erlbaum.

Tizard, J. (1975). Three dysfunctional environmental influences in development: malnutrition, non-accidental injury and child minding. In D. Baltrop (Ed.), *Pediatrics and the environment*. Unigate Paediatric Workshops No. 2 (1974) (pp. 19–27). London: Fellowship of Postgraduate Medicine.

Tizard, J. (1976). Psychology and social policy. *British Psychological Society Bulletin, 29,* 225–234. (Reprinted in A. D. B. Clarke & B. Tizard, 1983. *Child development and social policy: The life and work of Jack Tizard.* Leicester: British Psychological Society.)

Warr, P. (1987). *Work, unemployment and mental health.* Oxford: Clarendon Press.

Waters, E., Hay, D. & Richters, J. (1986). Infant–parent attachment and the origins of prosocial and antisocial behavior. In D. Olweus, J. Block & M. Radke-Yarrow (Eds), *Development of antisocial and prosocial behavior: Research theories and issues* (pp. 97–125). London: Academic Press.

Weinberger, D. R. (1987). Implications of normal brain development for the pathogenesis of schizophrenia. *Archives of General Psychiatry, 44,* 660–669.

Werner, E. E. (1985). Stress and protective factors in children's life. In A. R. Nicol (Ed.), *Longitudinal studies in child psychology and psychiatry: Practical lessons from research experience* (pp. 335–355). Chichester: Wiley.

Werner, E. E. & Smith, R. S. (1982). *Vulnerable but invincible: A longitudinal study of resilient children and youth.* New York: McGraw-Hill.

Wortman, C. B. & Silver, R. C. (in press). The myths of coping with loss. *Journal of Consulting and Clinical Psychology.*

Yarrow, L. J. (1961). Maternal deprivation: Toward an empirical and conceptual re-evaluation. *Psychological Bulletin, 58,* 459–490.

Zeitlin, H. (1986). *The natural history of disorder in childhood. Institute of Psychiatry/Maudsley Monograph* No. 29. Oxford: Oxford University Press.

■ 31

Archives of General Psychiatry, 1988, vol. 45, pp. 486–495

Epidemiological Approaches to Developmental Psychopathology

32. ■

Michael Rutter, FRS

● Developmental psychopathology as a research approach draws on both developmental and psychopathologic perspectives to tackle questions about causal mechanisms. Developmental perspectives are discussed in terms of the implications that flow from age differences in prevalence, age trends in remission of disorders, developmental appropriateness of psychiatric conditions, continuities and discontinuities in psychopathology between childhood and adult life, and age differences in the effects of psychiatric risk factors. Psychopathologic perspectives are considered in terms of continuities and discontinuities between normality and pathology and the contrasts between pervasive and situation-specific disorders, and by the differences between single variables and behavioral composites. The use of epidemiological data to examine causal processes is discussed, with attention to the need to consider development in its social context and to examine indirect, as well as direct, causal chains of connection.

(*Arch Gen Psychiatry* 1988;45:486-495)

Epidemiology, of course, is concerned with the study of the distribution of disorders in defined populations, together with an examination of the factors that influence that distribution. Often, cross-sectional approaches are combined with longitudinal research strategies because of the substantial additional leverage provided by a longitudinal or natural history component.[1,2] Epidemiological data are used for many purposes, including service planning[3,4] and the search for causes of diseases.[5] In psychiatry, as in other branches of medicine, case-control designs and cohort studies have been used for these ends through the familiar statistics of incidence, prevalence, relative risks, and odds ratios.[6] These methods have proved as applicable in child psychiatry as in the adult field, with the result that we know a great deal, albeit not enough, about the epidemiology of psychiatric disorders in childhood and adolescence.[7-11]

Accepted for publication Sept 10, 1987.
From the Medical Research Council Child Psychiatry Unit, Institute of Psychiatry, London.
Based on the Rema Lapouse Mental Health Epidemiology Award Lecture, 1986, given at the American Public Health Association 114th Annual Meeting, Las Vegas, Sept 30, 1986.
Reprint requests to MRC Child Psychiatry Unit, Institute of Psychiatry, De Crespigny Park, Denmark Hill, London SE5 8AF (Prof Rutter).

Nevertheless, the epidemiological approach in child psychiatry has involved some differences in emphasis that stem from the adoption of developmental psychopathology concepts. These concepts, however, apply across the life span and are relevant to adult as well as child psychiatry. In the present article I seek to outline some of the main features of these concepts. Empirical examples are used to illustrate the points but no attempt is made to review the research literature on each of the various topics used in illustration; instead, where possible, reference is made to books or articles that provide some appraisal of the relevant research findings. In short, my aim here is to introduce a perspective rather than to present a body of knowledge.

DEVELOPMENTAL PSYCHOPATHOLOGY

Developmental psychopathology comprises a set of research approaches that capitalize on developmental variations and psychopathologic variations to ask questions about mechanisms and processes.[12-15] Epidemiological data have proved invaluable when seeking to tackle these questions, but the research issues have been formulated in ways that depart in some respects from those that have been traditional in epidemiology. Most crucially, there is a focus on continuities and discontinuities rather than on rates of disorder as such. The developmental perspective is concerned with continuities and discontinuities over time, and the psychopathologic perspective with continuities and discontinuities over the span of behavioral variation. In both cases the findings are used to examine mechanisms and processes. In other words, the aim is to go beyond the identification of risk factors to the delineation of the chain of operations by which such factors lead to disorder.

Developmental Perspective

The developmental perspective takes age as a key variable in both research strategies and data analyses. Of course, age is an ambiguous variable in that it can mean so many different things.[16] Thus, age reflects the various different aspects of biologic maturation, cognitive level, social status, the duration of experiences, and the type of experiences encountered. However, it is the different aspects of age that make it so powerful a variable in research, provided it is broken down into its various components. The comparison of behaviors according to their correlates with different facets of age (such as stage of puberty, mental age, and measures of experience) may be used to test competing causal hypotheses. The assumption is that the asking and answering of questions about age differences may cast important light on causal processes. Such age differences may be apparent in several different ways. Thus, for example, there may be age differences in prevalence, as there are with depression, suicide, and attempted suicide.[17] Much research in recent years has concentrated on showing that depressive disorders of an adult type can and do arise in childhood and that when they occur their features are quite similar to those seen in adult patients. That is an important finding, but the developmental perspective demands the further inquiry into why depressive conditions appear to be so much *less* common in early life than in adulthood. What is it about childhood that protects or what is it about adult life that puts people at greater risk for depression?

Alternatively, age differences may be applied to rates of remission, a strategy that has been informative in the case of nocturnal enuresis.[18] A further approach is afforded by the subdivision of disorders according to age at onset. For example, the Isle of Wight study data showed that psychiatric disorders among adolescents varied markedly according to whether the disorders began during that age period or whether they represented the persistence of disorders that had their onset in earlier childhood.[19] Another research strategy is to subdivide conditions according to whether or not the phenomena are developmentally appropriate. Many psychiatric disorders in childhood, as with many in adult life, do not involve symptoms that are abnormal in themselves. The pathology lies in the severity, extent, or persistence of behaviors that in lesser degrees are part of normal functioning. Thus, everyone experiences fear and anxiety in some circumstances; what makes anxiety states into disorders is not so much the *form* of the anxiety as its severity and the social impairment to which it gives rise. In the case of psychiatric disorders arising in childhood we can ask the additional question of whether the particular types of symptoms would be regarded as developmentally appropriate were they milder in degree. Some kinds of fears are so common as to be a normal part of growing up. Fears of the dark and separation anxiety fall into that category. Others have no obvious and straightforward normal counterpart; for example, agoraphobia. It may be that this differentiation is of some diagnostic importance (not with respect to judgments on abnormality as such, but rather on what that abnormality may reflect or mean). Finally, age may be considered in terms of the extent and nature of continuities in psychopathology between childhood and adult life. These vary markedly according to psychiatric diagnosis; such variations in continuity may throw important light on the nature of the disorders and the differences between diagnostic groups.

Psychopathologic Perspective

The second major perspective, that of psychopathologic variation, takes different definitions of normality and abnormality as the key variables that are crucial to the research strategies employed. In psychiatry as a whole there has been much argument over how to define a "case."[20] Thus, disputes have raged over the differentiation of "true" depression, a hypothesized disease state, from "demoralization," conceptualized as a normal response to stressful or adverse life circumstances. As epidemiology is concerned with the study of the distribution of cases in different populations, it would seem crucial to decide in advance just what constitutes a "case." Developmental psychopathology rejects that view. There is no prior assumption that there is or is not a continuity between normality and illness. Rather there is a central focus on the question of the nature and extent of continuities and discontinuities. The "gray" area of doubt as to whether or not the behaviors are sufficient to meet the criteria for "caseness" becomes a crucial feature of the research and not just a methodologic problem to be circumvented.

This question of psychopathologic variation may be posed in several different ways. Thus, there is the immediate issue of continuities and discontinuities between normality and abnormality. Psychiatry is full of examples where that problem is central—severe dieting and anorexia nervosa, heavy drinking and alcoholism, ordinary misery and depressive illness, to mention but three. In addition, there is the closely related problem of how to subdivide abnormality. It is clear that schizophrenia is genetically associated with a broader range of personality disorders but it remains unclear just how this nonpsychotic phenotype should be defined.[21-23] Similarly, it seems that autism is genetically associated with a range of cognitive and social disabilities of types that do not fulfill the diagnostic criteria for autism.[24] But what differentiates the language and personality disorders that are part of the autistic "spectrum" from those that are not? Rather than predecide these issues to undertake genetic research, it is necessary to use epidemiologically sound genetic data to derive and test alternative definitions.

However, the normality-abnormality differentiation is not the only psychopathologic variation issue to consider. Epidemiological studies have shown the high frequency with which psychiatric disorders in childhood are situation-specific.[4] The same data have indicated that, at least so far as hyperactivity is concerned, there may be important differences between those disorders that are pervasive over situations and those that are specific to particular social contexts.[25] In addition, there is a need to examine the nature of situation specificity. What are the characteristics of the situations that elicit the abnormal behaviors, and which mechanisms are involved in the processes leading to situation specificity? A third issue concerns the differences between variables and composites. Much psychologic research is based on the premise that the key datum is the individual variable; analyses concern the statistical manipulation of particular behavioral features, such as activity level, mood, or aggression. Of course, factors may be derived from the correlations between several variables but these rely on the pattern of associations found in the population as a whole. In contrast, much psychiatric research assumes that the patterns of interest may be characteristic only of abnormal groups. The concept of schizophrenia, for example, is in no way based on evidence that the key behaviors used in diagnosis cluster together in the normal population; rather it is that clustering that defines the abnormal condition. In some instances it seems fairly obvious which approach is to be preferred but in others there is real doubt. The need in these cases is to focus on the contrast to determine what effect this has on the correlates and consequences of the behavior in question.

Focus on Mechanisms and Processes

The third characteristic of a developmental psychopathology perspective is a focus on developmental and psychopathologic mechanisms; the aim being to move from statistical associations to psychobiologic processes. One key way in which this objective is met is through the epidemiologically time-honored search for experiments of

■ 33

Archives of General Psychiatry, 1988, vol. 45, pp. 486–495

nature to test causal hypotheses.[5] However, there is a difference in emphasis, perhaps, in the rejection of the assumption that there is one basic cause that necessarily operates by establishing some pathologic process within the individual. That is one possibility, but there are others. There are many examples of causal processes that operate through their effects on interpersonal interactions; thus, certain temperamental features elicit negative reactions from other people,[26,27] reactions that in turn have consequences for the children. That observation brings out another aspect of research into mechanisms, namely, that often it is necessary to examine causal chains in which the end product is the result of many linkages over time rather than one event- or time-restricted causal mechanism. Attempts to delineate the various mechanisms involved in these chains of indirect connections underlying continuities and discontinuities in development are a hallmark of the developmental psychopathology approach to causal questions. It should be noted that because indirect linkages provide the opportunity for varied outcomes and for turning points in the life trajectory, the focus is as much on discontinuities as on continuities.

Developmental Psychopathology as a Unifying Theme

It is clear that developmental psychopathology does not constitute a theory, nor is it an approach that can sensibly be seen as providing an all-encompassing concept in psychiatry (although some of its proponents might wish that it did so). Rather, it serves as a means of bringing together a set of research strategies that have been little used until now and that carry the potential of throwing new light on old topics. As will be apparent from the examples to be given, these strategies overlap with those that derive from other starting points. Nevertheless, the perspectives' difference in emphasis is sufficient to warrant attention.

DEVELOPMENTAL PERSPECTIVES
Age Differences in Prevalence

The topic of age differences in prevalence provides an appropriate starting point. Depressive disorders constitute a good example of a psychiatric condition that shows marked variations in rate with age.[17] Both clinic and general population studies suggest that serious depressive conditions are relatively infrequent in early and middle childhood, become much more common during the years of adolescence, and probably reach a peak in late adolescence or early adult life. The data on these age trends are not as sound as one would like, and there are methodologic queries about the comparability of the measures used at different age periods. Nevertheless, there seems little doubt that depressive disorders do show a marked rise in prevalence during the teenage years. Several questions arise from this observation. First, the trends are not the same for all measures of affective disturbance. For example, whereas attempted suicide peaks at about 20 years of age, completed suicide does not peak until old age. Also, crying is most prevalent in infancy, irritability shows little change in frequency over the 5- to 15-year age span, and mood swings increase in adolescence.[28] Negative mood cannot be considered as a unitary phenomenon. We need to ask why different aspects show different age patterns. However, we also have to determine which processes underlie each age trend.

In the Isle of Wight study[19] we examined the possibility that the stage of puberty constituted the crucial determinant. The children were all 14½ to 15½ years of age so that there was little variation in chronological age; but within this single age cohort there was, as should be expected, marked individual variation in the timing of puberty. Sub-

jects in the sample were too old for us to examine the association with puberty in girls, as virtually all girls had reached their menarche. But, the association could be determined in boys. However it was measured, depression was most prevalent in those who had completed puberty and was least prevalent in those who had not yet entered puberty. The implication is that the hormonal changes of puberty may have been responsible for the increased vulnerability to depression. The finding needs replicating with better measures of depression than were available to us 20 years ago, before accepting it as a fact. Also, the association needs examining in girls, as the hormonal changes in females differ from those in males. In addition, it is necessary to keep in mind the possibility that it is not a direct hormonal effect at all but rather a psychologic response to the physical changes of puberty and to the social consequences that ensue.[29]

The need to consider age trends in male and female subjects separately is underlined by the evidence that there may be a change in the sex ratio of depressive disorders associated with puberty. In a study of psychiatric clinic patients, Pearce[30] found that whereas psychiatric disorders showing an operationally defined constellation of depressive symptoms were more common in boys before puberty, they were more frequent in girls after puberty. Other research, too, has shown that depressive disorders in younger children are equally common in the two sexes or are more common in boys, whereas those in later adolescence exhibit the female preponderance that is typical of depressive conditions in adult life.[31,32]

It will be appreciated that the finding of an age difference in the prevalence of any psychiatric disorder constitutes the beginning and not the end of the research enterprise. As already noted, age is an ambiguous variable with many different meanings. However, that very feature provides the means to test competing hypotheses on mechanisms just because the different facets of age do not proceed exactly in parallel. I have mentioned the possibility that hormonal factors influence the risk for depression, but it is also possible that the age variations in risk stem from cognitive factors (a degree of cognitive maturity is required to experience the cognitive components of depression such as feelings of hopelessness, self-depreciation, and guilt) or from experiential factors (perhaps young children are less likely to experience the loss events that tend to precipitate depression or perhaps they have more protective family supports).

Researchers into childhood depression have tended to stress that the characteristics closely parallel those associated with adult depression. The developmental perspective forces one to ask why depression nevertheless shows such a marked age trend. Obviously, the same question could be posed for the onset of autism in infancy, of anorexia nervosa in adolescence, and of numerous other age-diagnosis associations. It should be emphasized that the developmental perspective requires one to ask why certain adult psychiatric disorders usually do *not* have an onset in childhood as it is to focus on those that begin in early life.

Age Differences in Remission

Age trends may be examined for remission as well as for prevalence. The most obvious group of disorders in which this is relevant is developmental disorders. The general concept is that they represent the extreme end of the normal curve for the acquisition of various developmental milestones. It is known that there is individual variability in the rate of biologic maturation and it is also known that different parts of the brain mature at different rates. It

34 ■

seems a natural extrapolation to assume that the cause for an unusual delay in, for example, the acquisition of bladder control is a specific retardation in the maturation of the relevant section of the central nervous system. The expectation associated with this biologic maturation hypothesis is that there should be a clear-cut age curve for the acquisition of bladder control. At first sight, that is what epidemiological data suggest. The proportion of children becoming permanently dry rises steadily with age, as the Baltimore study[18] shows. However, the remission rate findings tell a somewhat different story. The likelihood that an enuretic child will become dry during any given 12-month period remains roughly constant, at approximately 15%, over the period from 4 to 10 years of age. If the explanation of the late acquisition of bladder control was delay in biologic maturation one might expect that the likelihood of remission should increase with age, but it does not. Epidemiological-longitudinal data also show that there is a slight *increase* in the prevalence of enuresis after starting school and that as many as one fourth of children who have acquired reliable bladder control subsequently lose it. It has been argued that because enuresis is, relatively speaking, so common in middle childhood, it should not be regarded as a disorder until at least 8 years of age.[33] However, data on prevalence provide a highly fallible guide to what is or is not pathology. Dental caries is exceedingly common but we do not regard it as normal for that reason; we consider it pathologic because it leads to tissue damage. The developmental trends for enuresis suggest that the factors associated with acquisition of bladder control after the age of 4 or 5 years are not identical with those that operate in infancy and early childhood. Of course, to some extent the findings may reflect a difference between primary and secondary enuresis (ie, between those who have never acquired control and those who have but who subsequently lose it), but the scanty available data suggest that this is unlikely to be the whole explanation. In any case, the point of the developmental perspective is to force one to ask what the findings on age differences in remission mean.

Similar issues arise with respect to other developmental disorders. We know that normal children vary greatly in the age at which they begin to speak. Some children do not begin until approximately 2 years of age yet subsequently progress entirely normally.[34] Yet others who are delayed in their acquisition of spoken language show all sorts of associated problems that persist long after they speak fluently; such problems include socio-emotional-behavioral abnormalities as well as reading and spelling difficulties. Developmental data on age variations regarding the likelihood of acquiring speech without psychologic sequelae would be helpful in determining what proportion of cases are likely to be due to simple maturational delay. Such data are not available, but they could be obtained. Equally, the data would focus attention on the nature of the group whose language retardation cannot be explained in that way. For example, does that group include cases due to some identifiable neurodevelopmental abnormality, and are the associated psychological problems consequences of the language disorder or do both stem from some underlying pathologic lesion of the brain?

Subdivision by Age at Onset

The third developmental strategy is to subdivide disorders according to the subjects' age at onset. The assumption is that at any one age, some disorders will have begun during that age period, whereas others will represent the persistence of conditions that began very much earlier. This is not a research approach that has been much employed, but

the Isle of Wight data[19] suggest that it can be very informative. Thus, most studies of psychiatric disorders in adolescents have either considered them as a group or have subdivided them according to diagnosis. Because the Isle of Wight survey of 15-year-old adolescents also represented a follow-up of the same cohort that had been studied similarly at 10 years of age, we were able to subdivide the disorders at 15 years of age into those already identified at 10 years of age and those that developed after that age. It was found that the persisting disorders of early onset had strong associations with various measures of family psychopathology and disruption, whereas this was not so for the disorders that had begun de novo during the early years of adolescence.

In part, this difference according to age at onset was a function of chronicity as the disorders beginning before 10 years of age that did not persist until age 15 also showed a lesser association with family adversity. However, that was not the explanation for the link between reading retardation and age at onset. Disorders beginning before 10 years of age showed a very strong association with specific reading difficulties, whereas young people whose psychiatric disorders that began after 10 years of age showed *no* increase in reading difficulties compared with the general population. The implication is that there is something rather different about emotional and conduct disorders with an onset in adolescence. We know a good deal about the correlates (and by extension, possibly, also the causes) of disorders of early onset but much less about those that begin in the adolescent years.

Subdivision by Developmental Appropriateness

The fourth developmental strategy, namely, making use of developmental appropriateness, has not been used systematically until now, but such data that are available suggest that it would be worthwhile to employ it more. Following are just two examples. School refusal, an emotional disorder in which the act of going to school is associated with severe anxiety often amounting to panic, is commonly held to be due to separation anxiety in many cases.[35] Anxiety over separation from parents is, of course, a normal phenomenon in early childhood. Hence, an exaggeration of that anxiety in the form of school refusal in the first few years of schooling might be considered to be developmentally appropriate. However, school refusal actually becomes more frequent during the adolescent age period, a developmental phase when fear over physical separation from parents is not normally expected. The very few data available[36,37] suggest that school refusal may have a much better prognosis in young children, in keeping perhaps with the suggestion of developmental appropriateness.

The data on delinquency indicate an opposite age trend. In the general population, minor delinquent acts by boys are most common during adolescence.[38] The prognosis is also best for delinquency that begins for the first time during that age period.[39,40] The greatest likelihood that crime will persist into adult life and that antisocial behavior will be followed by a persisting personality disorder is seen with antisocial behavior that begins in early childhood. In other words, the greatest chance that there will be a persistence of criminality into adulthood is seen with onsets that are furthest removed from the adult age period.

These two examples indicate that prognostic power does not lie in early or late onset per se. Whether the outlook is better or worse with an early onset depends on the particular disorder. The suggestion is that the key feature may be whether or not the behavior in question is developmentally appropriate. Traditionally, child psychiatrists

Archives of General Psychiatry, 1988, vol. 45, pp. 486–495

have differentiated between emotional disorders with an onset specific to childhood and adult-type anxiety or "neurotic" conditions, a differentiation present in both the *DSM-III*[41] and *ICD-9*.[42] Unfortunately, there is great uncertainty about the criteria to be used in making this differential diagnosis. The draft guidelines for the *ICD-10* suggest that developmental appropriateness should be the criterion, with adult-type disorders being those that do *not* represent an exaggeration of any usual developmental trend.[43] Research is needed to test the utility of this diagnostic criterion, but it seems worthy of further trial and testing.

Temporal Continuities and Discontinuities in Psychopathology

The fifth developmental research strategy involves the use of data on continuities and discontinuities in psychopathology between childhood and adult life. Empirical findings show that the patterns of linkage between these two age periods vary greatly across diagnostic groups.[44] However, surprisingly little use has been made of this important set of differences. The findings fall into several different patterns.

The first pattern is exemplified by the progression from antisocial disorders in childhood to sociopathy in adult life.[45] Almost all cases of sociopathy have been preceded by antisocial disturbance in childhood. Indeed, recent data from Zeitlin's[46] study of psychiatric patients treated both as children and adults, and from our own study of institution-reared women,[47,48] suggest that most (but not all) forms of adult personality disorder (and not just the antisocial or sociopathic varieties) have been preceded by conduct disorders in childhood. That finding throws doubt on the traditional subdivision of personality disorders.[49] The parallel observation that perhaps only one third of antisocial conditions in childhood go on to become personality disorders raises the further question of how these persistent varieties of conduct disturbance differ from those that do not last into adult life. The limited available evidence suggests that persistence is associated with an early onset, with overactive, inattentive behavior, and with marked family psychopathology.[29,39,40,50] Again, the findings suggest that a reconceptualization is needed for the subdivision of conduct disorders.

The second pattern is provided by depressive conditions.[17,46] These differ sharply from conduct disturbances in three key respects: (1) in the majority of cases the onset is in adult life, not childhood; (2) the childhood precursors are quite heterogeneous with no clearly definable pattern; and (3) in the minority of cases in which the onset of depression is in childhood there is a strong element of continuity into adult life despite a mixed and varying assortment of associated symptoms. The meaning of this rather complex set of findings remains uncertain at the moment. Among other things it raises the question of whether disorders should be defined according to the presence of key depressive symptoms, regardless of the presence of other symptoms, or whether it is the preponderant pattern that matters, with the depressive symptoms adding only a dysphoric coloring.

Emotional disorders in childhood show an important continuity with anxiety disorders in adult life in that, when there is persistence, the form of the disorder usually remains similar across age periods. However, most children with emotional disturbance become psychiatrically normal adults; also, anxiety conditions often have an onset in adult life. The unresolved question regarding both age periods is what differentiates or distinguishes those conditions that span the two age periods from those conditions that do not.

The fourth pattern is provided by schizophrenia, in which approximately one half of the patients with an onset of psychosis in adult life have shown nonpsychotic abnormalities in childhood.[12] The behavioral pattern in childhood is not one that is easy to recognize at the time, but it tends to be characterized by social oddities, aggressive or antisocial behavior in the home (but *not* group delinquency), attentional deficits, and neurodevelopmental abnormalities. There is a need to identify the key diagnostic features of this set of childhood precursors of schizophrenia. However, it is also important to ask what is different about schizophrenia that is preceded by abnormalities in childhood from schizophrenia in which the childhood behavior has been unremarkable.

It is evident that the data on continuities and discontinuities in psychopathology between childhood and adult life provide potentially useful ways of subdividing psychiatric disorders in both age periods. We know that each of the diagnostic groupings that have been discussed is likely to be etiologically heterogeneous; what is uncertain is how this heterogeneity is composed. Perhaps the use of findings on continuities provides one possible way forward. It is striking, for example, that almost no use has been made of this approach in genetic studies. The limited available empirical evidence suggests that genetic factors are more important in adult criminality than in juvenile delinquency.[50] On the other hand, in adult life genetic factors seem to play a greater role in minor than in major crime.[51] Perhaps it is that genetic influences have their main effect on personality disabilities associated with antisocial behavior that begins early and persists into adult life. It would be informative to examine the possibility that juvenile delinquency includes both transient antisocial behavior with a limited genetic component and persistent antisocial behavior in which genetic factors are much more influential. The point is that it would be useful to reexamine genetic data using continuity from childhood into adult life as a subdividing variable. Such data might well indicate that, as suggested by the few available longitudinal findings,[13] the unifying feature is abnormality in personality functioning rather than criminality as such.

PSYCHOPATHOLOGIC PERSPECTIVES
Age Differences in Operation of Risk Factors

The developmental perspective also emphasizes the need to consider the possibility that the consequences of psychiatric risk factors may vary according to the individual's age at the time the risk factors operate. Of course, some risk factors have similar effects regardless of age, but others do not. For example, hospital admission constitutes more of a stressor during the age period from 1 to 4 years than it does during either early infancy or later childhood.[52,53] Similarly, it appears that an institutional rearing has different consequences according to whether or not it operated during the first few years of life.[52,53] The same applies to the effects of social isolation in animals. Relative age specificity may also apply to the effects of neural damage. It is not so much that the effects are greater at one age period than another, as was once thought, but rather that they may be different in kind.[54,55] Thus, the psychological sequelae of perinatal brain damage differ somewhat in form from those following lateralized damage occurring in later childhood or adult life.[56] This difference probably arises from the contrast between the effect of damage on an established psychologic skill and that on a skill that is yet to develop. However, it may also be that age differences in outcome will also arise from age effects in the response of neural tissues to damage.

Thus, Goodman (R. Goodman, MRCPsych, unpublished data, 1987) has recently suggested that the sequelae of perinatal damage may be affected by the likelihood that anomalous connections may develop as a result of axonal regrowth, something that is less likely to occur with damage arriving later. Plomin[57] has also noted that for many psychological characteristics genetic influences increase with age during childhood and shared environmental influences decrease after middle childhood. Moreover, genetic factors play an important role in the pattern or course of psychological development as well as in the variance of characteristics. As with the other developmental considerations that I have noted, it is not that there is an accumulation of evidence on their importance. To the contrary, there has been very little investigation of these factors. It is simply that the few available findings suggest that it would be informative to pay greater attention to developmental considerations.

Continuities/Discontinuities Between Normality and Psychopathology

Let me turn now to the psychopathologic perspective and to a consideration of the continuities and discontinuities between normality and psychopathology, an issue that pervades most of psychiatry. Of course, it is often the case that both are present. Anorexia nervosa provides a case in point. There are many parallels with "normal" dieting and shape consciousness.[10] Thus, in both cases the onset typically occurs about the time of puberty; there is a marked female preponderance; both anorexia nervosa and dieting are much less prevalent in Afro-Asian communities than in white Anglo-American societies; and many of the phenomena are closely similar, as with dieting, severe exercise, and distortion of the self-concept. The implication is that anorexia nervosa may be just an extreme variant of the "normal" dieting of female adolescence. Yet, there are important differences as well. Purging and vomiting occur frequently in anorexia nervosa as means of losing weight but are rare in normal dieting[10]; the prognosis for even severe dieting is good, whereas anorexia nervosa carries with it a significant mortality.[58] Also, twin data suggest an important genetic component in anorexia nervosa[59]; it is uncertain whether the same applies to normal dieting.

Similar considerations apply to many other psychiatric disorders and it is clear that it would be informative to obtain a better definition of the nature of continuities and discontinuities between normality and psychopathology as they apply to different psychiatric conditions. For example, does the genetic influence in alcoholism apply to variations in patterns of drinking or rather to a categorical[18] condition that differs qualitatively from normality?[60] It should be added that the psychopathologic perspective suggests that it may be informative to examine causal influences separately according to the different dimensions or components of a disorder and not just in relation to the condition as a diagnostic entity. Thus, data suggest that environmental factors may be differentially associated with the symptoms of anxiety that so often accompany depression.[61]

Pervasiveness and Situation Specificity

A further approach to the psychopathologic dimension is provided by the distinction between pervasive and situation-specific disorders. The Isle of Wight data were used by Schachar and colleagues[62] to examine this matter in relation to hyperactivity. The findings showed that pervasive overactivity at 10 years of age carried a worse prognosis for continuing behavioral disturbance at 14 to 15 years of age than did situational overactivity. This was not just a general

characteristic of pervasiveness as the distinction did not apply in the presence of unsociability. In both cases pervasiveness was defined in terms of similar abnormal behaviors on both the teachers' and the parents' questionnaires. The situational-pervasiveness differentiation was even more marked in relation to associations with cognitive impairment. Nearly one fourth of the children with pervasive overactivity had a nonverbal IQ below 70, compared with only approximately 3% of those with situational overactivity. This epidemiological finding has been supported by other data from clinical studies, most of which agree in showing the need to define hyperkinetic or attention deficit disorders in terms of pervasiveness of the abnormality as well as other features.[25,63] It cannot be claimed that the value of the pervasive-situational distinction is established as yet, but it is clear that this way of subdividing disorders warrants more attention than it has received up to now. It should be added, however, that the finding that a particular situational context is needed to elicit a behavior does not necessarily mean that it does not have a strong intrinsic component. Thus, behavioral inhibition in monkeys requires a stress situation for it to be manifest, but this inhibition still has proved to be strongly stable over time and appears to be under the influence of genetic factors to a major degree.[64]

Single Variables vs Behavioral Composites

Hyperactivity again provides the example for another (somewhat related) distinction between single variables and behavioral composites. The data from Magnusson's[29] Swedish epidemiological longitudinal study showed that the prediction of adult criminality was more certain in the presence of both high aggression and high restlessness in childhood than in the presence of either variable alone. Nearly three fifths of the individuals with the combined behavioral characteristics had an adult crime record, against a base rate of 16%. Other studies have similarly shown that poor outcome is most strongly predicted by the combination of overactivity and aggression.[25]

The change in effect consequent to a combination of variables was, perhaps, even more striking in the case of restlessness and poor concentration with respect to the association with a low adrenalin response to stress in the Magnusson study.[29] Physiologic hyporesponsiveness has long been associated with criminality and especially with recidivism and sociopathy.[65] Magnusson's[29] data showed that young people with either poor concentration or high restlessness did not differ from normal persons in their levels of adrenalin as measured in a stress situation. However, the levels were significantly below normal when these two behavioral features were found in combination. It should be noted that this was not just an additive effect because *no* effect was found when poor concentration and high restlessness occurred on their own without the other characteristic. It seemed that the combination of behaviors changed the meaning of poor concentration and high restlessness and their correlates. The implication is that epidemiologists need to be alert to the need to look for meaningful patterns of psychopathology and that various ways of examining possible continuities between normality and psychopathology need to be used for that purpose.

DEVELOPMENTAL AND PSYCHOPATHOLOGIC MECHANISMS AND PROCESSES
Causal Connections

The final characteristic of developmental psychopathology concepts to consider is the attempt to elucidate mechanisms and processes. Of course, the first need, as in

■ 37

Archives of General Psychiatry, 1988, vol. 45, pp. 486–495

any epidemiological study using statistical associations, is to seek to test whether the associations represent truly causal connections. There are several ways in which causal hypotheses can be tested but there are many advantages to the use of experiments of nature.[5] The idea is to provide a naturalistic equivalent of the laboratory experiment in which the hypothesized causal variable can be introduced in a manner that allows the examination of changes over time.

The study of behavioral changes following a severe head injury provides a case in point. Brain damage cannot be induced experimentally but ordinary life circumstances, through road traffic accidents and the like, do this without the need for laboratory experiment. Measures of the children's preinjury behavior obtained immediately after the accident but before it can be known whether there will be sequelae provide an acceptable baseline. In our 2¼-year prospective study we compared the changes following severe head injury with those consequent to severe orthopedic injuries that did not involve trauma to the head or loss of consciousness.[66] There was a marked increase in the rate of psychiatric disorder following brain damage, an increase that greatly exceeded that found after orthopedic injuries. The demonstration of longitudinal *change* in behavior following the natural experiment of injury to the brain but not following the control condition of injury to the limbs provides strong support for the causal hypothesis that brain injury leads to psychiatric disturbance.

A second example is provided by an investigation of school influences on children's behavior and academic achievement.[67] Various studies,[68] including our own epidemiological-longitudinal study of 12 secondary schools in inner London,[69] had shown marked school effects. The demonstration of school differences in pupil progress following transfer from primary to secondary schools supported the causal hypothesis. However, it depended on the statistical adjustment for differences between schools in the characteristics of their pupil intake. An alternative approach is provided by the study of changes over time in a single school following a change in regime or practice. We followed this strategy in our investigation of what happened after the appointment of new principals in three secondary schools following concern about the poor performance of children in those schools.[70] In two of those schools there were important and substantial improvements in various indicators of pupil progress, with the changes in one school being major. For all three intellectual ability bands in that school there was a dramatic improvement in rates of attendance over the four years following the change in principal. Indeed, the school went from one of the worst attendance records in the area to one of the best. This change occurred, moreover, at a time when there was no alteration in catchment area and no substantial change in intake characteristics. The national examination scores in the same school similarly showed marked improvements in scholastic attainment in the middle and upper ability bands. Data over the same time period from other London secondary schools showed little shift in levels of attendance or attainment. Accordingly, it could be inferred that the improvements in pupil behavior and achievement were likely to be the result of some change in the school's functioning following change in the principal.

Interpersonal Interactions

A key feature of developmental psychopathology is a concern for viewing human behavior and development in its social context.[71] Because human beings are social animals, their behavior will have social consequences and will be subject to social influences. That fact raises the important possibility that some causal processes may be mediated through effects on social interactions rather than through intraindividual mechanisms as such.

The findings on the effects of temperamental differences provide an example of how an individual characteristic may have consequences for interpersonal interactions. The results from our prospective high-risk study of 4- to 7-year-old children being reared in families with a mentally ill parent are illustrative.[27] Family discord proved to be the single most important risk variable for psychiatric disorder in childhood.[47] However, discord did not impinge equally on all children in the same family. Some children tended to take the brunt of parental irritability and hostility, sometimes to the extent of becoming scapegoats. Others tended to be favored and protected so that they were relatively well dealt with even when parents were at a very low ebb and openly expressed their anger and frustration. This differential treatment was found to be a function in part of children's temperamental qualities. Those with an easy adaptive behavioral style tended to be favored, whereas those with difficult characteristics tended to be the focus of parental criticism and anger.

Lee and Bates'[26] data with younger children in a more normal population showed the same pattern. Children with difficult temperaments were involved in more parent-child conflicts and also were more likely to be the recipients of negative parental responses. Children's behavior influences how other people respond to them; these induced responses from others then have consequent further effects on the children.

Similar issues arise with respect to sex differences in the correlates and consequences of various forms of behavioral difficulties in childhood. For example, Stevenson-Hinde and colleagues[72] have found that shyness in boys tends to be associated with negative social interactions, whereas in girls the association tends to be with positive ones. Maccoby and Jacklin[73] have shown that the circular processes of mother-child interaction that are linked with the persistence of difficult behavior in boys do not seem to operate in girls. Maccoby[74] has also discussed the evidence that sex differences in peer group patterns may accentuate antisocial behavior in boys in ways that are less common with girls. The point is that people's individual behavior (which may be constitutionally determined to a considerable extent) has social consequences and that those social effects may in turn influence the psychopathologic implications of the behavior in question. Once more, it is not that the importance of interpersonal interactions has been well established but rather that the evidence suggests that it is likely to be worthwhile to examine the issues more systematically than has often been the case until now.

Causal Chain Mechanisms

The final issue to consider, causal chain mechanisms, takes the interaction point a stage further. Research findings are consistent in showing both individual variation in children's responses to stress and adversity and also variations in subsequent life course, with adverse sequelae being intensified over time in some children but ameliorated in others.[52] Causes cannot be dealt with in terms of risk effects that occur at one point in time. Rather it is necessary to delineate the mechanisms involved in both continuities and discontinuities brought about by a variety of vulnerability and protective processes operating at turning points in people's lives.[75,76] The research strategies that may be employed in attempts to unravel the causal skein may be illustrated by considering our follow-up into adult life of girls who had been reared in the institutional environment of group foster homes.[48,77]

The institution-reared sample was compared with a control group of girls brought up in their own families, with both groups coming from a socially disadvantaged area of London. The same measures were available for both samples in childhood and again at follow-up in early adult life. Not surprisingly, the institution-reared group fared significantly worse in terms of adult psychiatric disorder, criminality, and psychosocial adaptation generally. Nevertheless, there was substantial heterogeneity, with some women functioning well. The single most important factor associated with a good outcome was a harmonious marriage to a nondeviant man. On the face of it, this suggested a marked discontinuity between childhood and adult life with the adult experience of marriage having an effect that was sufficiently powerful to counter many of the ill effects stemming from adverse experiences in early life. However, this apparent discontinuity was misleading. The institution-reared women were much more likely than those in the comparison sample to have made poor marriages. The evidence suggested that this was largely due to their tendency to marry young, and impulsively, as a means of escape from an intolerable family situation. Not surprisingly, many of these hasty marriages for negative reasons broke down. However, some of the institutional group made successful marriages to men who were highly supportive. The question is how this came about: What made for the difference in marital outcome?

We approached the question by asking whether there were differences in the ways in which the women planned their lives. For this purpose we took two domains of life—marriage and work. In each case we sought to measure whether the women had exerted any form of positive planning in their choice of marriage partners and jobs. Our criteria for planning were quite undemanding: we required no more than that the women had made some sort of definite choice, with the selection being on positive grounds and not just as a result of external pressure or as a means of escape. The results showed a strong association between planning in these domains and overall social outcome, the association being largely mediated through effects on marriage. The protective effect seemed to have come about as a result of the women taking positive steps to deal with their life situations rather than allowing themselves to be swept along on the tide of fate.

Of course, that finding merely pushed the causal question back one stage further. What was it that enabled some girls to take active steps to plan their lives, whereas others merely reacted passively to the hazards and adversities that life presented? The findings showed that the most important factor was positive school experiences. Girls who had experienced pleasure and/or accomplishment in several aspects of their school lives (friendships, school responsibilities, sport, work, or arts and crafts) were significantly more likely to exert planning. The probable reason why school experiences had such an important effect was that the institution's policy was to disperse the children to a wide variety of schools so that there would not be a substantial institutional group in any one school. The consequence of this policy was that there was a marked dysjunction between their institutional experiences and their school lives, and that the girls varied greatly in their school experiences. This enabled schools to have a rather greater impact than they would ordinarily.

The findings were surprisingly clear cut in demonstrating some of the key links in the causal chain. Obviously, many questions remain and there also is a need for replication.

Nevertheless, the data from other studies by independent research groups[78,79] tell a broadly comparable story. My point, however, is not to argue for the specifics of the causal mechanisms that appeared important in one study but rather to emphasize the need to delineate causal chain processes. It is not sufficient to isolate risk factors; we must also go on to determine the ways in which they operate over time and the reasons why the outcomes vary from individual to individual.

The example given from our own work focused on psychosocial influences, but the need to consider causal chain processes is equally applicable to constitutional variables, as is well recognized in psychobiology[80] and as recent work in genetics and animal studies illustrates. Traditionally, genetic research has tended to concentrate on genetic and environmental influences as main effects. In many circumstances these are indeed the mechanisms of importance. However, sometimes it is the combination of the two that is crucial as, for example, is apparent with the individual characteristic of behavioral inhibition and the experience of separation as factors leading to emotional disturbance in monkeys.[81] Kendler and Eaves[82] have recently outlined the various types of gene-environment interactions as they might operate in psychiatry and have showed how these lead to contrasting patterns of familiality that are open to empirical testing. Such testing requires specification of the relevant environmental variable, but this is possible, for example, in the case of life events and long-term difficulties with depression,[83] perinatal complications with autism,[84] and family discord with conduct disorders.[85]

Scarr and McCartney[86] have also pointed out the need to consider the possibility that, to an important extent, people create their own environments; ie, the genotype shapes the environment. This can happen both because people respond to children on the basis of the children's characteristics and because children choose or modify environments so that they are conducive to the development of their genetic propensities (reactive and active genotype-environment correlations, respectively). The evidence that this process takes place is decidedly limited thus far because the matter has not been investigated deeply,[58] but recent evidence has begun to provide useful pointers. Thus, it seems that the frequency of adverse life events in adult life may be in part a function of people's behavior or experiences in childhood.[87,88] Similarly, it has been found that depressed patients show a familial loading for life events as well as for depressive disorders (P. McGuffin, PhD, R. Katz, PhD, P. Bebbington, PhD, unpublished data, 1987). The issue warrants further investigation.

CONCLUSIONS

Epidemiology constitutes a most versatile tool with which to tackle a wide range of research problems. It is especially effective when cross-sectional designs can be combined with longitudinal research strategies in child and general psychiatry, as well as in other branches of medicine. Nevertheless, the fact that children are developing organisms introduces a variety of special considerations that may be summarized by the set of concepts associated with developmental psychopathology. Because social development continues in adult life,[89] because adult functioning is influenced by earlier developmental processes, because the fact that adult psychiatric disorders differ in their continuities with childhood psychopathology is likely to carry meaning, and because the notions regarding person-environment interaction and causal chain mechanisms apply at all ages, developmental psychopathology concepts are as relevant for adult psychiatry as they are for child psychia-

■ 39

Archives of General Psychiatry, 1988, vol. 45, pp. 486–495

try. In particular, there is a need to examine continuities and discontinuities over the span of time—the developmental perspective—and over the span of behavioral variation—the psychopathologic perspective. Developmental variations may be examined by means of age differences in prevalence, remission, and time of onset, as well as by consideration of the developmental appropriateness of behavioral patterns and the continuities and discontinuities in psychopathology between childhood and adult life. Psychopathologic variations may be studied through investigation of the links between normality and abnormality, of the differences between situation-specific and pervasive psychiatric disorders, and of the contrasts between sample-wide variable-oriented approaches and those based on behavioral composites that apply only to subgroups of the population. Finally, developmental psychopathology emphasizes the need to focus on causal mechanisms and processes through the use of experiments of nature, the study of social interactions, and the delineation of causal chains. The approach is one that has scarcely begun to show what it can achieve but there is an abundance of leads that indicate potentially worthwhile avenues of investigation.

40 ■

This study was supported in part by the John D. and Catherine R. MacArthur Foundation Mental Health Research Network on Risk and Protective Factors in the Major Mental Disorders.

References

1. Robins LN: Epidemiological approaches to natural history research: Antisocial disorders in children. *J Am Acad Child Psychiatry* 1981;20:566-580.

2. Rutter M: Epidemiological-longitudinal approaches to the study of development, in Collins WA (ed): *The Concept of Development: Minnesota Symposium on Child Psychology*. Hillsdale NJ, Lawrence Erlbaum Assoc Inc Publishers, 1982, vol 15, pp 105-144.

3. Gould MS, Wunsch-Hitzig R, Dohrenwend BP: Formulation of hypotheses about the prevalence, treatment and prognostic significance of psychiatric disorders in children in the US, in Dohrenwend BS, Gould MS, Link B, Neugebauer R, Wunsch-Hitzig R (eds): *Mental Illness in the United States: Epidemiological Estimates*. New York, Praeger Publishers, 1980, pp 9-45.

4. Rutter M, Tizard J, Whitmore K (eds): *Education, Health and Behaviour*. London, Longman, 1970 (reprinted Melbourne, Fla, Robert E. Krieger Publishing Co Inc, 1981).

5. Rutter M: Epidemiological/longitudinal strategies and causal research in child psychiatry. *J Am Acad Child Psychiatry* 1981;50:513-544.

6. Stein Z, Susser M: Methods in epidemiology. *J Am Acad Child Psychiatry* 1981;20:444-461.

7. Earls F: Epidemiological child psychiatry: An American perspective, in Purcell EF (ed): *Psychopathology of Children and Youth: A Cross-Cultural Perspective*. New York, Macy Foundation, 1980.

8. Graham PJ: Epidemiological studies, in Quay HC, Werry JS (eds): *Psychopathological Disorders of Childhood*, ed 2. New York, John Wiley & Sons Inc, 1977, pp 185-209.

9. Links PS, Community surveys of the prevalence of childhood psychiatric disorders: A review. *Child Dev* 1983;54:531-548.

10. Rutter M, Sandberg S: Epidemiology of child psychiatric disorder: Methodological issues and some substantive findings. *Child Psychiatry Hum Dev* 1985;15:209-233.

11. Yule W: The epidemiology of child psychopathology, in Lahey BB, Kazdin AE (eds): *Advances in Clinical Child Psychology*. New York, Plenum Publishing Corp, 1981, vol 4, pp 1-51.

12. Rutter M, Garmezy N: Developmental psychopathology, in *Mussen's Handbook of Child Psychology*, ed 4. New York, John Wiley & Sons Inc, 1983, vol 4; Hetherinwend EM (section ed): *Socialization, Personality and Social Development*, pp 775-911.

13. Rutter M: Child Psychiatry: The interface between clinical and developmental research. *Psychol Med* 1986;16:151-160.

14. Rutter M: The developmental psychopathology of depression: Issues and perspectives, in Rutter M, Izard C, Read P (eds): *Depression in Young People: Developmental and Clinical Perspectives*. New York, Guilford Press, 1986, pp 3-30.

15. Stroufe LA, Rutter M: The domain of developmental psychopathology. *Child Dev* 1984;55:17-29.

16. Rutter M: Age as an ambiguous variable in developmental research: Some epidemiological considerations from developmental psychopathology. *Int J Behav Dev*, in press.

17. Rutter M, Izard C, Read P (eds): *Depression in Young People: Developmental and Clinical Perspectives*. New York, Guilford Press, 1986.

18. Oppel WC, Harper PA, Rider RV: The age of attaining bladder control. *Pediatrics* 1968;42:614-626.

19. Rutter M: *Changing Youth in a Changing Society*. Cambridge, Mass, Harvard University Press, 1980.

20. Wing JK, Bebbington P, Robins LN (eds): *What Is a Case? The Problem of Definition in Psychiatric Community Surveys*. Boston, Blackwell Scientific Publications Inc, 1981.

21. Kendler KS, Gruenberg AM, Strauss JS: An independent analysis of the Copenhagen sample of the Danish adoption study of schizophrenia: II. The relationship between schizotypal personality disorder and schizophrenia. *Arch Gen Psychiatry* 1981;38:982-984.

22. Kendler KS, Gruenberg AM: An independent analysis of the Danish adoption study of schizophrenia: IV. The relationship between psychiatric disorders as defined in *DSM-III* in the relatives and adoptees. *Arch Gen Psychiatry* 1985;44:555-564.

23. Torgerson G: Genetic and nosological aspects of schizotypal and borderline personality disorders. *Arch Gen Psychiatry* 1984;41:546-554.

24. Folstein S, Rutter M: Autism: Familial aggregation and genetic implications, in Schopler E, Mesibov G (eds): *Diagnosis and Assessment in Autism*. New York, Plenum Press Publishing Corp, 1987, pp 83-105.

25. Rutter M: Attention deficit disorder/hyperkinetic syndrome: Conceptual and research issues regarding diagnosis and classification, in Sagvolden T, Borchgrevink HM, Archer T (eds): *Attention Deficit Disorder and Hyperkinetic Syndrome*. Hillsdale, NJ, Lawrence J Erlbaum Assoc Inc Publishers, in press.

26. Lee CL, Bates JE: Mother-child interaction at age 2 years and perceived difficult temperament. *Child Dev* 1985;56:1314-1325.

27. Rutter M: Family, area and social influences in the genesis of conduct disorders, in Hersov L, Berger M, Shaffer D (eds): *Aggression and Antisocial Behaviour in Childhood and Adolescence*. Elmsford, NY, Pergamon Press Inc, 1978, pp 95-133.

28. Shepherd M, Oppenheim B, Mitchell S (eds): *Childhood Behaviour and Mental Health*. London, University of London Press, 1971.

29. Magnusson D: *Paths Through Life*. Hillsdale, NJ, Lawrence J Erlbaum Assoc Inc Publishers, 1987, vol 1, Magnusson D: *Individual Development in an Interactional Perspective*.

30. Pearce J: *Childhood Depression*, thesis. London, University of London, 1974.

31. Kovacs M, Feinberg TL, Crouse-Novak HA, Paulauskas SL, Finkelstein R: Depressive disorders in childhood: I. A longitudinal perspective study of characteristics and recovery. *Arch Gen Psychiatry* 1984;41:229-237.

32. Weissman MM: Psychopathology in the children of depressed and normal parents: Direct interview study, in Dunner DL, Gershon ES (eds): *Relatives at Risk for Mental Disorders*. New York, Raven Press, in press.

33. Verhulst FC, van der Lee JH, Akkerhuis GW, Sanders-Woudstra JAR, Timmer FC, Donkorst ID: The prevalence of nocturnal enuresis: Do *DSM-III* criteria need to be changed? A brief research report. *J Child Psychol Psychiatry* 1985;26:989-993.

34. Yule W, Rutter M (eds): *Language Development and Disorders*. Boston, Blackwell Scientific Publications Inc, 1987, pp 382-399.

35. Hersov L, School refusal, in Rutter M, Hersov L (eds): *Child and Adolescent Psychiatry: Modern Approaches*, ed 2. Boston, Blackwell Scientific Publications Inc, 1985, pp 382-399.

36. Rodriguez A, Rodriguez M, Eisenberg L: The outcome of school phobia: A follow up study based on 41 cases. *Am J Psychiatry* 1959;116:540-544.

37. Hersov L, Berg O (eds): *Out of School: Modern Perspectives in Truancy and School Refusal*. New York, John Wiley & Sons Inc, 1985.

38. Farrington DP: Age and crime, in Tonry M, Morris N (eds): *Crime and Justice*. Chicago, University of Chicago Press, 1986, vol 7, pp 189-250.

39. Loeber R: The stability of antisocial and delinquent child behaviour: A review. *Child Dev* 1982;53:1431-1446.

40. Loeber R, Dishon TJ: Boys who fight: Familial and antisocial correlates. *J Consult Clin Psychol* 1984;52:759-768.

41. American Psychiatric Association, Committee on Nomenclature and Statistics: *Diagnostic and Statistical Manual of Mental Disorders*, ed 3. Washington, DC, American Psychiatric Association, 1980.

42. World Health Organization: *International Classification of Diseases (9th revision)*. Geneva, World Health Authority, 1978.

43. Rutter M: Child psychiatric disorders in ICD-10. Read before the 11th International Congress on Child and Adolescent Psychiatry and Allied Professions, Paris, July 23, 1986.

44. Rutter M: Psychopathology and development: I. Childhood antecedents of adult psychiatric disorder. *Aust NZ J Psychiatry* 1984;18:225-234.

45. Robins LN: Sturdy childhood predictors of adult antisocial behavior: Replications from longitudinal studies. *Psychol Med* 1978;8:611-622.

46. Zeitlin H: *The Natural History of Psychiatric Disorder in Childhood*. New York, Oxford University Press Inc, 1986.

47. Rutter M, Quinton D: Long term follow-up of women institutionalized in childhood: Factors promoting good functioning in adult life. *Br J Dev Psychol* 1984;2:191-204.

48. Quinton D, Rutter M: *Parental Breakdown: The Making and Breaking of Intergenerational Links*. Aldershot, England, Gower Publishing Co Ltd, in press.

49. Rutter M: Temperament, personality and personality disorder. *Br J*

Psychiatry 1987;150:443-458.

50. Rutter M, Giller H: *Juvenile Delinquency: Trends and Perspectives.* Harmondsworth, England, Penguin Books Ltd, 1983.

51. Vandenberg SG, Singer SM, Pauls DL: *The Heredity of Behavior Disorders in Adults and Children.* New York, Plenum Publishing Corp, 1986.

52. Rutter M: *Maternal Deprivation Reassessed,* ed 2. Harmondsworth, England, Penguin Books Ltd, 1981.

53. Rutter M: Continuities and discontinuities from infancy, in Osofsky J (ed): *Handbook of Infant Development,* ed 2. New York, John Wiley & Sons Inc, 1987, pp 1256-1296.

54. Rutter M: Developmental neuropsychiatry: Concepts, issues and prospects. *J Clin Neuropsychol* 1982;4:91-115.

55. Goodman R: The developmental neurobiology of language, in Yule W, Rutter M (eds): *Language Development and Disorders.* Boston, Blackwell Scientific Publications, 1987, pp 129-145.

56. Goldman-Rakic PS, Isseroff A, Schwartz M, Bugbee NM: The neurobiology of cognitive development, in *Mussen's Handbook of Child Psychiatry,* ed 4. New York, John Wiley & Sons Inc, 1983, pp 281-344, vol 2; Haith MM, Campos JJ (section eds): *Infancy and Developmental Psychobiology,* pp 281-344.

57. Plomin R: *Development, Genetics and Psychology.* Hillsdale, NJ, Lawrence J Erlbaum Assoc Inc Publishers, 1986.

58. Abrahams SF, Mira M, Beumont PJV, Sowerbutts TD, Llewellyn Jones D: Eating behaviours among young women. *Med J Aust* 1983;2: 225-228.

59. Holland AJ, Hall A, Murray R, Russell GFM, Crisp AH: Anorexia nervosa: The study of 34 twin pairs and one set of triplets. *Br J Psychiatry* 1984;145:414-419.

60. McGuffin P: Genetic influences on personality, neurosis and psychosis, in McGuffin P, Shanks ME, Hodgson RJ (eds): *The Scientific Principles of Psychopathology.* New York, Grune & Stratton, 1984, pp 190-226.

61. Kendler KS, Head AC, Martin NG, Eaves LJ: Symptoms of anxiety and symptoms of depression: Same genes, different environments? *Arch Gen Psychiatry* 1987;44:451-461.

62. Schachar R, Rutter M, Smith A: The characteristics of situationally and pervasive hyperactive children: Implications for syndrome definition. *J Child Psychol Psychiatry* 1981;22:375-392.

63. Taylor EA (ed): *The Overactive Child.* Philadelphia, JB Lippincott, 1986.

64. Suomi SJ: Social development in rhesus monkeys: Considerations of individual differences, in Oliverio A, Zappella M (eds): *The Behaviour of Human Infants.* New York, Plenum Publishers, 1984.

65. Hare RD, Shalling D (eds): *Psychopathic Behaviour: Approaches to Research.* New York, John Wiley & Sons Inc, 1978.

66. Rutter M, Chadwick O, Shaffer D: The behavioural and cognitive sequelae of head injury, in Rutter M (ed): *Developmental Neuropsychiatry.* New York, Guilford Press, 1983, pp 83-111.

67. Maughan B: School experiences as risk/protective factors, in Rutter M (ed): *Studies of Psychosocial Risk: The Power of Longitudinal Data.* New York, Cambridge University Press, in press.

68. Rutter M: School effects on pupil progress: Research findings and policy implications. *Child Dev* 1983;54:1-29.

69. Rutter M, Maughan B, Mortimore P, Ouston J, Smith A: *Fifteen Thousand Hours: Secondary Schools and Their Effects on Children.* Cambridge, Mass, Harvard University Press, 1979.

70. Ouston J, Maughan B, Rutter M: *Innovation and Change in Six Secondary Schools.* Report to the Department of Education and Science.

London, DES reference No. P81/139/03, 1985.

71. Bronfenbrenner U: *Ecology of Human Development: Experiments by Nature and Design.* Cambridge, Mass, Harvard University Press, 1979.

72. Stevenson-Hinde J, Hinde RA: Changes in associations between characteristics and interactions, in Plomin R, Dunn J (eds): *The Study of Temperament: Changes, Continuities and Challenges.* Hillsdale, NJ, Lawrence J Erlbaum Assoc Inc Publishers, 1986, pp 115-130.

73. Maccoby EE, Jacklin CN: The 'person' characteristics of children and the family as environment, in Magnusson D, Allen V (eds): *Human Development: An Interactional Perspective,* Orlando, Fla, Academic Press Inc, 1983, pp 75-91.

74. Maccoby EE: Social groupings in childhood: Their relationship to prosocial and antisocial behavior in boys and girls, in Olweus D, Block J, Radke-Yarrow M (eds): *Development of Antisocial and Prosocial Behavior: Research, Theories and Issues.* Orlando, Fla, Academic Press Inc, 1986, pp 263-284.

75. Rutter M: Resilience in the face of adversity: Protective factors and resistance to psychiatric disorder. *Br J Psychiatry* 1985;147:598-611.

76. Rutter M: Psychosocial resilience and protective mechanisms, in Rolf J, Masten A, Cicchetti D, Nuechterlein K, Weintraub S (eds): *Risk and Protective Factors in the Development of Psychopathology.* New York, Cambridge University Press, in press.

77. Quinton D, Rutter M, Liddle C: Institutional rearing, parenting difficulties and marital support. *Psychol Med* 1984;14:107-124.

78. Brown GW, Harris TO, Bifulco A: The long term effects of early loss of parent, in Rutter M, Izard CE, Read P (eds): *Depression in Young People: Clinical and Developmental Perspectives.* New York, Guilford Press, 1986, pp 251-296.

79. Parker G, Hadzik-Pavlovic D: Modification of levels of depression in mother-bereaved women by parental and marriage relationships. *Psychol Med* 1984;14:125-135.

80. Rutter M: Meyerian psychobiology, personality development and the role of life experiences. *Am J Psychiatry* 1986;143:1077-1087.

81. Suomi S: Uptight and laidback monkeys: Individual differences in response style and risk for developing psychopathology. Presented at the Institute of Psychiatry, London, June 18, 1987.

82. Kendler KS, Eaves LJ: Models for the joint effect of genotype and environment on liability to psychiatric illness. *Am J Psychiatry* 1986;143: 279-289.

83. Brown GW, Harris TO: *Social Origins of Depression: A Study of Psychiatric Disorders in Women.* London, Tavistock Publications Ltd, 1978.

84. Tsai LY: Pre-, peri- and neonatal factors in autism, in Schopler E, Mesibov GB (eds): *Neurobiological Issues in Autism.* New York, Plenum Publishing Corp, 1987, pp 179-189.

85. Rutter M: Family and school influences on behavioural development. *J Child Psychol Psychiatry* 1985;26:349-368.

86. Scarr S, McCartney K: How people make their own environments: A theory of genotype-environmental effects. *Child Dev* 1983;54:424-435.

87. Robins LN: The consequences of conduct disorder in girls, in Olweus D, Block J, Radke-Yarrow M (eds): *Development of Antisocial and Prosocial Behavior: Research, Theories and Issues.* Orlando, Fla, Academic Press Inc, 1986, pp 385-414.

88. Kandel DB, Davies M: Adult sequelae of adolescent depressive symptoms. *Arch Gen Psychiatry* 1986;43:255-262.

89. Rutter M: Psychopathology and development: II. Childhood experiences and personality development. *Aust NZ J Psychiatry* 1984;18: 314-327.

■ 41

Part II
Genetics

British Journal of Psychiatry, 1997, vol. 171, pp. 209–219

Opportunities for psychiatry from genetic findings

MICHAEL RUTTER and ROBERT PLOMIN

Background The opportunities for psychiatry deriving from available or likely genetic advances are reviewed.

Method Clinical implications are considered in the context of both the misconceptions and benefits associated with relevant genetic findings.

Results Misconceptions include that: heritability estimates have a 'true' fixed value; a high heritability means that environmental interventions will be ineffective; a high heritability within groups means that differences between groups will also be due to genes; genetic effects are determinative; 'genetic' means single abnormal genes; genes associated with disease must be bad and justify eugenic measures; gene therapy will be widely applicable; and genetic screening of the general population will be useful. The benefits include demonstrations that: both genes and environment have an ubiquitous influence; some prevailing diagnostic assumptions are mistaken; genes influence development; the effects of nature and nurture are not separate; and environmental effects tend to be person-specific. The potential value of molecular genetics lies in elucidation of causal processes as they apply to both brain systems and nature–nurture interplay; improving diagnosis and genetic counselling; and the development of improved pharmacological interventions.

Conclusion Advances in genetics will make a major impact on clinical psychiatry, and should bring practical benefits for both prevention and treatment.

The extensive quantitative evidence of the role of genetic influences in all manner of psychiatric disorders (McGuffin *et al*, 1994; Plomin *et al*, 1997), together with the growing awareness of the power of molecular genetics (Lander & Schork, 1994; Risch & Merikangas, 1996), and the progress in mapping and sequencing human and non-human genomes (Lander, 1996; Schuler *et al*, 1996) has meant that genetics now has a firm place on the psychiatric research agenda (Rutter, 1994). However, this has been accompanied by the increasing expression of concerns that this will lead to a neglect of environmental influences on mental disorder (Pelosi & David, 1989) and on psychological development more generally (Baumrind, 1993). In addition, fears have been expressed about genetic determinism and the medicalisation of normal behaviours (Rose, 1995); about the risks regarding misuse of genetic data to deny people health insurance or exert discrimination in employment (Pokorski, 1995; Lapham *et al*, 1996; Marshall, 1996; Masood, 1996); about the problems of genetic screening (Nuffield Council on Bioethics, 1993; Andrews *et al*, 1994); and about the misuse of genetics for eugenic purposes (Gottesman & Bertelsen, 1996; Weber, 1996). Responsible voices have rightly urged that psychiatry tackle these ethical and moral issues seriously (Farmer & Owen, 1996).

That need is great. It raises complex issues about which views are divided, and those warrant extended discussion. It is good that they are being addressed by both the Institute of Medicine in the USA and the Nuffield Council on Bioethics in the UK. Nevertheless, it is clear that the concerns being expressed represent a complex mixture of important ethical questions and serious misunderstandings of what genetics can and cannot accomplish, as well as both an excessive optimism and an unwarranted pessimism about the potential clinical implications of genetic discoveries. This essay seeks to address the latter topics by providing a succinct summary of what is known about the opportunities for psychiatry that are likely to derive from genetic findings as they emerge from future research. The research techniques used in both quantitative genetics (Rutter *et al*, 1990*a*) and molecular genetics (Owen & McGuffin, 1993; Lander & Schork, 1994; Risch & Merikangas, 1996) have been the subject of previous non-technical reviews and will not be considered here. Similarly, there are several comprehensive reviews of the substantive specific genetic research findings as they apply to psychiatric disorders (Rutter *et al*, 1990*b*; McGuffin *et al*, 1994; Simonoff & Rutter, 1996; Simonoff *et al*, 1996; Plomin *et al*, 1997) and these will also not be reconsidered. In addition, this paper will not deal with the various false starts and premature claims in psychiatric genetics (although we need to learn from them – Rutter, 1994; Plomin *et al*, 1997), or with the numerous parallel problems in medical genetics more generally (Cookson, 1994). Instead, the focus is on the general misconceptions, messages and clinical implications of genetic knowledge as available now and as is likely to become available in the near future.

SOME MISCONCEPTIONS ABOUT GENETICS

Before proceeding to discuss the many important opportunities that arise from genetic findings, it is necessary to start with a number of misconceptions that are rife in both the literature and in the response of the media to genetic findings.

Heritability estimates have a 'true' fixed value for each trait

The first misconception is that there is a 'true' figure for the heritability of each trait and disorder that applies generally over time and across populations. That is completely mistaken (Plomin *et al*, 1997). Estimates of heritability apply only to the population studied at that particular time, and under the environmental conditions that prevail at that point. That is not just an academic quibble or caution but is an inherent feature of what heritabilities mean. They have nothing to say about individuals or fixed features of a disorder. That is, they do not indicate, in any one person, how much of their schizophrenia is genetically determined and how much environmentally determined.

■45

British Journal of Psychiatry, 1997, vol. 171, pp. 209–219

Rather, the heritability estimate indicates, on average, how much of individual variations in the liability to schizophrenia in a particular population at a particular time is due to genetic influences. If circumstances change, the heritabilities will also alter.

The same qualification applies to variations according to when a particular disease or trait is examined. For example, it would make little sense to ask about the heritability of reaching the menopause because all women, if they live long enough, have a menopause. On the other hand, it *would* make sense to enquire about the extent to which genetic factors play a role in the age at which one reaches the menopause. The same applies to diseases. For example, Alzheimer's disease is infrequent at the age of 70 but it is very common at the age of 90. It is not likely that the role of genetic heritability would be the same at both ages (Blacker *et al*, 1997), quite apart from the evidence that different genetic factors operate with early onset familial varieties of the disease.

A high heritability means that environmental interventions will be ineffective

A second misconception is that a very high heritability means that it is not likely that environmental interventions will have much effect. This message was, for example, one of the controversial points in Jensen's (1969) article arguing that high heritability for IQ meant that preschool programmes to improve children's mental performance were doomed to failure. That implication was, and still is, mistaken. Even a heritability as high as 90% carries no implications that environmental effects will not bring about big changes. Height constitutes the obvious example, where there is a heritability of about 90%, but where there has been a huge increase in height during this century, almost certainly as a result of improved nutrition (Tizard, 1975). It follows from this feature that there are no necessary policy or practice implications that follow from variations in heritability within a very broad range indeed. Geneticists have occasionally wished to emphasise that a certain trait has a heritability of, say, 60% whereas another has a heritability of only 30% but, in fact, there are no implications for the likely impact of environmental intervention from this difference in heritability.

Genetic effects on disease are unaffected by environmental interventions

A related misconception is that the effects of a genetically determined abnormality cannot be changed by environmental manipulations. Again, that is wrong even with single gene diseases. The example of the inherited metabolic disorder phenylketonuria (PKU) illustrates the point well (Simonoff *et al*, 1996). The biochemical abnormality, which means that the individual cannot handle the intake of phenylalanine in the diet (a normal substance in all ordinary diets), is indeed fully genetically determined. On the other hand, its effects, in leading to mental retardation, are almost entirely reversible by the simple expedient of keeping the levels of phenylalanine in the diet low. Whether or not the ill effects of genetic mutations can, or cannot, be altered by environmental manipulations entirely depends on how the genes work. With respect to psychiatric disorders, there are good reasons for supposing that many genetic factors operate, at least in part, by creating a vulnerability to environmental risks (Plomin, 1994; Rutter *et al*, 1997a). That seems to be the case, for example, with respect to both depressive (Kendler *et al*, 1995a) and antisocial disorders (Cadoret *et al*, 1995; Bohman, 1996). Accordingly, environmental manipulation may be most beneficial for individuals who have an increased genetic vulnerability.

A high heritability within populations means that differences between populations will also be genetically determined

Another misconception is that when the evidence indicates that a particular characteristic has a strong genetic contribution in two populations, then differences in the mean level of that characteristic between the two populations must be genetically determined. That, too, was the implication of Jensen's 1969 paper and it was wrong (Morton, 1974; Block, 1995). The reasons why populations vary in the mean level of a characteristic may be the same as those causing variations within that population or they may be entirely different (Rutter & Smith, 1995). It is quite invalid to generalise from the findings within one population to assumptions about the reasons for differences between populations.

Genetic effects are determinative

There is the assumption that genes are directly determinative such that if you have a particular gene, you will inevitably get the disorder with which it is associated. In the great majority of cases, that is not so. There are, of course, rare genetic disorders in which the underlying disease state is inherited directly without any other genetic or environmental factors being involved, for example, Huntington's disease, a dominant Mendelian disorder leading to dementia in middle age. Nevertheless, even with these conditions, there may be a more uncertain route from the genetically determined disease state to the actual disability suffered by the individual. For example, tuberous sclerosis is a disease caused directly by one or other of two genes (Simonoff *et al*, 1996). Nevertheless, although the disease is inherited directly, there is an extraordinarily wide variation in the ways in which it manifests in the individual. Thus, some people have learning disabilities, have epilepsy, and have calcified masses in their brain. By contrast, others have just skin lesions that are detectable only by an expert. The reasons for this considerable variation remain unknown at the moment.

But the vast majority of medical conditions are not like that at all. Instead, they are multifactorially determined, meaning that they arise from the interplay among a mixture of genetic and environmental risk and protective factors. That would be the case, for example, with diseases such as diabetes, hypertension, asthma and coronary artery disease. With only a few exceptions, it also applies to psychiatric disorders. There are several in which genetic factors play a very large role and in some cases they seem to predominate. Nevertheless, in most cases, environmental factors also play a substantial, often major, role. Accordingly, genetic effects are probabilistic rather than deterministic in their effects (see Plomin & Rutter, 1997). Indeed, genetic research has been particularly important in showing that the popular assumption that genetic effects are largely deterministic is mistaken.

A closely related concern is that if there is a strong genetic influence on a behaviour or a disorder, this necessarily requires a denial of free will and of individual responsibility. Clearly, that is not the case. To begin with, no person can be reduced to a mere vehicle of the disorder from which they suffer. Even when the disease is completely genetically determined and associated with

46 ■

severe disability, as with Down's syndrome or Huntington's disease, that does not mean that the disease controls the whole of the individual's behaviour. That is even more the case with most psychiatric disorders in which the genetic effects are only contributory and operate in indirect ways. It should be added, however, that although we all act on the assumption that we, and others, have free will and individual responsibility, it is an assumption and not a fact open to scientific testing (Glover, 1996). There are good reasons for acting on the basis of that assumption and, if anything, the finding that the vast majority of genetic effects are probabilistic increases the plausibility, rather than detracting from it.

'Genetic' means single abnormal genes

A misconception abetted by the media is that evidence for genetic influence means that a single abnormal gene is responsible. When evidence is found for genetic influence on a disorder, the media often translates this to headlines about *the* gene for the disorder. Although there are thousands of rare disorders that show clear patterns of single-gene inheritance, most common medical and psychiatric disorders show no signs of single-gene or even major gene effects. Evidence from many quarters, including animal models, converges on the conclusion that most genetic influence on common and complex disorders involves multiple genes of varying effect size that contribute probabilistically to risk. Moreover, most of these genes are normal variations and not abnormal mutations. The recognition that complex traits involve multiple 'susceptibility' genes, often involving variations on normal dimensions such as temperamental features or physiological reactivity, has led to new conceptions of molecular genetic strategies referred to as 'qualitative trait loci' (QTL) (Plomin *et al*, 1994).

A related misconception is that if a susceptibility gene is discovered for some behaviour, then that necessarily 'medicalises' it. The discovery of a susceptibility gene has nothing whatsoever to do with medicine *per se*. There are susceptibility genes for all forms of human behaviour and not just for those that involve diseases. It would be seriously mistaken to equate the discovery of a susceptibility gene with any implication that the gene is pathological or that the behaviour should now be seen in medical terms. It is a very common misunderstanding, but it

represents a serious misconception of what is involved in the operation of genetic influences.

Genes associated with disease must be bad

A sixth misconception is that the genes associated with disease are necessarily bad and that, once the genes have been discovered, the next step should be to seek to get rid of them. That too is wrong. In the first place, some genes operate protectively, rather than as a risk factor. For example, that applies to the gene in many Asiatic people that causes a flushing response with alcohol and which serves to protect them to a considerable extent against alcoholism (McGue, 1993). Also, however, the same genetically influenced behaviour may serve as a risk factor for some outcomes but a protective factor for others. For example, behavioural inhibition is a risk factor for anxiety disorders (Biederman *et al*, 1995) but a protective factor against antisocial behaviour (Lahey *et al*, 1995). In addition, some genetically influenced behaviours may depend on particular environmental circumstances in order for them to lead to disorder. For example, novelty seeking is an indirect risk factor for antisocial behaviour (Cloninger *et al*, 1996) but it seems likely that this may be a positive trait in some circumstances, although it is a risk factor in others. In other words, genetic factors associated with disease are neither necessarily good nor bad.

'Bad' genes justify both eugenic programmes and termination of pregnancy

A further misconception is that when a gene that is undoubtedly bad in most of its effects has been found, the next step will ordinarily be to try to remove the gene from the population. That was the rationale behind eugenics programmes in the past. However, the implication, although it may seem logical, is seriously mistaken. To begin with, some genetic anomalies and mutations are not inherited. Thus, that is usually so with Down's syndrome and about half the cases of tuberous sclerosis (Simonoff *et al*, 1996). But, more importantly, the rationale is wrong because most genes are not only probabilistic in their effects but also constitute just one of many risk factors. Almost everybody carries risk genes that they do not realise they have got because they have not led to any particular disease. They have not done so either because the individual has

only some of the risk genes that are necessary or because the person has not experienced the risk environments that are necessary along with the risk genes. To get rid of risk genes in the population would mean getting rid of most of the world's population!

The same considerations mean that the discovery of susceptibility genes for mental disorders should not provide the basis for a major expansion of the grounds for termination of pregnancy. Four considerations predominate. First, in the majority of cases, susceptibility genes play only a contributory role in the causative processes. Their presence means that the *relative* risk for disorder is substantially raised but the absolute probability of the disorder may still be quite small. Second, it is most unlikely to be ethically acceptable to terminate a pregnancy on the basis of a disorder that may leave the person functioning well for much of their life. Thus, for example, for most people, it would not be ethically acceptable to consider termination simply because someone's risk for having a depressive disorder at some time in their life was increased. The situation is different for lifelong conditions involving major disability (such as severe mental retardation). Third, the genetic liability may lie in a dimensional characteristic on which there is no single point above which the risk arises. Fourth, even when the presence of a mutant gene carries a high level of risk for a major disabling condition, the response may be the development of effective treatments, rather than therapeutic abortion. Thus, the former was the response in the case of PKU.

Gene therapy will be widely applicable

Alternatively, there is the possibility of replacing a mutant gene with a normal gene that will correct some basic pathophysiological disturbance. In certain circumstances, gene therapy will prove useful (Birnstiel, 1996), although there are still very considerable practical problems to be overcome if it is to prove clinically feasible and effective (Crystal, 1995). Thus, for example, clinical trials are underway with the monogenic disorder cystic fibrosis (Knowles *et al*, 1995). It may also have a place in the treatment of some of the single gene disorders associated with severe learning disability (Fletcher, 1995; Moser, 1995). It is much more doubtful, however, whether gene therapy will have any significant place in the treatment of most multifactorial

■47

British Journal of Psychiatry, 1997, vol. 171, pp. 209–219

psychiatric disorders in which several genes, each of small effect, are implicated. Not only would gene replacement be unlikely to be effective in such a situation, but also genetic findings may well lead to effective (and less heroic) interventions of other kinds. Although it would be wrong to assume that gene therapy could have no place in the treatment of psychiatric disorders, it seems a rather distant prospect of uncertain value.

Genetic screening

The last major misconception is that the prime purpose of molecular genetic findings will be the development of genetic screening of the general population. This prospect raises serious ethical issues (Nuffield Council on Bioethics, 1993; Andrews et al, 1994), including the possible misuses for denial of health insurance or for discrimination in employment. Even in the medical arena, there are quite tricky ethical, as well as practical, dilemmas (for example, with respect to screening children for disorders with an onset in adult life, or screening at any age for diseases that are currently untreatable).

In some respects the situation with respect to susceptibility genes for multifactorial disorders is more straightforward in that the predictions at an individual level are so much weaker that, if dealt with rationally, they should be less open to misuse. Nevertheless, in practice, the problems may be greater simply because of the lack of appreciation that this is so. As already discussed, it is likely that virtually everyone in the general population has genes that are involved in the liability to some multifactorial disorder. That is both because some are extremely common (such as short sight or hay fever in the domain of somatic diseases and depression or anxiety in the domain of mental disorders) but it is also because most multifactorial disorders will involve the operation of several susceptibility genes. Sometimes these may be required in combination for the disease or disorder to develop and in other cases a varied assortment of genes may suffice. Either way, all of us will have quite a complex set of varied genetic risk and protective factors. But, most of all, genetic screening in the field of multifactorial disorders cannot have quite the same meaning as with monogenic disorders because the risks are probabilistic and often they may be contingent on the occurrence of some parallel set of environmental risk

factors. All of these considerations mean that there are very severe constraints on both the practicality and the utility of genetic screening.

There is one further point that requires emphasis with respect to actuarial predictions based on genetic screening for either insurance purposes or genetic counselling (Masood, 1996). The initial findings on the risks associated with a particular susceptibility gene are likely to stem from unusual samples (chosen deliberately for their advantages in localising genes). Thus, they may derive from families with an unusually heavy concentration of affected members or from clinical samples in which the patients have severe typical disorders. The risks associated with susceptibility genes may be substantially lower in other samples. Also, it is important to bear in mind that the risks may vary by racial group, by environmental circumstances, or by associations with other genes. It is necessary to exercise considerable caution in estimating genetic risks and to appreciate that they are relative, and not absolute.

THE VALUE OF QUANTITATIVE GENETICS

Given all these misconceptions, it might be thought that the use of quantitative genetics to determine the relative importance of genetic and environmental influences on particular behaviour or particular diseases has been a waste of time. That is clearly not the case, however. To the contrary, it has been hugely important in at least five different ways.

Ubiquitous influence of both genes and environment

The first important finding from quantitative genetics that has a pervasive influence on how we think about the role of genetic factors is that there is a genetic contribution to virtually all complex human traits and behaviours (Plomin et al, 1997). The same evidence, however, also shows that environmental factors are similarly ubiquitous in their effects. Although both conclusions would now be generally accepted by almost everyone, it is necessary to note that it does represent a marked departure from the past in which much time was spent in sorting out behaviours that were supposedly due to nature and those that were supposedly due to nurture. The finding that genetic influences are ubiquitous is, of course, not really

a surprise to anyone who approaches the matter from a biological perspective. The workings of the mind have to be based on the functioning of the brain and all human structures and functions exhibit individual variation that is, at least in part, subject to genetic influences. It would be very surprising indeed if human behaviour constituted an exception to this general tendency. There are, however, three very important consequences of this first finding.

First, it is necessary that we get away from thinking that genetic factors apply only to diseases and, instead, take on board the fact that they apply to all aspects of human functioning. Second, it is necessary to appreciate that it is likely that many genetically influenced dimensional characteristics will play a role in the risk for diseases. That is to say, the risks may derive from someone's level on some perfectly normal dimensional attribute rather than their possession of some abnormal trait. For example, in the field of somatic medicine, cholesterol levels are systematically related to the risk of coronary artery disease at all points on the distribution, and not just at the so-called 'pathological' end of the scale (Chen et al, 1991). It is virtually certain that the same will apply to psychological characteristics such as temperamental variations, or reactivity to stress, or cognitive skills (Plomin et al, 1991). Third, genetic influences extend to what seem to be environmental risk factors (Plomin & Bergeman, 1991; Plomin, 1994; Kendler, 1996; Plomin et al, 1997). At first sight that sounds counter-intuitive in that, for obvious reasons, there cannot be DNA in the environment. Nevertheless, the finding is both real and important and it arises in three main ways. To begin with, many measures of the environment rely on people's perceptions of their experiences. This would be so, for example, with family members' ratings of discord or warmth or hostility. In so far as such ratings derive from their own attitudes and biases and perceptions, the measures may say more about the people making the ratings than about the events, experiences or circumstances that the measures are meant to reflect. When that is the case, the 'environmental measure' is not a measure of the environment at all.

An alternative way in which environments reflect a genetic influence arises from the fact that environments are not randomly distributed (Rutter et al, 1995). Whether or not someone experiences divorce or a breakup of a longstanding friendship, or a lack of

48

social support, will be in part determined by their own ways of behaving. In this case, the measures truly reflect the environment but individual differences in the likelihood of experiencing those risk environments are influenced, in part, by genetic factors.

The third possibility is that although the environmental risk is real, the main impact arises from its association with genetic risk. For example, many studies have shown that parental mental disorder is accompanied by an increased likelihood of many different sorts of risk experiences (Rutter, 1989). Nevertheless, it remains an important empirical question whether the risks associated with parental mental disorder reflect the risk environments engendered by that disorder or rather a direct passing on of genes.

Some prevailing diagnostic conventions are mistaken

Genetic findings have also been important in showing that, not only does the strength of genetic influence vary according to the type of psychiatric disorder, but so also does the degree of diagnosis-specificity. Thus, for example, genetic factors predominate in accounting for population variance in the underlying liability to such psychiatric disorders as autism (Rutter *et al*, 1997*a*), schizophrenia (McGuffin *et al*, 1994), and bipolar affective disorder (McGuffin & Sargeant, 1991), as well as hyperkinetic disorder symptoms (Silberg *et al*, 1996*a,b*). In each of these cases, too, there is a degree of diagnostic specificity for the genetic contribution. The strength and relative specificity of the genetic contribution makes these strong candidates for molecular genetic studies. By contrast, there are other psychiatric disorders where the effects seem more indirect and not diagnosis-specific. It is important to appreciate that many genetic factors have quite diverse, pleiotropic effects (Plomin, 1991). For example, the genetic contribution to anxiety disorders and depressive disorders seems to be the same in large part (Kendler *et al*, 1995*a*). Possibly, it is mediated, to a considerable extent, through genetic effects on the temperamental characteristic of neuroticism or emotionality. Because this temperamental feature itself shows very substantial heritability, it, too, provides a good candidate for molecular genetic studies.

Twin, adoptee, and family studies have been crucially informative in their indication that some of the prevailing diagnostic assumptions in psychiatry are, at least

partially, mistaken. For example, many clinicians have tended to assume that schizophrenia constituted a qualitatively distinct abnormal disease or disorder category that had no continuity with normal variations. Quantitative genetic studies have, however, shown that the genetic liability to schizophrenia also extends to a liability to schizotypal personality disorders and other conditions that are now conceptualised as part of a broader 'schizophrenic spectrum' (Kendler *et al*, 1993, 1995*b*; Erlenmeyer-Kimling *et al*, 1995). It remains unclear whether this means that the liability to schizophrenia operates through normal dimensions of personality or whether, by contrast, it is simply that the diagnostic concept needs to be very much broadened, although not extended into normal variations. Exactly comparable issues arise with respect to autism and the extension of the genetic liability to related social and communicative abnormalities occurring in individuals of normal intelligence (Bailey *et al*, 1996). In much the same way, the genetic liability for oppositional defiant disorder and conduct disorder seems to be the same (Eaves *et al*, 1997). There is also substantial overlap with the genetic liability for hyperkinetic disorder (Silberg *et al*, 1996*a,b*). Although the evidence is not quite perhaps as clear-cut, it has been generally supposed that the genetic liability to Tourette's syndrome incorporates at least some forms of multiple tics and obsessive–compulsive disorder (Pauls *et al*, 1991, 1995; Simonoff & Rutter, 1996). Molecular genetic research will obviously take us very much further in understanding the patterning of disorders (see below) but it is already clear that there needs to be something of a rethink on diagnostic conventions and psychiatric classification.

Just as genetic findings have indicated that some disorders are more broadly based than previously appreciated and that some of the finer diagnostic distinctions may not be justifiable, so also genetic findings have indicated that some broadly based psychiatric diagnostic categories may need to be subdivided. For example, it is clear that the genetic contribution to bipolar affective disorder and to the most severe unipolar disorders is very substantial, whereas environmental factors seem to predominate in the liability to the much more common milder varieties of depression (McGuffin & Katz, 1986). Similarly, it is clear that antisocial behaviour includes varieties (such as those associated with hyperactivity) that have a

very strong genetic contribution, and varieties (such as the milder forms of antisocial behaviour that so frequently constitute a temporary phase in adolescence) that are largely environmental in origin (Silberg *et al*, 1996*a*).

Genes influence the course of development

Because all the genes are in place at the time of birth, sometimes it is assumed that all genetic effects must also be operative then. A moment's thought makes it clear that that cannot be the case. Not only do some genetic diseases (such as Huntington's) not have an onset until mid-life, but also genetic effects on the timing of maturational transitions such as puberty are strong (see Rutter & Rutter, 1993). Genetic factors play a role, too, in the ups and downs of normal development – that is in the patterning and course of psychological growth (Matheny, 1989, 1990). The effects of genes are dynamic, not static.

The same wrong assumption has led to the expectation that genetic effects should be maximal at birth and decrease progressively thereafter as environmental influences progressively exert their power. In fact, the evidence suggests that the reverse tends to be the case, at least for some traits (Plomin, 1986). This, at first-sight counter-intuitive finding, probably arises through several different mechanisms (Rutter *et al*, 1997*a*). For example, genetic effects on the same behaviours as shown at different ages tend to be the same, whereas the environmental effects are often different; as a consequence, there is more opportunity for genetic effects to be cumulative. Also, insofar as genetic effects shape either individual differences in environmental risk exposure or sensitivities to environmental risks (see below) their input will tend to increase over time. This may be relevant, for example, in relation to the rise in depressive disorders in females over the period of adolescence, and to the suggestion that this is associated with an increasing genetic influence (Thapar & McGuffin, 1994).

The effects of nature and nurture are not separate

In some respects, one of the most fundamental contributions of quantitative genetics has been the demonstration that nature and nurture are no way near so separate as once used to be assumed (Scarr, 1992; Plomin *et al*, 1997; Rutter *et al*, 1997*a*).

British Journal of Psychiatry, 1997, vol. 171, pp. 209–219

The evidence is clear that there are important, and sometimes quite strong, associations between genetic risks and environmental risks (gene–environment correlations). For example, the forms of parental mental disorder or psychopathology that entail the passing on of genes creating a liability to the same disorders in the offspring, are also ones that are associated with a much increased likelihood of environments carrying psychiatric risk (because of the increased rate of family discord, divorce and separation, impaired parenting, etc. – see Rutter, 1989). Also, people's own characteristics play a substantial role in eliciting particular behaviours in other people (evocative gene–environment correlations). Thus, the work of Patterson (1982) and his colleagues showed the extent to which aversive behaviour by children (which is likely to be genetically influenced to some degree) tends to evoke coercive negative responses from other family members. Also, people's own characteristics will play a substantial role in their selection and shaping of their own environments and experiences (active gene–environment correlations). Finally, some genetic effects operate through rendering individuals more vulnerable than other people to risk environments (gene–environment interactions). These features appear to be particularly important in the field of antisocial behaviour (Rutter, 1997), mild learning disability (Rutter *et al*, 1996), unipolar depression (Rutter *et al*, 1997*b*) and possibly schizophrenia (Tienari *et al*, 1994). At present, the best data are available on person–environment interplay rather than on the specific role of genetic factors in such interplay. Nevertheless, this body of work has already been important in emphasising various indirect ways in which many genetic factors operate. That necessarily has an impact on how we need to think about genetic risk and on what we do with findings about the importance of genetic factors.

Environmental effects tend to be person-specific

Finally, genetic findings have been influential in forcing a major change in the ways in which we have to think about environmental influences (Plomin & Daniels, 1987; Dunn & Plomin, 1990). The key finding is that, in general (but with some important exceptions) most environmental influences tend to serve to make children growing up in the same family different

rather than similar in their characteristics. The strong implication is that the study of environmental risk factors needs to pay much more attention to person-specific features than has been the case in the past. That is to say, for example, we need to determine the extent to which family conflict actually impinges on each child in the family rather than relying on global measures of the extent to which the family as a whole is characterised by discord (Reiss *et al*, 1995; Rutter *et al*, 1997*c*). This relative specificity of the impact of environmental risks does not, of course, mean that family-wide risk features (such as discord or divorce or poverty or overcrowding) do not create any significant risk. Rather, what the findings mean is that the extent to which children are embroiled in these family-wide risks shows considerable individual variation; the impact will also be influenced by the ways in which they think and feel about their experiences; the impact may also vary according to their age, gender, or particular environmental risks (as a result of past experiences or constitutional features).

Implications for the future

It is sometimes assumed by enthusiasts for the new opportunities of molecular genetics that the field of quantitative genetics is strictly for the past and not for the future. As is explicit in this discussion of the contributions of quantitative genetics, new areas are still being opened up in which quantitative genetics has a lot to offer. It is true that there is now limited scope for studies primarily concerned with quantifying the genetic contribution to yet another human trait or disorder (although there are still some conditions where this information is needed because we know so little). The greatest potential is in terms of the specifics outlined above and, especially, in the various complex mechanisms involved in the interplay between nature and nurture. Molecular genetics will take these matters further forward (see below) but there is still a very considerable need for quantitative genetics and, most particularly, for the integration of quantitative and molecular genetic strategies with epidemiological and developmental perspectives. The crucial qualification that needs to be added, however, is that such research will only fulfil its potential if genetic designs include high quality, discriminating, measures of putative environmental risk factors. That has been a

most notable lack in most genetic studies that have been undertaken up to now.

THE VALUE OF MOLECULAR GENETICS

Most of the issues raised with respect to quantitative genetics can be tackled better if specific susceptibility genes can be identified (Plomin & Rutter, 1997). The most important contribution of molecular genetics, however, is novel in that it opens the way for a more direct study of causal processes. Because the contribution of molecular genetics to psychiatry is only just beginning to be evident, it is inevitable that this section is more of a promissory note than an account of accomplishments with proven clinical implications. Nevertheless, it is obvious that these are likely to be forthcoming very soon as findings with respect to schizophrenia (Peltonen, 1995), affective disorder (Detera-Wadleigh *et al*, 1996) and dyslexia (Grigorenko *et al*, 1997) all show.

Elucidation of causal processes: brain systems

Without doubt, much the most important purpose of molecular genetic research lies in its potential as a crucial step in the understanding of the processes involved in the causation and course of mental disorders. Even with mental disorders where there is good evidence to suppose that there are abnormalities in basic aspects of brain functioning, as would be the case with both schizophrenia (Mednick & Hollister, 1995) and autism (Bailey *et al*, 1996), biological research up to now has been surprisingly unhelpful in showing the nature of the specific pathophysiology involved in the causation of these conditions. Where these disorders have been shown to have a strong genetic component (as is the case with schizophrenia and autism), there is every reason to suppose that identification of the susceptibility genes will, in time, lead on to a much greater understanding of the basic causal processes. What needs to be understood, however, is that the identification of susceptibility genes marks the beginning of the research endeavour, and not its end. The discovery that a susceptibility gene is located at some particular site on a certain chromosome is of very limited value in its own right. Indeed, given modern technology, it is not unfair to state that finding the gene location is the easy bit (difficult though it has proved to be in the past). The real challenge is identifying the gene itself, finding out how it works and determining what it actually does in order to bring about the disorder of concern.

The research required to delineate the causal pathway from gene to mental disorder involves several rather different steps spanning quite disparate scientific domains (Lander, 1996). The first step in linkage studies is showing that a particular psychiatric disorder (or behavioural dimension predisposing to it) is connected with a locus on a particular chromosome (Lander & Schork, 1994). Typically, the specified locus includes many genes and the next step of identifying the actual gene responsible involves cloning and sequencing the genes in that region (Antonarakis & Scott, 1996) and identifying associations between specific mutations and the disorder in question. Human research constitutes the main focus in this step but very important leads may be provided by what is known about genes in other species, particularly the mouse whose genome closely parallels that of humans.

The next step of finding the function of the gene product requires experimental approaches with animals. In essence, gene function must be manipulated experimentally by techniques such as inserting, or 'knocking out', genes in order to determine what happens when this is done (Capecchi, 1994; Crabbe *et al*, 1994; Sibilia & Wagner, 1996). There are problems, however, in that the altered gene in the mouse may not result in a recognisable, or even detectable, behavioural picture. Alternatively, the animal model for the disorder being studied may differ from that in the human in key respects. In addition to genetic manipulation, however, there is a need to study protein structure and function directly – a field of science that requires the expertise of biochemists and biophysicists. The need to integrate information across different fields has led to the new field of bioinformatics (the use of computing techniques in the collection, storage and interpretation of biological information). At present we know much more about how to go from gene to protein structure than we do about how to proceed from structure to function, but this last step is a crucial one in the causal pathway.

This research road is a long and difficult one with many problems to be overcome. Nevertheless, what is needed with respect to single gene disorders is relatively straightforward compared with what is required for multifactorial disorders. At present, molecular biology tends to be extremely reductionist, so that the focus is on the elucidation of mechanisms at the molecular level, although it is appreciated that there is a need to understand the structure and function of supermolecular complexes and of protein–protein interactions. With multifactorial disorders, it will also be essential to move on to the role of these proteins in complex systems with multiple interacting components. That is already happening in immunology and metabolic regulation and it will have to happen, too, with behavioural systems.

The research challenge is considerable but it can be met. To begin with, connections with other bodies of knowledge are likely to be very helpful. For example, the apoliprotein E, which is a gene for cholesterol transport, was discovered to be associated with Alzheimer's disease, so far the only common confirmed genetic risk factor. It was found to be a functional polymorphism and although its mechanism at first seemed to be puzzling, its possible role in the amyloid cascade theory coalesced (Hardy & Higgins, 1992; Hardy & Hutton, 1995). Moreover, finding this susceptibility gene for Alzheimer's disease has revolutionised research in this field and may well have effects on clinical practice in the future. Nevertheless, it is necessary to be realistic in recognising that sometimes it may take a considerable time to find out just how particular susceptibility genes do work. Progress will be enhanced, by ensuring that genetics is well integrated with other branches of science.

Elucidation of causal processes: nature–nurture interplay

Across the range of psychiatric disorders, there will be immense variation in the sorts of causal mechanisms that will have to be considered. With respect to a few conditions, such as schizophrenia and autism, the main focus may well need to be on the persistent abnormal functioning of brain systems. In other cases, by contrast, the focus may need to be much more on the interplay between genes and environment. For example, although it will clearly be useful to know more about the brain mechanisms involved in susceptibility traits such as novelty seeking or emotionality, it is very probable that the risks lie less in what goes on in the brain all the time than in what a particular form of brain functioning does

when the person is having to deal with environmental risks of various kinds.

For this reason, it also follows that one of the main gains that will come from identification of susceptibility genes is the much greater power to study both environmental risk mechanisms and the interplay between nature and nurture (Plomin & Rutter, 1997). Thus, for example, quantitative genetic research has been helpful in showing that, even when full account has been taken of genetic risk, there are valid and important associations between environmental risk factors and various types of mental disorder. But research has been much less helpful in the elucidation of how environmental risk mechanisms operate and in determining what the experience of environmental risks does to the organism. In other words, we know little about how the results of environmental risk exposure are carried forward in time through their effects on a person's functioning (whether in terms of neuroendocrine functioning, styles of thinking, or habits of behaviour).

There is the further difficulty that it has proved extremely difficult in practice to separate the effects of deviant behaviour of the child on environmental functioning, from the effects of environmental risks predisposing to the child's disorder. For example, clearly there is likely to be a two-way interplay between family discord and disruptive behaviour in the child but it proved difficult to go beyond that truism to a precise elucidation of how this two-way process actually works in practice. The research into environmental risk mechanisms will be greatly aided by the discovery of the susceptibility genes so that it will be possible to identify the individual risk in advance of the development of the disorder. In this way, the operation over time of environmental risk factors can be studied in a much more satisfactory fashion (Plomin & Rutter, 1997).

In the same sort of way, the study of nature–nurture interplay will be greatly facilitated by identification of susceptibility genes. It is all very well to be able to say that there is a strong genetic component to some form of psychopathology (for example, schizophrenia) but it is quite another thing to be able to assess the particular genetic risk in a given individual. That is what quantitative genetics cannot do, but molecular genetics can. It is obvious, therefore, that the study of gene–environment correlations and interactions will be able to be undertaken directly and meaningfully on a person by

British Journal of Psychiatry, 1997, vol. 171, pp. 209–219

person basis once susceptibility genes have been discovered (Plomin & Rutter, 1997).

Diagnosis

Quantitative genetic findings have demonstrated the extent to which the genetic liability for many psychiatric disorders is far from coterminous with the traditional diagnostic boundaries. Thus, for example, it has been shown that some schizotypal personality disorders are associated with the genetic liability for schizophrenia (e.g. Kendler *et al*, 1993, 1995*b*; Erlenmeyer–Kimling *et al*, 1995) and that some social and communicative deficits are associated with the genetic liability for autism (Bailey *et al*, 1996). But the same research has also indicated that these broader patterns of disorder also include many instances in which the disorder seems completely separate from schizophrenia or autism or whatever psychiatric condition is being considered (Bailey *et al*, 1996). Molecular genetic findings should be very helpful in sorting out, within this broader pattern of disorder, which individuals do and which do not have the liability to the traditional diagnosis. There is no doubt that that will help immensely in sorting out diagnostic boundaries and patterns in a much more satisfactory way than is possible now. Exactly the same applies with respect to the elucidation of the mechanisms involved in the co-occurrence of two supposedly separate psychiatric conditions – a very common circumstance indeed (Caron & Rutter, 1991). Some psychiatrists undertaking research in the biology of disorders have gone further in their hope that molecular genetic research will lead to diagnostic tests for mental disorders. Nowadays, in somatic medicine, it is usual for there to be laboratory tests to confirm or disconfirm clinical diagnoses. There is no longer a need to rely entirely on patterns of signs and symptoms. Thus, for example, conditions such as diabetes or thyrotoxicosis can be diagnosed precisely as a result of laboratory findings, in a way that is not possible at all at the moment in relation to virtually all forms of psychiatric disorder. Clearly, it would indeed be most useful to have such tests in the field of psychiatry. Nevertheless, a careful consideration of the issues makes it apparent that our expectations in that connection must be quite modest. To begin with, most diagnoses in medicine are based on particular patterns of abnormal physiology or chemistry and not on the

identification of a single basic cause. That is because most medical diseases are multifactorial and, therefore, do not have a single basic cause, any more than psychiatric disorders do. Accordingly, the identification of a susceptibility gene will not, in itself, usually lead to a diagnostic test. On the other hand, if such identification leads on to an understanding of the basic abnormal processes within the body that lead to the disorder in question, that could proceed to the development of a useful diagnostic test. Whether or not that takes place, however, will be dependent, not so much on the identification of the gene, but rather on whether the identification of the gene leads to the hoped-for understanding of the causal processes.

The identification of a gene is much more likely to lead to a diagnostic test in the case of monogenic disorders where the genetic mutation constitutes a necessary and sufficient cause of the underlying disease process (although as discussed above, not necessarily of the disorder itself, as it is shown in the form of behaviour). Even with Mendelian disorders, however, there is the quite important added complication that in many, probably most, cases the same disorder may be due to several different genes or a large number of mutations of the same gene. Such genes are not interchangeable but they provide alternative single gene routes to the disease in question. Thus, for example, it is known that tuberous sclerosis may be due to one or other of two genes and several different genes are involved with fragile X anomaly (Simonoff *et al*, 1996). In these circumstances, the identification of a known single gene that operates in Mendelian fashion does provide certainty on the diagnosis. The problem comes with what you do with a negative finding. That is, if a person is shown *not* to have a particular gene, that may simply mean that there is another gene involved in that Mendelian disorder, the nature of which has still be discovered.

With respect to multifactorial disorders, it could still be the case that a genetic factor is a necessary predisposing feature, although not a sufficient one. For example, that could prove to be the case with schizophrenia. Although the genetic component in schizophrenia does not account for all the variance in liability, it has not so far proved possible to identify any environmental risk that leads to schizophrenia in the absence of a genetic liability. It is not that that possibility has been ruled out (see, for example, the findings with

respect to risks during pregnancy – McGrath *et al*, 1995; Wyatt, 1996) but so far, it does appear that in most instances a genetic predisposition is required. In such cases, although the discovery of susceptibility genes will not indicate that the person is certain to develop schizophrenia it could mean that if they do not have any of the susceptibility genes, then the likelihood of their developing schizophrenia is either very low or perhaps even absent. Much more commonly, probably, a multifactorial pattern of causation will involve genetic factors that play a substantial role in susceptibility but that are neither necessary nor sufficient. In that case, there will be an inevitably high proportion of both false negatives and false positives. The information deriving from the identification of susceptibility genes will be of huge help in understanding risk processes and in estimating risks but they will be of quite limited use for the purpose of individual diagnosis.

Genetic counselling

At the moment, genetic counselling in the field of psychiatric disorders is quite severely constrained both by the uncertainties over diagnostic boundaries and uncertainties over how genetic factors operate. As already indicated, molecular genetic findings are likely to help in both connections. One specific way in which molecular genetic findings have already been informative is in their identification of novel, hitherto unappreciated, genetic mechanisms. One of the puzzles in the family findings with respect to the fragile X anomaly was that the pattern did not seem to follow any of the known modes of genetic transmission (Simonoff *et al*, 1996). There was also appreciation that carriers of the gene sometimes themselves had milder disabilities of one kind or another and it was not clear quite what that meant. The discovery that the basis of the fragile X anomaly lay in a much expanded set of trinucleotide repeat sequences, that a lesser degree of expansion occurred in the preceding generation, and that the transmission of the genetic anomaly across generations led to the expansion solved the riddle. Since then, several other neuropsychiatric disorders, including Huntington's disease, have been found to have somewhat similar expanding sequences (Petronis & Kennedy, 1995). The ways in which this works differ somewhat in detail among the various disorders but the findings are already of considerable help in genetic counselling. The discovery of so-called genomic imprinting (Nicholls, 1994), by which consequences of a genetic anomaly differ according to whether the transmission is through the mother or the father (a phenomenon seen, for example, with the Prader–Willi syndrome and Angelman's syndrome), provides a somewhat comparable example (Simonoff *et al*, 1996).

Gene identification will also be enormously valuable with respect to personalising risks. Thus, quantitative genetic findings allow estimates of the risk that, say, a child born to a schizophrenic parent will themselves develop schizophrenia. But that is simply a population average. The identification of susceptibility genes allows the crucial step of proceeding to the risks for that particular individual, based on their genetic make-up. The increase in precision provided by the ability to calculate risks on an individual by individual basis will be of huge clinical benefit. Nevertheless, as already discussed, great care will be needed in their use because the true risk will be dependent on other factors, many of which may be unknown. Even so, it is clear that molecular genetic findings will immensely enhance what will be possible in genetic counselling, with respect to both precision and, through the elucidation of causal mechanisms, knowledge on how risks may be reduced.

Medication

It is quite likely that elucidation of the causal processes underlying psychiatric disorders will, in some cases, lead to the development of medication that may be helpful in either prevention or treatment or both. The development of effective methods of drug treatment does not necessarily depend on an understanding of causal processes but, for obvious reasons, the rational development of pharmacological treatments is immensely helped by an understanding of causal processes. Thus, for example, at the present time there are no drugs that have a major specific beneficial effect in the case of autism, although there are many such drugs that are useful in the treatment of schizophrenia. A better understanding of the causal processes involved in autism might well lead to improved pharmacological treatments. On the other hand, it would be a mistake to assume that that will ordinarily be the case. Much depends on what the causal process is. For example, if the genetically influenced liability operates through normal traits, it does not follow

that manipulation of trait levels through drugs would be the treatment of choice. Instead, the focus may be on the interactions with environmental risks. Also, drugs that affect key processes may carry with them serious undesirable side-effects. For example, there are many drugs that have been shown to be effective in the reduction of anxiety but the risks of dependence on those drugs has meant that their utility is substantially constrained and long-term treatment involves quite major risks (Petursson & Lader, 1984).

There are also quite tricky issues involved when a pharmacological approach is the treatment of choice. For example, the stimulant drug methylphenidate has been shown to be effective in improving attention in normal individuals, and in those with other psychiatric disorders as well as in children who show the specific seriously disabling syndrome of hyperkinetic disorder (Taylor, 1994). But that does not necessarily mean that it would be sensible and appropriate to put everyone on this drug because it improves their attention to some small degree. Similarly, although it appears that selective serotonin reuptake inhibitors have beneficial effects across a wide span of affective disorders, it does not mean that everyone should take such drugs on the grounds that everyone feels depressed sometimes (although that has been suggested – Kramer, 1994). In summary, an understanding of causal processes brought about by molecular genetic advances will be helpful in the development of new pharmacological treatments but this will be so in only some cases.

CONCLUSIONS

It is evident that advances in genetics will make a major impact on clinical psychiatry and that there are several ways in which the practical benefits should be very considerable. Most especially, these apply to the implications for improved prevention and treatment that should stem from a better understanding of the causal processes involved. The relevant causal mechanisms need to be considered in relation to both the functioning of brain systems and the interplay between nature and nurture as played out in people's social lives. In addition, there should be real gains with respect to diagnosis, genetic counselling and the development of improved pharmacological treatments. However, what molecular genetics should *not* bring about is either biological determinism

or the 'medicalisation' of either normal variations in behaviour or maladaptive responses to psychosocial stress or adversity. Any appreciation of the real benefits and opportunities that will derive from genetic advances requires a recognition of the numerous misconceptions and false hopes associated with genetic findings.

REFERENCES

Andrews, L. B., Fullarton, J. E., Holtzman, N. A., et al (1994) *Assessing Genetic Risks: Implications for Health and Social Policy.* Report of the Committee on Assessing Genetic Risks, Institute of Medicine. Washington, DC: National Academy Press.

Antonarakis, S. E. & Scott, H. S. (1996) The human genome project and its impact in medicine. *European Review,* **4**, 415–426.

Bailey, A., Phillips, W. & Rutter, M. (1996) Autism: Towards an integration of clinical, genetic, neuropsychological, and neurobiological perspectives. *Journal of Child Psychology and Psychiatry Annual Research Review,* **37**, 89–126.

Baumrind, D. (1993) The average expectable environment is not good enough: A response to Scarr. *Child Development,* **64**, 1299–1317.

Biederman, J., Rosenbaum, J. F., Chaloff, J., et al (1995) Behavioral inhibition as a risk factor for anxiety disorders. In *Anxiety Disorders in Children and Adolescents* (ed. J. L. March), pp. 61–81. New York: Guilford.

Birnstiel, M. L. (1996) Gene therapy. *European Review,* **4**, 335–356.

Blacker, D., Haine, J. L., Rodes, L., et al (1997) ApoE-4 and age at onset of Alzheimer's disease: The NIMH Genetics Initiative. *Neurology,* **48**, 139–147.

Block, N. (1995) How heritability misleads about race. *Cognition,* **56**, 99–128.

Bohman, M. (1996) Predisposition to criminality: Swedish adoption studies in retrospect. In *Genetics of Criminal and Antisocial Behaviour. Ciba Symposium No. 194* (eds G. R. Bock & J. A. Goode), pp. 99–114. Chichester: Wiley.

Cadoret, R. J., Yates, W. R., Troughton, E., et al (1995) Genetic–environmental interaction in the genesis of aggressivity and conduct disorders. *Archives of General Psychiatry,* **52**, 916–924.

Capecchi, M. R. (1994) Targeted gene replacement. *Scientific American,* **270**, 34–41.

Caron, C. & Rutter, M. (1991) Comorbidity in child psychopathology: Concepts, issues and research strategies. *Journal of Child Psychology and Psychiatry,* **32**, 1063–1080.

Chen, Z., Peto, R., Collins, R., et al (1991) Serum cholesterol concentration and coronary heart disease in population with low cholesterol concentrations. *British Medical Journal,* **303**, 276–282.

Cloninger, C. R., Adolfsson, R. & Svrakic, N. M. (1996) Mapping genes for human personality. *Nature Genetics,* **12**, 3–4.

Cookson, W. (1994) *Gene Hunters: Adventures in the Genome Jungle.* London: Aurum Press.

Crabbe, J. C., Belknap, J. K. & Buck, K. J. (1994) Genetic animal models of alcohol and drug abuse. *Science,* **264**, 1715–1723.

Crystal, R. G. (1995) Transfer of genes to humans: Early lessons and obstacles to success. *Science,* **270**, 404–410.

Detera-Wadleigh, S. D., Badner, J. A., Goldin, L. R., et al (1996) Affected-sib-pair analyses reveal support of prior

■ 53

British Journal of Psychiatry, 1997, vol. 171, pp. 209–219

evidence for a susceptibility locus for bipolar disorder on 21-Q. *American Journal of Human Genetics*, **58**, 1279–1285.

Dunn, J. & Plomin, R. (1990) *Separate Lives: Why Siblings Are So Different*. New York: Basic Books.

Eaves, L. J., Silberg, J. L., Meyer, J. M., et al (1997) Genetics and developmental psychopathology: 2. The main effects of genes and environment on behavioural problems in the Virginia Twin Study of Adolescent Behavioural Development. *Journal of Child Psychology and Psychiatry*, in press.

Erlenmeyer-Kimling, L., Squires-Wheeler, E., Adamo, U. H., et al (1995) The New York High-Risk Project: Psychoses and Cluster A personality disorders in offspring of schizophrenic parents at 23 years of follow-up. *Archives of General Psychiatry*, **52**, 857–865.

Farmer, A. & Owen, M. J. (1996) Genomics: the next psychiatric revolution? *British Journal of Psychiatry*, **169**, 135–138.

Fletcher, J. C. (1995) Gene therapy in mental retardation: Ethical considerations. *Mental Retardation and Developmental Disabilities Research Reviews*, **1**, 7–13.

Glover, J. (1996) The implications for responsibility of possible genetic factors in the explanation of violence. In *Genetics of Criminal and Antisocial Behaviour. Ciba Foundation Symposium No. 194* (eds G. R. Bock & J. A. Goode), pp. 237–243. Chichester: Wiley.

Gottesman, I. I. & Bertelsen, A. (1996) Legacy of German psychiatric genetics: hindsight is always 20/20. *American Journal of Medical Genetics*, **67**, 317–322.

Grigorenko, E. L., Wood, F. B., Meyer, M. S., et al (1997) Susceptibility loci for distinct components of dyslexia on chromosomes 6 and 15. *American Journal of Human Genetics*, **60**, 27–39.

Hardy, J. A. & Higgins, G. A. (1992) Alzheimer's disease: The amyloid cascade hypothesis. *Science*, **256**, 184–187.

___ & Hutton, M. (1995) Two new genes for Alzheimer's disease. *Trends in Neuroscience*, **18**, 436.

Jensen, A. R. (1969) How much can we boost IQ and scholastic achievement? *Harvard Education Review*, **39**, 1–123.

Kendler, K. S. (1996) Parenting: A genetic–epidemiologic perspective. *American Journal of Psychiatry*, **153**, 11–20.

___, McGuire, M., Gruenberg, A., et al (1993) The Roscommon Family Study: III. Schizophrenia-related personality disorders in relatives. *Archives of General Psychiatry*, **50**, 781–788.

___, Kessler, R. C., Walters, E. E., et al (1995a) Stressful life events, genetic liability, and onset of an episode of major depression in women. *American Journal of Psychiatry*, **152**, 833–842.

___, Neale, M. C. & Walsh, D. (1995b) Evaluating the spectrum concept of schizophrenia in the Roscommon Family Study. *American Journal of Psychiatry*, **152**, 749–754.

Knowles, M. R., Hohneker, K. W., Zhou, Z., et al (1995) A controlled study of adenoviral-vector-mediated gene transfer in the nasal epithelium of patients with cystic fibrosis. *New England Journal of Medicine*, **333**, 823–831.

Kramer, P. D. (1994) *Listening to Prozac*. Harmondsworth, Middlesex: Penguin.

Lahey, B. B., McBurnett, K., Loeber, R., et al (1995) Psychobiology of conduct disorder. In *Conduct Disorders in Children and Adolescents: Assessments and Interventions* (ed. G. P. Sholevar), pp. 27–44. Washington, DC: American Psychiatric Press.

Lander, E. S. (1996) The new genomics: Global views of biology. *Science*, **274**, 536–639.

___ & Schork, N. J. (1994) Genetic dissection of complex traits. *Science*, **265**, 2037–2048.

Lapham, E. V., Kozma, C. & Weiss, J. O. (1996) Genetic discrimination: perspectives of consumers. *Science*, **274**, 621–624.

Marshall, E. (1996) The genome program's conscience. *Science*, **274**, 488–490.

Masood, E. (1996) Gene tests: Who benefits from risk? *Nature*, **379**, 389–392.

Matheny, A. P., Jr (1989) Children's behavioral inhibition over age and across situations: Genetic similarity for a trait during change. *Journal of Personality*, **57**, 215–235.

___ (1990) Developmental behavior genetics: Contributions from the Louisville Twin Study. In *Developmental Behaviour Genetics: Neural, Biometrical, and Evolutionary Approaches* (eds M. E. Hahn, J. K. Hewitt, N. D. Henderson, et al), pp. 25–39. New York: Oxford University Press.

McGrath, J., Castle, D. & Murray, R. (1995) How can we judge whether or not prenatal exposure to influenza causes schizophrenia? In *Neural Development and Schizophrenia* (eds S. A. Mednick & J. M. Hollister), pp. 203–214. New York: Plenum.

McGue, M. (1993) From proteins to cognitions: the behavioral genetics of alcoholism. In *Nature Nurture and Psychology* (eds R. Plomin & G. E. McClearn), pp. 245–268. Washington, DC: American Psychological Association.

McGuffin, P. & Katz, R. (1986) Nature, nurture and affective disorder. In *The Biology of Depression* (ed. J. F. W. Deakin), pp. 26–52. London: Royal College of Psychiatrists.

___ & Sargeant, M. P. (1991) Genetic markers and affective disorder. In *The New Genetics of Mental Illness* (eds P. McGuffin & R. Murray), pp. 165–181. Oxford: Butterworth-Heinemann.

___, Owen, M. J., O'Donovan, M., et al (1994) *Seminars in Psychiatric Genetics*. London: Gaskell.

Mednick, S. A. & Hollister, J. M. (eds) (1995) *Neural Development and Schizophrenia*. New York: Plenum Press.

Morton, N. E. (1974) Analysis of family resemblance. I. Introduction. *American Journal of Human Genetics*, **26**, 318–330.

Moser, H. W. (1995) A role for gene therapy in mental retardation. *Mental Retardation and Developmental Disabilities Research Reviews*, **1**, 4–6.

Nicholls, R. D. (1994) New insights reveal complex mechanisms involved in genomic imprinting. *American Journal of Human Genetics*, **54**, 733–740.

Nuffield Council on Bioethics (1993) *Genetic Screening: Ethical Issues*. London: Nuffield Foundation.

Owen, M. J. & McGuffin, P. (1993) Association and linkage: Complementary strategies for complex disorders. *Journal of Medical Genetics*, **30**, 638–639.

Pauls, D. L., Raymond, C. L., Stevenson, J. M., et al (1991) A family study of Gilles de la Tourette syndrome. *American Journal of Human Genetics*, **48**, 154–163.

___, Alsobrook, J. P., Goodman, W., et al (1995) A family study of obsessive–compulsive disorder. *American Journal of Psychiatry*, **152**, 76–84.

Patterson, G. R. (1982) *Coercive Family Process*. Eugene, OR: Castalia Publishing Company.

Pelosi, A. & David, A. (1989) Ethical implication of the new genetics for psychiatry. *International Review of Psychiatry*, **1**, 315–320.

Peltonen, L. (1995) Schizophrenia: All out for chromosome six. *Nature*, **378**, 665–666.

Petronis, A. & Kennedy, J. L. (1995) Unstable genes – unstable mind? *American Journal of Psychiatry*, **152**, 164–172.

Petursson, H. & Lader, M. (1984) *Dependence on Tranquillizers. Maudsley Monographs 28*. Oxford: Oxford University Press.

Plomin, R. (1986) *Development, Genetics, and Psychology*. Hillsdale, NJ: Erlbaum.

___ (1991) Genetic risk and psychosocial disorders: links between the normal and abnormal. In *Biological Risk Factors for Psychosocial Disorders* (eds M. Rutter & P. Casaer), pp. 101–138. Cambridge: Cambridge University Press.

___ (1994) *Genetics and Experience: The Interplay Between Nature and Nurture*. Thousand Oaks, CA: Sage.

___ & Daniels, D. (1987) Why are children in the same family so different from one another? *Behavioral and Brain Sciences*, **10**, 1–15.

___, Rende, R. & Rutter, M. (1991) Quantitative genetics and developmental psychopathology. In *Rochester Symposium on Developmental Psychopathology, Vol. 2: Internalizing and Externalizing Expressions of Dysfunction* (eds D. Cicchetti & S. Toth), pp 155–202. Hillsdale, NJ: Erlbaum.

___ & Bergeman, C. S. (1991) The nature of nurture: Genetic influences on "environmental" measures. *Behavioral and Brain Sciences*, **14**, 373–386.

___, Owen, M. J. & McGuffin, P. (1994) The genetic basis of complex human behaviours. *Science*, **264**, 1733–1739.

___, DeFries, J., McClearn, G. E., et al (1997) *Behavioral Genetics* (3rd edn). New York: W. H. Freeman.

___ & Rutter, M. (1997) Child development, molecular genetics and what do we do with genes once they are found. *Child Development*, in press.

Pokorski, R. J. (1995) Genetic information and life insurance. *Nature*, **376**, 13–14.

Reiss, D., Hetherington, M., Plomin, R., et al (1995) Genetic questions for environmental studies: Differential parenting and psychopathology in adolescence. *Archives of General Psychiatry*, **52**, 925–936.

Risch, N. & Merikangas, K. (1996) The future of genetic studies of complex human diseases. *Sciences*, **273**, 1516–1517.

Rose, S. (1995) The rise of neurogenetic determinism. *Nature*, **373**, 380–382.

Rutter, M. (1989) Psychiatric disorder in parents as a risk factor for children. In *Prevention of Mental Disorders, Alcohol and Other Drug Use in Children and Adolescents* (eds D. Shaffer, I. Philips & N. B. Enzer, et al), pp. 157–189. OSAP Prevention Monograph 2. Rockville, MD: Office for Substance Abuse Prevention, US Department of Health & Human Services.

___ (1994) Psychiatric genetics: Research challenges and pathways forward. *American Journal of Medical Genetics (Neuropsychiatric Genetics)*, **54**, 185–198.

___ (1997) Nature–nurture integration: The example of antisocial behavior. *American Psychologist*, **52**, 390–398.

___, Bolton, P., Harrington, R., et al (1990a) Genetic factors in child psychiatric disorders. I. A review of research strategies. *Journal of Child Psychology and Psychiatry*, **31**, 3–37.

___, Macdonald, H., Le Couteur, A., et al (1990b) Genetic factors in child psychiatric disorders. II. Empirical findings. *Journal of Child Psychology and Psychiatry*, **31**, 39–83.

___ & Rutter, M. (1993) *Developing Minds: Challenge and Continuity Across the Life Span*. Harmondsworth, Middlesex: Penguin; New York: Basic Books.

___, Champion, L., Quinton, D., et al (1995) Understanding individual differences in environmental risk exposure. In *Examining Lives in Context: Perspectives on the Ecology of Human Development* (eds P. Moen, G. H. Elder, Jr & K. Lüscher), pp. 61–93. Washington, DC: American Psychological Association.

___ & Smith, D. J. (eds) (1995) *Psychosocial Disorders in Young People: Time Trends and their Causes*. Chichester: Wiley.

___, Simonoff, E. & Plomin, R. (1996) Genetic influences on mild mental retardation: Concepts, findings and research implications. *Journal of Biosocial Science*, **28**, 509–526.

54

___ , **Bailey, A., Simonoff, E., et al (1997a)** Genetic influences and autism. In *Handbook of Autism* (eds F. Volkmar & D. Cohen), pp. 370–387. New York: Wiley.

___ , **Dunn, J., Plomin, R., et al (1997b)** Integrating nature and nurture: Implications of person–environment correlations and interactions for developmental psychopathology. *Development and Psychopathology,* in press.

___ , **Maughan, B., Meyer, J., et al (1997c)** Heterogeneity of antisocial behavior: Causes, continuities, and consequences. In *Nebraska Symposium on Motivation: Vol. 44: Motivation and Delinquency* (Series ed. R. Dienstbier & Vol. ed. D. W. Osgood). Lincoln, NE: University of Nebraska Press, in press.

Scarr, S. (1992) Developmental theories for the 1990s: Development and individual differences. *Child Development,* **63**, 1–19.

Schuler, G. D., Boguski, M. S., Stewart, E. A., et al (1996) A gene map of the human genome. *Science,* **274**, 540–546.

Sibilia, M. & Wagner, E. F. (1996) Transgenic animals. *European Review,* **4**, 371–392.

Silberg, J., Meyer, J., Pickles, A., et al (1996a) Heterogeneity among juvenile antisocial behaviours: findings from the VTSABD. In *Genetics of Criminal and Antisocial Behaviour. Ciba Symposium No. 194* (eds G. Bock & J. Goode), pp. 76–86. Chichester: Wiley.

___ , **Rutter, M., Meyer, J., et al (1996b)** Genetic and environmental influences on the covariation between hyperactivity and conduct disturbance in juvenile twins. *Journal of Child Psychology and Psychiatry,* **37**, 803–816.

Simonoff, E., Bolton, P. & Rutter, M. (1996) Mental retardation: Genetic findings, clinical implications and research agenda. *Journal of Child Psychology and Psychiatry,* **37**, 259–280.

___ **& Rutter, M. (1996)** Autism and other behavioral disorders. In *Emery and Rimoin's Principles and Practice of Medical Genetics* (3rd edn) (eds D. L. Rimoin, J. M. Connor, R. E. Pyeritz, et al), pp. 1791–1806. New York: Churchill Livingstone.

Taylor, E. (1994) Syndromes of attention deficit and overactivity. In *Child and Adolescent Psychiatry: Modern Approaches* (3rd edn) (eds M. Rutter, E. Taylor & L. Hersov), pp. 285–307. Oxford: Blackwell.

Thapar, A. & McGuffin, P. (1994) A twin study of depressive symptoms in childhood. *British Journal of Psychiatry,* **165**, 259–265.

Tienari, P., Wynne, L. C., Moring, J., et al (1994) The Finnish adoptive family study of schizophrenia: Implications for family research. *British Journal of Psychiatry,* **164** (suppl. 23), 20–26.

Tizard, J. (1975) Race and IQ: The limits of probability. *New Behaviour,* **1**, 6–9.

Weber, M. W. (1996) Ernst Rudin, 1874–1952: a German psychiatric geneticist. *American Journal of Medical Genetics,* **67**, 323–331.

Wyatt, R. J. (1996) Commentary: Neurodevelopmental abnormalities and schizophrenia: A family affair. *Archives of General Psychiatry,* **53**, 11–14.

MICHAEL RUTTER, FRCPsych, MRC Child Psychiatry Unit and Social, Genetic and Developmental Psychiatry Research Centre; ROBERT PLOMIN, Social, Genetic and Developmental Psychiatry Research Centre

Correspondence: Professor Sir Michael Rutter, Institute of Psychiatry, Denmark Hill, London SE5 8AF

(First received 9 January 1997, final revision 14 April 1997, accepted 16 April 1997)

■55

Part III
Assessment

Journal of Child Psychology and Psychiatry, 1965, vol. 6, pp. 71–83

CLASSIFICATION AND CATEGORIZATION IN CHILD PSYCHIATRY*

MICHAEL RUTTER

Institute of Psychiatry, Maudsley Hospital, London

■59

INTRODUCTION

A GENERALLY acceptable classification of psychiatric disorders which occur in childhood is urgently needed and the lack of such a classification has been a severe obstacle to progress in child psychiatry. A classification is a kind of language which facilitates communication between different professional workers. In its absence communication is likely to be beset with misunderstandings and misinterpretations; the comparison of psychiatric observations and the interchange of ideas will be seriously hampered. Without a common terminology and ordering of material, studies at different clinical or research centres cannot be compared one with the other. Until a disorder can be identified and characterized it cannot be adequately studied. This means that we cannot wait for more information to become available before we develop a classification. Indeed, if we do wait, such information is not likely to be forthcoming.

The classification of adult mental disorders is unsatisfactory (Stengel, 1959) but the situation in child psychiatry is worse. Child psychiatry is still a relatively new discipline without the accumulated knowledge necessary for a classification which will stand the test of time. However, that in no way lessens the need for a tentative classification as a beginning. From this better schemes can be developed as further knowledge becomes available.

The increasing recognition of this need is reflected in the recent publication by the American Psychiatric Association of a report on "Diagnostic Classification in Child Psychiatry" (Jenkins and Cole, 1964). This includes a classification derived from the deliberations of the Group for the Advancement of Psychiatry (Langford, 1964), which constitutes a decided improvement over most previous schemes. Unfortunately, it is, to some extent, still based on a mixture of phenomenology and theoretical assumptions. It also contains some bewildering contradictions—such as 'anxious personality' as the first subcategory of 'personality disorders . . . with minimal subjective anxiety'. However, what is important are not the details of the scheme but rather the evidence that it provides of a developing concern with the issues of classification.

There are several reasons why child psychiatrists have failed to agree on a common classification. Some have felt that there is little point in distinguishing between different conditions (Szurek, 1956) or that classification tends to obscure

*Lecture given as part of the Course of Child Psychiatry, Central University of Venezuela, Caracas, Venezuela, in March, 1965.

Accepted manuscript received 2 June 1965.

individual differences and prevent a more penetrating understanding of disorders (Huschka, 1941). Of course, it is very important to consider each patient as a unique individual with his own particular attributes and life history. But, it is also necessary to consider those characteristics which he shares with others, and it would be a retrograde step to regard every patient as *entirely* individual (Kanner, 1959). A diagnostic classification should be able to convey important and relevant information about the patient, but one should not expect it to say all that is relevant or important. Classification is not the same as a diagnostic formulation. An adequate formulation should include statements about the type of disorder, the manner of its development, its aetiology, prognosis, and likely response to treatment, but clearly all this cannot be encompassed in a classification which has only the more modest aim of ordering the material in such a way that it can be communicated to others.

Some workers have tried to base classification on a theoretical framework such as psychoanalysis; Anna Freud has produced a diagnostic categorization based on the child's libidinal development (Freud, 1962). Other theories have led to other classifications. For example, Eysenck (Eysenck, 1960, Eysenck and Rachman, 1965), on the basis of learning theory, has attempted to classify disorders in terms of personality variables such as neuroticism or extraversion. In support of his classification he has cited factor analytic studies of symptoms. However, there is no satisfactory evidence to suggest that the symptom clusters are measures of enduring aspects of personality rather than measures of a temporary disorder of behaviour which may have little relationship to the child's temperament. Furthermore, at the moment, the theoretical construct used lacks experimental support as far as children are concerned and it is not generally accepted. A theoretical basis for classification is certainly desirable, but as yet no theory has gained sufficient general support for it to be used as the basis of a diagnostic scheme. Alternative approaches must be taken.

Other psychiatrists, such as the late Dr. Kenneth Cameron, have produced ways of categorizing children according to their symptomatology (Cameron, 1955 and 1958). His scheme allowed a ready description of the child's disorder, and this marked an advance. However, this grouping of disorders was not based on any known relationship between symptoms, and although the scheme categorized various aspects of the child and his disturbance, it did not provide any overall classification of the disorder.

If we accept that it is imperative to have a classification we must search for information about disorders in childhood from which a classification can be derived, and that is my purpose in this paper. The present aim is to discuss some of the research findings upon which an acceptable classification might be based, and not to provide such a classification.

The principles of classification have been clearly outlined by Hempel (1961) and the advantages and disadvantages of different approaches were fully discussed by Jaspers (1962) in his classical text. The factors which could provide the structure for an ideal diagnostic scheme are undecided and are a function of the purposes for which the classification will be employed (Rutter, 1963). Two points must be made clear at the outset. Firstly, there is no 'natural' scheme, and secondly, classification in no way implies the existence of disease entities (Jaspers, 1962). Continua of personality characteristics or tempo of maturation may be classified just as 'illnesses' are. The child is a developing organism and it is essential that the classification take this into account. Maturation sometimes causes the same abnormality to manifest itself in different ways at different ages. For example, children who are severely *over*active at age 7 years are often *under*active at 17 years (Rutter, 1965). An additional problem is that what is abnormal at one age may be normal at another (e.g. enuresis).

Although aetiology is probably an indispensable part of any adequate diagnostic scheme it is unlikely to be sufficient in itself. For example, a classification of fractures based only on the causative agent would have failed to encompass the crucial distinctions between injuries where there is disruption of the skin, or trauma to internal organs, and those where there is not. It is also certain that disorders can be defined before the aetiology is known. John Snow made his classical study of cholera well before the cholera vibrio had been discovered. Indeed, one might go farther and say that advances in our knowledge about aetiology are likely to be slow until we can identify and classify disorders. A further problem with a purely aetiological classification is that the same agent may lead to very different outcomes (e.g. tertiary syphilis). In our present state of knowledge it is likely that any classification will have to be largely based on behavioural manifestations, but it should be noted that the same clinical picture may be due to many different aetiological factors (e.g. dementia).

■ 61

Finally, before proceeding to a survey of relevant research findings three principles must be stated:

1. If the classification is to be acceptable it must be based on facts not concepts, and it must be defined in operational terms.
2. If it is to be useful it must convey information relevant to the clinical situation and it must have predictive value.
3. The aim is to classify disorders, *not* to classify children. Just as children may have measles one year and scarlet fever the next, equally it is possible that children may have one kind of psychiatric disorder at 5 years and another at 12 years.

SYMPTOM CLUSTERS

Of all the diagnostic distinctions made in child psychiatry, perhaps the most universal has been between 'conduct problems' by which is meant antisocial or aggressive behaviour, and 'personality problems' which refer to emotional or neurotic disorders (e.g. Ackerson, 1931 and 1942; Becker *et al.*, 1962; Paynter and Blanchard, 1929; Peterson, 1960 and 1961). The terms are somewhat unfortunate in that there is no good reason to suppose that neurosis is much more closely related to personality than is antisocial behaviour (Kanner, 1957). Nevertheless, although the terms may be somewhat misleading the distinction between neurotic disorders and antisocial disorders has appeared in nearly all symptom cluster or factor analytic studies (Peterson, 1961; Collins *et al.*, 1962; Eysenck and Rachman, 1965), and it has been argued that if symptoms tend to correlate or 'go together' they should be classified together. The distinction has been shown to be important in relation to delinquency (Mulligan *et al.*, 1963). Whereas delinquent boys have a strikingly high rate of aggressive symptoms, they do not differ from the normal population in terms of neurotic type maladjustment.

Diagnostic groupings based on symptom cluster studies have also been shown to be important in relation to the family background. On the basis of intercorrelations between symptoms, Hewitt and Jenkins (1946) distinguished three types of disorder:

1. 'over-inhibited behaviour' (a neurotic type disorder);
2. 'socialized delinquency', where the child stole and truanted but was on good terms with his peers, and
3. 'unsocialized aggressive behaviour'.

Unsocialized aggression was found to be associated with parental rejection, socialized delinquency with neglect and bad company, and neurotic behaviour with parental repression and constraint. These relationships were confirmed in a subsequent and separate study by Lewis (1954).

Unfortunately there are one or two drawbacks associated with the Hewitt and Jenkins classification. Habit disorders were excluded so that this group was not studied. Even so, many children still did not fall into any of the three categories. Further, the criteria for 'unsocialized aggressive behaviour' and 'socialized delinquency' were somewhat changed in the replication study (Jenkins and Glickman, 1946) so that the differentiation between the two antisocial categories is slightly dubious. However, the clear distinction between neurotic disorders and antisocial disorders remains.

RESPONSE TO TREATMENT

The same distinction appears in studies of the short-term response to treatment. Eisenberg and his colleagues found that 2 out of 3 children with neurotic symptoms improved significantly following a brief course of supportive psychotherapy, in comparison with a much smaller proportion of hyperkinetic or antisocial children (Cytryn *et al.*, 1960; Eisenberg *et al.*, 1961). Thus, children with antisocial and neurotic disorders were again distinguished, but in addition a hyperkinetic group was also separated from neurotic disorders. Amphetamine sulphate sometimes produces a remarkable tranquillizing effect on hyperkinetic children (Bradley and Bowen, 1941; Eisenberg, 1964). It is likely that this too is a feature which distinguishes hyperkinetic from neurotic or antisocial disorders, but reliable comparisons have not been made.

Child psychosis is differentiated from all other psychiatric disorders by its much worse response to treatment.

LONG-TERM PROGNOSIS

The long-term prognosis is also relevant to problems of classification. Neurotic disorders usually carry a good prognosis, whereas children with aggressive antisocial disorders do much less well with a significant proportion continuing as delinquents or becoming schizophrenic (Morris *et al.*, 1954; Morris *et al.*, 1956). The most comprehensive long-term follow-up study was carried out by O'Neal and Robins (1958 and 1960). They examined several hundred adults who had attended child guidance clinics in the United States some 30 to 35 years earlier. They also examined a smaller number of adults who, as far as was known, had presented no problems of behaviour in childhood. On the basis of the original clinic records the patients were divided into 3 groups: (1) neurotic children, (2) delinquents and (3) antisocial children who had not come before the Courts. These three 'abnormal' groups were compared with the fourth 'control' group, those who had not had any psychiatric disorder in childhood. Approximately 3 out of 5 control subjects were considered psychiatrically normal as adults as against 2 out of 5 neurotic children, 1 out of 3 antisocial and 1 in 4 delinquent children. In the main, delinquent children became criminal or sociopathic adults with a high rate of social and marital difficulties (over half were divorced). The antisocial children who had not been before the Courts at the time they attended the child guidance clinic, also included an excess of criminal and sociopathic adults, but the proportion was less than for the delinquent children. More striking was the fact that 1 in 5 had become psychotic, although few of these had received psychiatric care. The outcome for the neurotic children was similar to that for the controls except that there was a slightly higher proportion of adults who had been neurotic as children in each of the abnormal categories. However, it was particularly noteworthy that the proportion of adult neurotics was quite similar for those who were neurotic and for those who were normal as children. Thus, again children with neurotic and antisocial disorders were clearly distinguished. In addition, there appeared to be a sub-group of antisocial children who developed into schizophrenic adults. However, it should be noted that schizophrenia tends to include a wider range of disorders in the U.S.A. than it does in England, and the authors have not yet published details of the kind of abnormalities shown by those adults who were antisocial in childhood.

A slightly different approach to the same general problem has been followed by Pritchard and Graham (1965). They compared, within a group of patients who had attended the Maudsley Hospital both as children and as adults, the type of disorder present on the two occasions. They found that the majority of the neurotic children had become neurotic adults, and the majority of delinquent children presented with some form of antisocial or psychopathic behaviour in adult life. Nevertheless, there was some overlap in that a number of antisocial children developed depressive or neurotic reactions in later life. Also, in contrast to the O'Neal and Robins study very few antisocial children developed schizophrenia. This finding may reflect diagnostic differences between Great Britain and the United States. By definition, all the children had psychiatric disorder as adults, so that no conclusion can be drawn concerning the incidence of adult mental illness among people who have attended child guidance clinics. However, what is clearly shown is that *if* the children develop psychiatric disorder in adult life it is usually (but not always) of a type similar to that which they exhibited as children. Again, the distinction between neurotic and antisocial disorders appears.

Child psychosis is also very clearly distinguished from other disorders by the long-term prognosis. With our present treatment facilities very few psychotic children recover, a larger number achieve some kind of social adjustment but nearly half remain in a long-stay institution (Eisenberg, 1957; Rutter, 1965). About 2 out of 5 fail to gain any useful speech and those whose speech does improve are often left with abnormalities of articulation. A further differentiating feature is that a proportion, 1 in 6 in one study (Rutter, 1965), develop epileptic fits—usually in early adolescence. Of all the psychiatric disorders of childhood, psychosis is the most clearly differentiated from all others by long-term outcome. The course of child

■63

Journal of Child Psychology and Psychiatry, 1965, vol. 6, pp. 71–83

psychosis which develops in early childhood is also very different from the adult-type schizophrenia which begins in adolescence (Rutter, 1965).

AETIOLOGY

We are still far from the situation where specific disorders can be related to specific aetiological factors. Most research has emphasized the very diverse consequences of factors harmful to the child's behavioural development. The stereotypes of the 'brain damaged' child, and of 'affectionless psychopathy' as the usual end-result of prolonged maternal deprivation have had to be abandoned (cf. Bowlby *et al.*, 1956; Birch, 1964).

Nevertheless, aetiological studies have provided some data which are relevant for classification. The association between parental variables and the type of disorder shown by the children, which was found in the Hewitt and Jenkins (1946) study, has already been mentioned. Disruption of the home by death, divorce or separation of the parents is sometimes associated with the development of psychiatric disorder in the children. Most studies have shown that when this occurs the child usually develops an antisocial disorder rather than a neurotic disorder (Wardle, 1961).

There are no behavioural disorders which are invariably associated with cerebral dysfunction or 'brain damage', but two—child psychosis and the hyperkinetic syndrome—are distinguished from other psychiatric disorders in childhood by the high frequency of their association with neurological abnormality. About 1 in 2 psychotic children have evidence of cerebral dysfunction, although the evidence does not always appear until late childhood. Sometimes the dysfunction is shown by the development of epileptic fits in early adolescence (Rutter, 1965).

The situation with regard to the hyperkinetic syndrome is somewhat similar. However, there are the added difficulties that overactivity is found in many disorders and that a high level of activity is normal in young children. Some psychiatrists refer to any disorder with overactivity as 'hyperkinetic', but what is meant here is a syndrome characterized by *severe* and disorganized overactivity together with impulsiveness and a very short attention span and often extreme distractibility. Aggressive behaviour is also frequently part of the clinical picture. This kind of disorder is often associated with epilepsy or other evidence of neurological abnormality (Ingram, 1956). Differences in the photo-metrazol threshold have been described (Laufer *et al.*, 1957) and abnormalities in intellectual functioning are common (Eisenberg, 1964). It seems very likely that brain dysfunction or damage is an important aetiological factor in many, if not most, cases of hyperkinetic disorder. However, it has been argued that the symptoms are merely those appropriate to the child's mental age and are thus related not to brain damage, but to low intelligence (Pond, 1965). This argument has force in that in most hyperkinetic children the intelligence level is rather low, but there are two main objections to it. In the first place, children of normal or even above normal intelligence can have a hyperkinetic disorder at an age when overactivity is clearly inappropriate for the mental or chronological age. In the second place, among subnormal children, hyperkinesis is usually found in those who have evidence of brain damage as well, *not* among those without such evidence (Rutter and Graham, 1965).

To summarize so far, symptom clusters separate neurotic and antisocial disorders. The two groups also differ somewhat in aetiology, and both can be distinguished from child psychosis and the hyperkinetic syndrome in which brain damage is frequently an important causal factor. Response to treatment also differentiates these four groups. The hyperkinetic syndrome and child psychosis are dissimilar not only in symptomatology but also in long-term course, child psychosis carrying the worse prognosis.

EPIDEMIOLOGY

Findings important for classification purposes also come from epidemiological studies. All investigations have shown the very high prevalence of individual symptoms such as fears, temper tantrums and enuresis (Mensch *et al.*, 1959; Lapouse and Monk, 1958) so that psychiatric abnormality should not be inferred on the basis of single items of behaviour.

Perhaps the most important result of these investigations has been the finding that several items of behaviour which have been thought to be indicators of maladjustment, are not. Developmental conditions such as enuresis or speech disorder have been found to have no significant association with psychiatric disorder (Mensch *et al.*, 1959; Tapia *et al.*, 1960). No significant relationships were found between enuresis and an overall measure of maladjustment nor between enuresis and any other symptom. Similarly thumb-sucking and fears were also unrelated to maladjustment. Among children attending a psychiatric clinic these symptoms are often part of a general disorder but this is a function of the biased sample of children that we see at clinics. These epidemiological findings suggest that certain developmental disorders such as enuresis and speech disorders, when they occur in isolation, should be classified separately from neurotic, antisocial and other disorders.

AGE AND SEX TRENDS

Different kinds of disorders present at different age-periods in childhood (Macfarlane *et al.*, 1954; Grant, 1958). The existence of large differences in prevalence and in age-trends suggest the need for differences in classification. Developmental disorders such as enuresis, speech disorders, and sleep disturbances are characteristic of early childhood. They become increasingly rare among older children, with the main decline in frequency occurring before the age of 6 years. In contrast, delinquency and sexual abnormalities are much more characteristic of later childhood and adolescence. Overt neurotic disorders are also much commoner among elder children. On the other hand, tearfulness and jealousy are disorders of young children, while shyness and fears are at their peak in middle childhood.

Nearly all psychiatric disorders are considerably more common among boys than girls (Ullman, 1952; Lapouse and Monk, 1958). The main exceptions to this general sex-difference are timidity and fears, which occur with about the same frequency in the sexes or are slightly commoner among girls (Lapouse and Monk, 1959).

Of the age and sex differences the most important for purposes of classification is the age trend for developmental disorders (i.e. a decrease with increasing age) which stands in sharp contrast to the increasing incidence with age of many other disorders, especially neurosis and delinquency.

65

Journal of Child Psychology and Psychiatry, 1965, vol. 6, pp. 71–83

MENTAL SUBNORMALITY AND EDUCATIONAL RETARDATION

Two large groups of disorders have not yet been mentioned—mental subnormality and educational retardation. Both are very important conditions for the child psychiatrist but attention in this paper has been confined to behavioural disorders. Mental subnormality is not a single condition but rather a heterogeneous group of conditions. The chief distinction, in terms of the approaches considered, between mental subnormality and disorders of behaviour is the importance of both specific and general abnormalities of the brain in the aetiology of subnormality, especially severe subnormality (Kirman, 1965). Mental subnormality may be associated with any of the psychiatric disorders already considered.

Educational retardation is also an admixture of different disorders. Even 'specific' varieties of retardation such as reading disability form a very heterogeneous group. Retardation may be genetically determined, it may be associated with various perceptual defects, it may follow injury to the brain, it may form part of a psychiatric disorder, or be the result of cultural or educational deprivation, or other unknown factors (Money, 1962). Thus, many neurotic and delinquent children are significantly retarded in their educational progress but also it is probable that most educationally retarded children do not have any psychiatric disorder. The classification of varieties of educational retardation is still very unsatisfactory but it is clear that there is a sizeable group of children who are backward in their schooling but who are not neurotic, delinquent, or intellectually subnormal (Money, 1962). The size of this group is unknown but it should be distinguished from mental subnormality and from other psychiatric disorders.

SEVERITY AND DURATION OF DISORDERS

The severity and duration of disorders have been little explored in relation to prognosis or response to treatment, but clearly severity is a necessary parameter in any classification. Its utility has been most evident with respect to mental subnormality, where the distinction between an I.Q. below 50 and one above this point is of proven value (Penrose, 1949; Tizard, 1965). 'Organic' pathology of the brain is much more important in the aetiology when the subnormality is severe, and the distinction is also of considerable predictive value in terms of response to training, education, and employment. It is scarcely necessary to add that although in this connection an I.Q. score of about 50 is a most useful cut-off point on the continuum of measured intelligence, it is an arbitrary point on a continuum and distinctions in the area immediately around whatever cut-off point is used are necessarily weak.

The level of intelligence is also of predictive value in relation to child psychosis, both in terms of social adjustment in adult life and in terms of speech development (Rutter, 1965). Again an I.Q. score of about 50 seems the most useful place to draw the line—the prognosis is much better for children with measured abilities above this level. Of course, in part, this may be a function of currently available services which are usually much better for the more able child who can be retained within the school system. Another measure of 'severity'—the presence of useful speech at the age of 5 years has also been found to have predictive value (Eisenberg, 1957), although this may be partly due to the positive correlation between I.Q. and speech development (Rutter, 1965).

Fish has developed a typology of child psychiatric disorders in which 'severity of integrative defect' forms the major variable. Preliminary findings suggest that this may have value in the prediction of responses to drug treatment (Fish and Shapiro, 1964).

Every clinician distinguishes between mild neurotic, antisocial or other disorders which are only a little outside the limits of normality, and more serious disorders of rather similar symptomatology but a worse prognosis. The milder conditions have sometimes been classified under terms such as 'situational reactions' or 'reactive disorders'. However, even the severest disorders may have developed in response to environmental stresses and, conversely, mild disorders may be associated as much with factors in the child as with the environmental situation (Rutter *et al.*, 1964). The American Group for the Advancement of Psychiatry laid emphasis on the absence of 'internalized conflict' to define the milder disorders (Langford, 1964) but this presupposes an acceptance of a particular theoretical framework and thus violates the first principle suggested earlier, namely, that to be acceptable a classification must be based on observable behavioural signs, not concepts.

■67

Studies utilizing behavioural questionnaires (Mensch *et al.*, 1959; Mulligan, 1964) have shown that the number of symptoms gives some measure of severity, but it is a crude and not altogether satisfactory measure. Duration of symptoms has been shown to be important (Mulligan, 1964) and clinical experience suggests that, especially in the older child, it is necessary to take personality characteristics into account.

Enough is known to suggest that severity and/or duration of disorder should form one parameter in any adequate diagnostic classification but it is not yet clear what is the best way of measuring severity.

CONCLUSIONS

In summary, symptom cluster and factor analytic studies, investigations of treatment, of long-term prognosis, and of aetiology, epidemiological studies, and investigations of age and sex trends in behavioural development, have all produced findings which are relevant to the production of a classification of child psychiatric disorders. A few studies of each kind have been briefly considered.

Although I am not putting forward a detailed or complete classification, I would like to try to draw together the main findings in the form of an outline which might form the basis for such a classification.

1. *Neurotic disorders* can be differentiated in terms of symptom clusters, response to treatment, long-term prognosis, family background and aetiology from the other large group—that of:

2. *Antisocial or conduct disorders*. The differentiation between these two groups appears so often that it seems very likely that the distinction is of fundamental importance. It should be emphasized that the differentiation occurs when overt behaviour is considered. Delinquency may occasionally be secondary to a frank neurotic disorder and it may sometimes have a neurotic basis in terms of unconscious conflict (Glover, 1960), but the findings strongly suggest an important dichotomy between neurotic and antisocial disorders. Although most children present with a preponderantly neurotic or preponderantly antisocial clinical picture there is an overlap which necessitates a

Journal of Child Psychology and Psychiatry, 1965, vol. 6, pp. 71–83

3. *Mixed group* in which neither neurotic nor antisocial symptoms predominate.

4. *Developmental disorders* such as enuresis or speech abnormalities (sometimes called habit disorders) can be differentiated in terms of epidemiological findings and age-trends. These disorders may be part of a neurotic or antisocial disturbance, but when they occur in isolation they should be classified separately. It should be noted that this category is itself rather heterogeneous and in need of further subdivision.

5. *The hyperkinetic syndrome* can be distinguished in terms of response to treatment and its association with neurological abnormality.

6. *Child psychosis*, with an onset before pubescence, stands out as different from other psychiatric disorders by its response to treatment, long-term course, and its association with cerebral dysfunction. Psychosis has some similarities to the hyperkinetic syndrome, but, apart from differences in symptomatology, the long-term outcome differentiates the two conditions. It is also different from

7. *Psychosis developing at or after puberty* which is similar to schizophrenia as it occurs in adult life. In addition

8. *Mental subnormality* and

9. *Educational retardation as a primary problem* should be distinguished. Both categories require further subdivision. To what extent it is justifiable to separate

10. *Depression* and

11. *Adult-type neurotic illnesses* from the neurotic behaviour disorders remains uncertain. They are rather different in their phenomenology and the age at which they occur but the differences in long-term course remain largely unexplored.

This outline of a classification is purely phenomenological and operational definitions could easily be provided for each of the groups. Accordingly it would be relatively simple to apply to the individual case. However, it is probable that most of the categories require further subdivision and the scheme is no more than a basis for a classification which is likely to be superseded as further information becomes available. What value it has now lies in its utility as a means of communication and of ordering material. The groupings convey information about the type of disorder, its prognosis and the factors which may have been important in its development. This is likely to be useful in planning treatment although there is no direct and invariable relationship between diagnosis and the type of therapy. The most scientific interest is likely to be found in discrepancies in the classification which may form the basis for posing further clinical and research questions (Jaspers, 1962), which should themselves lead to better classifications.

SUMMARY

The need for a classification of child psychiatric disorders is emphasized and the principles of classification are briefly discussed. Research findings concerning symptom clusters, response to treatment, long-term prognosis, aetiology, epidemiology, age and sex trends, and severity and duration of disorders are reviewed in relation to their implications for classification. An outline for a possible classification is suggested.

REFERENCES

ACKERSON, L. (1931) *Children's Behaviour Problems*, Vol. 1. University Press, Chicago.

ACKERSON, L. (1942) *Children's Behaviour Problems*, Vol. 2. University Press, Chicago.

BECKER, W. C., PETERSON, D. B., LURIA, Z., SHOEMAKER, D. J., HELLMER, L. A. (1962) Relations of factors derived from parent interview ratings to behaviour problems of five-year-olds. *Child Dev.* **33**, 509-536.

BIRCH, H. G. (1964) (Ed.) *Brain Damage in Children: the biological and social aspects*. Williams and Wilkins, Baltimore.

BOWLBY, J., AINSWORTH, M., BOSTON, B., ROSENBLUTH, D. (1956) The effects of mother-child separation: a follow-up study. *Br. J. med. Psychol.* **29**, 211–249.

BRADLEY, C. and BOWEN, M. (1941) Amphetamine (Benzedrine) therapy of children's behaviour disorders. *Am. J. Orthopsychiat.* **11**, 92–103.

CAMERON, K. (1955) Diagnostic categories in child psychiatry. *Br. J. med. Psychol.* **28**, 67–71.

CAMERON, K. (1958) Symptom classification in child psychiatry. *Revue Psychiat. Infantile* **25**, 241–245.

COLLINS, L. F., MAXWELL, A. E., CAMERON, C. (1962) A factor analysis of some child psychiatric clinic data. *J. ment. Sci.* **108**, 274–285.

CYTRYN, L., GILBERT, A. EISENBERG, L. (1960) The effectiveness of tranquillizing drugs plus supportive psychotherapy in treating behaviour disorders of children. *Am. J. Orthopsychiat.* **30**, 113–129.

EISENBERG, L. (1957) The course of childhood schizophrenia. *Archs Neurol. Psychiat., Lond.* **78**, 69–83.

EISENBERG, L., GILBERT, A., CYTRYN, L., MOLLING, P. A. (1961) Effectiveness of psychotherapy alone and in conjunction with perphenazine and placebo. *Am. J. Psychiat.* **117**, 1088–1093.

EISENBERG, L. (1964) Behavioural manifestations of cerebral damage in childhood. *Brain Damage in Children: the biological and social aspects*, Birch, H. G. (Ed.). Williams and Wilkins, Baltimore.

EYSENCK, H. J. (1960) Classification and problem of diagnosis. *Handbook of Abnormal Psychology*, Eysenck, H. J. (Ed.). Pitman Medical, London.

EYSENCK, H. J. and RACHMAN, S. J. (1965) The application of learning theory to child psychiatry. *Modern Perspectives in Child Psychiatry*, Howells, J. G. (Ed.). Oliver and Boyd, Edinburgh.

FISH, B. and SHAPIRO, T. (1964) A descriptive typology of children's psychiatric disorders: II, A behavioural classification. Diagnostic Classification in Child Psychiatry, Jenkins, R. L. and Cole, J. O. (Eds.). *Am. Psychiat. Ass. Psychiat. Res. Rep. No.* 18.

FREUD, A. (1962) Assessment of child disturbances. *Psychoanal. Study Child* **17**, 149–158.

GLOVER, E. (1960) *The Roots of Crime*. Imago, London.

GRANT, Q. A. F. R. (1958) D.P.M. Dissertation, Univ. London. *Age and Sex Trends in the Symptomatology of Disturbed Children*.

HEMPEL, C. G. (1961) Some problems of taxonomy. *Field Studies in the Mental Disorders*, Zubin, J. (Ed.). Grune and Stratton, N.Y. and London.

HEWITT, L. E. and JENKINS, R. L. (1946) *Fundamental Patterns of Maladjustment—The Dynamics of their Origin*. Michigan Child Guidance Institute, Illinois.

HUSCHKA, M. (1941) Psychopathological disorders in the mother. *J. nerv. ment. Dis.* **94**, 76–83.

INGRAM, T. T. S. (1956) A characteristic form of overactive behaviour in brain damaged children. *J. ment. Sci.* **102**, 550–558.

JASPERS, K. (1962) *General Psychopathology*. Trans. Hoenig, J. and Hamilton, M. W. Manchester Univ. Press.

JENKINS, R. L. and GLICKMAN, S. (1946) Common syndromes in child psychiatry: I. Deviant behaviour traits. II. The schizoid child. *Am. J. Orthopsychiat.* **16**, 244–261.

JENKINS, R. L. and COLE, J. O. (Eds.) Diagnostic classification in child psychiatry. *Am. Psychiat. Ass. Psychiat. Res. Rep. No.* 18.

KANNER, L. (1957) *Child Psychiatry*. Charles C. Thomas, Springfield, Illinois.

KANNER, L. (1959) The thirty-third Maudsley lecture: Trends in Child Psychiatry. *J. ment. Sci.* **105**, 581–593.

KIRMAN, B. (1965) The Aetiology of Mental Subnormality. *Modern Perspectives in Child Psychiatry*, Howells, J. G. (Ed.). Oliver and Boyd, Edinburgh.

LANGFORD, W. S. (1964) Reflections on classification in child psychiatry as related to the activities of the committee on Child Psychiatry of the Group for the Advancement of Psychiatry. Diagnostic

69

Journal of Child Psychology and Psychiatry, 1965, vol. 6, pp. 71–83

Classification in Child Psychiatry. Jenkins, R. L. and Cole, J. O. (Eds.) *Am. Psychiat. Ass. Psychiat. Res. Rep. No.* 18.

LAPOUSE, R. and MONK, M. A. (1958) An epidemiologic study of behaviour characteristics in children. *Am. J. publ. Hlth* **48**, 1134–1144.

LAPOUSE, R. and MONK, M. A. (1959) Fears and worries in a representative sample of children. *Am. J. Orthopsychiat.* **29**, 803–818.

LAUFER, M. W., DENHOFF, E., SOLOMONS, G. (1957) Hyperkinetic impulse disorder in children's behaviour problems. *Psychosom. Med.* **19**, 38–49.

LEWIS, H. (1954) *Deprived Children*. Oxford Univ. Press, London.

MACFARLANE, J. W. *et al.* (1954) *A Developmental Study of the Behaviour Problems of Normal Children between 2½ and 14 Years*. Univ. California Press.

MENSCH, I. N., KANTOR, M. B., DOMKE, H. R., GILDEA, M. C.-L. and GLIDEWELL, J. G. (1959) Children's behaviour symptoms and their relationships to school adjustment, sex and social class. *J. Social Issues* **15**, 8–15.

MONEY, J. (1962) (Ed.) *Reading Disability: Progress and Research Needs in Dyslexia*. The Johns Hopkins Press, Baltimore.

MORRIS, D. P., SOROKER, E. and BURRUSS, G. (1954) Follow-up studies of shy, withdrawn children —I. Evaluation of later adjustment. *Am. J. Orthopsychiat.* **24**, 743–754.

MORRIS, H. H., ESCOLL, P. J. and WEXLER, R. (1956) Aggressive behaviour disorders of childhood— a follow-up study. *Am. J. Psychiat.* **112**, 991–997.

MULLIGAN, G. (1964) *Some Correlates of Maladjustment in a National Sample of School Children*. Unpublished Ph.D. Thesis, London Univ.

MULLIGAN, G., DOUGLAS, J. W. B., HAMMOND, W. A., TIZARD, J. (1963) Delinquency and symptoms of maladjustment: the findings of a longitudinal study. *Proc. R. Soc. Med.* **56**, 29–32.

O'NEAL, P. and ROBINS, L. N. (1958) The relation of childhood behaviour problems to adult psychiatric status: a 30 year follow-up study of 150 subjects. *Am. J. Psychiat.* **114**, 961–969.

O'NEAL, P., BERGMAN, J., SCHAFER, J. and ROBINS, L. N. (1960) The relation of childhood behaviour problems to adult psychiatric status: a 30 year follow-up study of 262 subjects. *Scientific Papers and Discussions—Am. Psychiat. Ass. District Branches Publication*, pp. 99–117.

PAYNTER, R. H. and BLANCHARD, P. (1929) *Educational Achievement of Problem Children*. The Commonwealth Fund, New York.

PENROSE, L. S. (1949) *The Biology of Mental Defect*. Sidgwick and Jackson, London.

PETERSON, D. R. (1960) The age generality of personality factors derived from ratings. *Educ. psychol. Measur.* **20**, 461–474.

PETERSON, D. R. (1961) Behaviour problems of middle childhood. *J. consult. Psychol.* **25**, 205–209.

POND, D. A. (1965) The neuropsychiatry of childhood. *Modern Perspectives in Child Psychiatry*, Howells, J. G. (Ed.). Oliver and Boyd, Edinburgh.

PRITCHARD, M. and GRAHAM, P. (1965) Personal communication.

RUTTER, M. (1963) Some current research issues in American child psychiatry. *Milbank meml Fund q. Bull.* **41**, 339–370.

RUTTER, M. (1965) In preparation.

RUTTER, M. (1965) The influences of organic and emotional factors in the origins, nature and outcome of childhood psychosis. *Dev. med. Child Neurol.* (in press).

RUTTER, M., BIRCH, H. G., THOMAS, A. and CHESS, S. (1964) Temperamental characteristics in infancy and the later development of behavioural disorders. *Br. J. Psychiat.* **110**, 651.

RUTTER, M. and GRAHAM, P. (1965) In preparation.

STENGEL, E. (1959) Classification of mental disorders. *Bull. Wld Hlth Org.* **21**, 601–663.

SZUREK, S. A. (1956) Psychotic episodes and psychotic maldevelopment. *Am. J. Orthopsychiat.* **26**, 519–543.

TAPIA, F., JEKEL, J. and DOMKE, H. (1960) Enuresis: an emotional symptom? *J. nerv. ment. Dis.* **130**, 61–66.

TIZARD, J. (1965) Mental subnormality and child psychiatry. Submitted to *J. Child Psychol. Psychiat.*

ULLMAN, C. A. (1952) Identification of Maladjusted School Children. *Publ. Hlth Monogr No. 7.*
WARDLE, C. J. (1961) Two generations of broken homes in the genesis of conduct and behaviour disorders in childhood. *Br. med. J.* **ii**, 349–354.

■71

British Journal of Psychiatry, 1981, vol. 138, pp. 456–465

Psychiatric Interviewing Techniques
IV. Experimental Study: Four Contrasting Styles

M. RUTTER, A. COX, S. EGERT, D. HOLBROOK and B. EVERITT

72 ■

Summary: The development and definition of four contrasting interview styles is described. The four styles were designed using different permutations of techniques which, on the basis of an earlier naturalistic study, appeared to be most effective in eliciting either factual information or feelings. A 'sounding board' style utilized a minimal activity approach; an 'active psychotherapy' style actively sought to explore feelings and to bring out emotional links and meanings; a 'structured' style adopted an active cross-questioning approach; and a 'systematic exploratory' style aimed to combine a high use of both fact-oriented and feeling-oriented techniques. Quantitative measures based on video-tape and audio-tape analysis showed that two experienced interviewers could be trained to adopt these four very different styles and yet remain feeling and appearing natural. An experimental design to compare the four styles is described.

Our naturalistic study of the initial interviews between psychiatric trainees and the parents of children referred to a psychiatric out-patient clinic showed a variety of statistically significant associations between interview styles or techniques on the one hand and outcome in terms of information obtained or emotions elicited on the other (Rutter and Cox, 1981; Cox, Hopkinson and Rutter, 1981, II; Hopkinson, Cox and Rutter, 1981). The results suggested that some interview techniques were likely to be more effective than others in eliciting detailed factual information, whereas other rather different techniques seemed to be optimal for eliciting emotions and feelings. The patterns of findings, especially with respect to active fact-oriented techniques strongly suggested that the associations represented causal influences, namely that the different interview techniques had caused different informant responses. However, because the study was non-experimental in design the causal inference was necessarily based on circumstantial evidence which could result only in tentative conclusions. This paper and its two companions report an experimental study testing the causal hypothesis directly (Cox, Rutter and Holbrook, 1981, V; Cox, Holbrook and Rutter, 1981, VI).

In planning the investigation, it was important to deal with various other limitations of the naturalistic study. Firstly, although the techniques associated with more effective fact-gathering were rather different from those associated with the more effective eliciting of emotions, there seemed to be no incompatability between the two. Indeed, in the naturalistic study, interviews with good factual coverage tended also to have rather above average levels of expressed feelings (Cox *et al*, 1981, II). Earlier work designing research interviews had indicated that it ought to be possible to combine both sorts of techniques (Brown and Rutter, 1966; Rutter and Brown, 1966). However, the effects of combining techniques had still to be systematically tested. Accordingly, there was a need to compare the effects of interviews with combined techniques as against interviews aimed exclusively to be optimal for either fact gathering or eliciting emotions, but not both.

Secondly, comparisons in the naturalistic study had to rely on the assumption that each interviewer had a broadly similar group of informants. While in general this appeared to be the case, it was decided to ensure that each experimental style was employed with the same informants.

Thirdly, in the naturalistic study the possibility could not be entirely ruled out that the interviewer behaviour was a result rather than a cause of the informant's response. This problem could be met by deliberately altering the interview style, in experimental fashion, to determine if this had the predicted effect on informant response. This required that both the styles to be compared should be used with each informant.

Fourthly, it had not been possible in the naturalistic enquiry to differentiate clearly between the style of interview and the interviewer's skills and competence. This limitation could be met by utilizing experienced interviewers each of whom would be trained to employ all the defined experimental styles.

Fifthly, the inferences to be drawn from the naturalistic study were complicated by the fact that some interviews were joint (i.e. with both parents) and some were individual (i.e. with just one parent). It was decided, therefore, to simplify the experimental comparisons by using only individual interviews with the mother of the child referred.

These five requirements formed the basis of the experimental design. By systematically varying interview techniques so that each informant was interviewed twice, once with one style and once with another it should prove possible to test the causal inferences. If the interview style was having a causal effect on the informant's responses, the variations in interview technique should lead to predictable and regular consequences in terms of the factual formation obtained and the feelings elicited. To maintain relevance for normal practice, however, the study needed to be in a clinical setting and the styles had to be ones which were actively used in ordinary practice and acceptable to both clients and clinicians.

Methods

Choice of style

The naturalistic study (Cox *et al*, 1981 II; Hopkinson *et al*, 1981) had suggested the importance of three active techniques designed to elicit factual information (a high rate of floorholdings and of topics first raised by the interviewer, a high rate of probes per topic, and many requests for detailed descriptions); and five active techniques designed to elicit emotional feelings (a high ratio of open to closed questions, and a high number of interpretations, of expressions of sympathy, of requests for feelings, and of pick-ups of emotional cues). Four experimental styles derived from these findings, based on combinations of high and low usage of these two sets of active techniques (see Table I).

However, for the experimental study (necessarily involving parents of children referred to a psychiatric clinic as part of routine practice) to be ethically acceptable it was essential to have four styles, all of which could be used naturally and convincingly and all of which followed good interview practice. The aim was to compare different techniques, not to compare good and bad interviewing. Further, for the results to be clinically useful it was essential to compare styles which were advocated by experts in the field and were being used in psychiatric practice. In short, it was necessary to consider how the naturalistic study findings could be linked with clinical teaching and practice, and how both the use *and* the non-use of active techniques could form part of an acceptable and sensible interview style. Four styles were identified which fulfilled these criteria and are described in terms of their most obvious characteristics: (a) *sounding board;* (b) *active psychotherapy;* (c) *structured;* and (d) *systematic exploratory.*

(a) *Sounding board style*

The sounding board technique approximates to the style based on a low use of both types of active techniques and it is nearest to the psychiatric interviewing methods advocated by Finesinger (1948) who urged the value of 'minimal activity' because it allows 'the patient to talk more freely in meaningful areas'. Psychiatrists were warned against the temptation to use active techniques such as provocative interpretations or rapid probing because 'when successful, these methods tend to emphasize the doctor's omnipotence and magic powers. When unsuccessful, they . . . may give the patient feelings of guilt and inadequacy'.

■73

TABLE I
Experimental styles deriving from naturalistic study

		Interviewer use of active fact-oriented techniques	
		Low use	High use
Interviewer use of active feeling oriented techniques	Low use	Low/low	Low feeling oriented: High fact oriented
	High use	High feeling oriented: Low fact oriented	High/high

British Journal of Psychiatry, 1981, vol. 138, pp. 456–465

In our procedure the interviewer started by asking in an open fashion about the informant's concerns, complaints or worries. The mother was allowed to decide what was important and the interviewer followed her lead. In order to keep her talking he used encouragements (mm-mm, yes, etc.), repetitions of her last words with a rising inflection, elaborations of the last word (e.g. 'you mentioned pain'), mild commands (e.g. 'tell me some more about that') and non-verbal cues (nods, smiles and so forth). The interviewer aimed to be warm, caring and interested but made minimal use of active techniques to elicit emotions; thus, interpretations, expressions of sympathy and emotional reflections were to be very little used. The interviewer was allowed to ask a direct question to introduce each major area (child symptoms, parental health, marital relationship, etc.) and to use checks to keep the informant talking, but otherwise should not probe, cross question or ask for specific examples. The general rationale of the style was to be non-intrusive and non-directive, to follow what the mother said and to allow her to make the running and decide what was relevant and important.

(b) *'Active psychotherapy' style*

The active psychotherapy technique approximates to the style based on a low use of active fact-oriented techniques and a high use of active feeling-oriented techniques. It is nearest to the diagnostic approach advocated by psychotherapists such as Balint (Balint and Balint, 1961) and Gill (Gill, Newman and Redlich, 1954). There is "the absolute necessity . . . of establishing a personal relationship between doctor and patient" (Balint and Balint, 1961). For the informant, 'the interview should be an impressive experience of being given the opportunity of revealing himself, of being understood, and of being helped to see himself—his past and present problems—in a new light' (Balint and Balint, 1961). The style was similar to the sounding board, in its aim to let the mother tell her story in her own fashion without cross-questioning, detailed probing or systematic coverage of predetermined areas. It was also similar in its use of encouragements to keep talking and its aim to follow the mother's lead. However, it was quite different in its intentions to actively intervene to explore feelings and bring out emotional links and meanings. To this end there was extensive use of open questions, reflective interpretations, requests for feelings and for self-disclosures, and expressions of sympathy. The interviewer sought to clarify the issues raised by the informant through picking up cues and through the use of open questions and responses to feelings, but there was no structured questioning in relation to fact gathering.

(c) *'Structured' style*

The structured style was, in a sense, the opposite of the active psychotherapy style in being based on a high use of active fact-oriented techniques. It was closest to the 'present state examination' interview developed by Wing and his colleagues (1967, 1977). The interviewer starts questioning with a firm set of ideas on the clinically important areas to be systematically covered. Thus, in contrast to the first two styles he is actively in charge of the factual content of the interview from the outset and directs the questions accordingly. He is warm, courteous, concerned and attentive to what the informant says; he picks up cues when they are relevant to his task but he provides the leads. The procedure is extremely flexible and nothing at all like a questionnaire. The wording and order of questions are adapted to the needs of each interview and whenever possible the informant's own words and ways of expressing things are used in formulating further probes. However, the interviewer's task is to cover pre-determined areas systematically and in all areas to obtain sufficient detail for him to judge whether any abnormality is present. This means that after the informant has described something in his own words, a process of clinical cross-examination is followed, using probes, asking for detailed descriptions and examples, and clarifying the situation by a variety of specific questions. Many closed questions are used and the interviewer actively directs the proceedings. On the other hand, the main verbal focus is on factual information and there is less direct concern with eliciting spontaneous feelings. Accordingly, very little use is made of interpretations, expressions of sympathy, requests for feelings and open questions generally. It is considered that feelings will be expressed more freely by a focus on what actually happened or was experienced rather than by a direct assault on the informant's emotions by trying to bring covert feelings to the surface.

(d) *'Systematic exploratory' style*

The fourth style approximates to one based on a high use of fact-oriented *and* feeling-oriented techniques. It is fairly close to a manner of interviewing which has many advocates but which may be exemplified by the techniques developed by Brown and Rutter (Brown and Rutter, 1966; Rutter and Brown, 1966; Quinton, Rutter and Rowlands, 1976) and it combines many of the features of both the active psychotherapy style and the structured approach.

In practice, the informant is first encouraged to tell things in her own words. She makes the running initially and the interviewer aims to establish from the beginning (through the use of interpretations, expressions of sympathy and requests for feelings) that he is interested in emotions and attitudes as well as events and activities. Open questions are used liberally to encourage free expression and the interviewer aims to obtain as much information as possible by following up the informant's leads, rather than through specific questioning on new topics which he himself has to introduce. However, the interviewer is expected to get ample detailed descriptions and must use active questioning whenever required to ensure either systematic coverage of topics or sufficient detail on each topic to make an adequate clinical evaluation. In this respect there is no essential difference from the structured style. The contrast lies largely in its emphasis on feelings as well as facts, on style of questions (a greater use of open questions) and on its aim to explore emotional meaning as well as observed behaviour.

Experimental design

When comparing two or more different interview styles in an experimental design, tight control is only possible when each informant is interviewed with every style to be compared. In this way the style is varied but the informant remains the same so allowing the effect of the former on the latter to be systematically studied. However, it would be impractical to interview each informant four times. Accordingly, a decision had to be taken on which comparisons were to have priority in the first instance. Because the naturalistic study findings provided clearer guidance and more straightforward hypotheses on active fact-oriented techniques it was decided to make these the basis of the paired comparisons. This choice was also guided by the view that whereas it was most unlikely that the use of feeling-oriented techniques would interfere with fact gathering, it was quite possible that systematic probing and detailed questioning could impede the expression of feelings. The design chosen allowed this latter possibility to be examined and is shown in Table II. Six mothers received the structured style first and the sounding board second (group A); six had these two interviews in the reverse order; six had the systematic exploratory style first and the active psychotherapy second; and six had these two interviews in the reverse order. Mothers were randomly allocated to the four conditions. Two experienced interviewers were used and each did an equal number of first and second interviews, and an equal number

■ 75

TABLE II
Experimental design

Group			Interviewer order	Number of cases	Occasion of interview	
					I	II
A.	Style Order	ST–SB	$I_1 - I_2$	3	I_1 ST	I_2 SB
			$I_1 - I_1$	3	I_2 ST	I_1 SB
		SB–ST	$I_1 - I_2$	3	I_1 SB	I_2 ST
			$I_2 - I_1$	3	I_2 SB	I_1 ST
B.	Style Order	SE–AP	$I_1 - I_2$	3	I_1 SE	I_2 AP
			$I_2 - I_1$	3	I_2 SE	I_1 AP
		AP–SE	$I_1 - I_2$	3	I_1 AP	I_2 SE
			$I_2 - I_1$	3	I_2 AP	I_1 SE

I_1 = Interviewer 1; I_2 = Interviewer 2; ST = Structured style; SB = Sounding-board style; SE = Systematic-exploratory style; AP = Active psychotherapy style.

British Journal of Psychiatry, 1981, vol. 138, pp. 456–465

of interviews with each style. For each pair of styles a three factor, repeated measures, analysis of variance was performed to test for differences between styles and between interviewers and for order effects.

Because the pairing was made on the basis of active fact-oriented techniques, the effects of active feeling-oriented techniques could be examined only by comparisons across groups (see Table II: Group A versus Group B). The effects of informant variability are necessarily much greater in this analysis because the comparisons have to be made between—rather than within—informants. This constraint needs to be borne in mind in interpreting the findings.

To make the interviews as comparable as possible in duration, the interviewers attempted to keep all interviews to one hour. Whenever the first interview departed from this the other interviewer was instructed to try to lengthen or shorten the second interview so that the lengths of the paired interviews would be as similar as possible.

Again, in order to maintain comparability, the interviewers were told to regard the same information areas as a priority in all interview styles. The techniques to obtain them were, of course, different but the aims were similar and the scoring for data obtained referred only to these high priority areas. These consisted of the same list of child symptoms used in the naturalistic study, the type and quality of relationships within the nuclear family, the composition of the nuclear family and the characteristics of the home, the mental health and behaviour of both parents, and the styles of child-rearing used.

Clinical procedure

Unlike the naturalistic study, it was made a requirement that all interviews should be with the mother on her own, so avoiding the necessity of comparing mothers with fathers or dyads with triads. This required a much more substantial and complex liaison with the teams working in the clinic and also a much more careful preparation of the mothers since in most cases the interviewers were not going to be the therapists involved in the case after the two diagnostic interviews. Carefully designed letters were sent to all selected mothers inviting their co-operation. As in the naturalistic study, families were excluded where the parents were immigrant or where colloquial English was not the usual language spoken at home. In addition, in order to ensure greater comparability between interviews, referrals made for second opinions, or to consider admission to hospital were excluded, as were cases of isolated educational difficulty or those where psychosis, mental retardation or organic disorders were suspected. There were 14 boys (58 per cent) and 10 girls (42 per cent). The age range was

1 year 10 months to 15 years 7 months, with a mean of 9 years 10 months. The majority (75 per cent) were referred by General Practitioners. The remainder came mostly from educational sources (17 per cent) with one self-referral, and one from a community physician. A third (8) presented with conduct disorders; 7 (29 per cent) with emotional disorders; 7 (29 per cent) with disorders involving a mixture of emotional and conduct problems; and 2 (8 per cent) with enuresis or encopresis.

Of the mothers approached, approximately half decided not to participate in the project; these families were assessed and taken on for treatment in the usual way without going through the experimental interviews. In epidemiological studies high non-co-operation rates can cause an important bias (Cox *et al*, 1977). However, this was not a distorting effect in the present experimental study as the aim was to compare effects *within* the sample rather than to draw any conclusions about the sample characteristics as a whole. The effects of the contrasting interview techniques could be validly examined within the sample of mothers who agreed to participate since they were randomly assigned to style and interviewer.

The two experimental interviews took place during the usual waiting period for a diagnostic appointment and at the end of the second interview the father and the referred child (plus other members of the family where relevant) were seen in the usual way by the ordinary clinic team. With the mother's consent in all cases, the data obtained during the experimental interviews was made freely available to the clinicians seeing each family.

The interviews took place not less than a week and not more than three weeks apart: the usual gap was two weeks. Immediately before the first interview the interviewer explained the procedures to the mother and obtained her written consent to video recording. At the end of each experimental interview one of the research team (who was not an interviewer) gave the mother a questionnaire which asked about her perceptions of the interview and her feelings about it. When the questionnaire had been completed after the second experimental interview, the mother was encouraged to make free comments contrasting the two approaches and whenever possible expressing a preference.

Training of interviewers

Before the experimental study started there was an intensive period of training for the two interviewers. First, they both calibrated their own natural technique by undertaking a video and audiotape recorded interview with a mother of a newly-referred child patient. The pattern of techniques they used was then compared with a constructed ideal profile for each of the four experimental styles so that each interviewer could determine how their natural style needed to be modified in order to fulfil the study criteria.

The interviewers then practised each of the four experimental styles by means of role play interviews with colleagues. The filming and recording procedures were adapted for these interviews in order to give as rapid as possible feedback on those techniques crucial to the style being followed. The experimental study proper began only when both interviewers were thoroughly comfortable and at ease with the styles and were using them in a satisfactory fashion.

Results

Style differences on fact-oriented techniques

Table III summarizes the differences in fact-oriented techniques which were found between styles. All the differences were large, statistically significant and in the intended direction, i.e. that the usage of these techniques should be greater in the structured and systematic exploratory styles than in either the active psychotherapy or sounding board styles. Thus, in the former two styles the interviewers had a higher number of floorholdings, asked three or four times as many closed questions, first raised new symptoms ten times as often, first raised new family topics 5 to 10 times as often, used considerably more probes per topic, and more often asked for detailed descriptions. As intended, the structured and systematic exploratory styles were much more active, directive and probing than the other two styles. It had proved possible to utilize radically different interview styles and maintain their consistency across a heterogeneous range of informants. Moreover, there were no significant differences between the two

experimental interviewers or between first and second interviews on any of these fact-oriented techniques.

On the other hand, the interviewers were to a substantial extent influenced by the characteristics of the mothers they interviewed. This was shown by the finding that there were significant product moment correlations within pairs for both floorholdings (r = .80 within systematic exploratory-active psychotherapy pairs and .59 within structured-sounding board pairs) and number of closed questions (r = .72 in the former pairings and .68 in the latter). Interviewers remained highly consistent in their use of styles (as shown by the analysis of various findings) but nevertheless some mothers demanded more use of questions and interventions than did others. Interviewers needed to be and were flexible and responsive to the needs of particular informants but this did not interfere with the maintenance of clearly differentiated styles.

Style differences on feeling-oriented techniques

Table IV summarizes the differences in feeling-oriented techniques which were found between styles. In this case the key comparison is between the systematic exploratory and active psychotherapy styles, where the use of feeling-oriented techniques should be high, and the structured and sounding board styles where they should be low. Again, the differences were generally large, statistically significant and in the intended direction. Thus, in the former two styles the interviewers were twice as likely to respond to feeling cues, used fewer closed questions, and gave twice as many requests for feelings, interpretations and expressions of sympathy.

One additional item, requests for self-disclosures,

■77

TABLE III

Style differences on fact-oriented techniques

	Styles					
Techniques	A Structured	B Systematic expl.	C Act. psychoth.	D Sounding board	Analysis of variance (A+B vs C+D; df 1, 16)	
	Mean (S.D.)	Mean (S.D.)	Mean (S.D.)	Mean (S.D.)	F ratio	P
No. floorholdings (per 60 mins)	154 (62)	160 (50)	100 (48)	83 (39)	68.62	< .0001
No. closed questions (per 60 mins)	62 (29)	73 (31)	15 (12)	19 (11)	110.70	< .0001
No. open questions (per 60 mins)	27 (13)	27 (13)	15 (11)	17 (13)	24.06	< .0002
No. symptoms first raised by interviewer	5.6 (2.6)	5.3 (1.8)	0.6 (1.0)	0.2 (0.4)	104.08	< .0001
No. family topics first raised by interviewer	3.8 (1.9)	4.9 (2.6)	0.8 (0.9)	0.5 (0.9)	60.00	< .0001
No. probes per child symptom	8.3 (3.4)	9.3 (3.4)	4.5 (2.1)	3.3 (2.2)	52.12	< .0001
No. requests for detailed descriptions	6.1 (4.2)	3.7 (2.7)	2.6 (2.8)	4.1 (3.2)	4.44	< .05

British Journal of Psychiatry, 1981, vol. 138, pp. 456–465

i.e. emotionally laden factual information, was included in the table because of its relevance to the eliciting of feelings. Its use should have been (and was) greater in the active questioning styles because it constituted questioning on factual information, but it might influence the expression of feelings.*

* We did not know at the start of the experimental study whether or not it would, because this was a measure added after the naturalistic study as a direct result of that study's findings.

Unlike the situation with fact-oriented techniques some differences between the experimental interviewers were found with respect to feeling-oriented techniques (see Table V). Especially in the structured and systematic exploratory styles, interviewer A made more requests for feelings/expressions of sympathy/interpretations whereas interviewer B made more requests for self-disclosures. Interviewer B used a higher proportion of open questions but, except in the structured style, the two did not differ in the proportion of feelings responded to.

TABLE IV

Style differences on feeling-oriented techniques

| | Styles | | | | | |
| | A Structured | B Systematic expl. | C Act. psychoth. | D Sounding board | Analysis of variance (B+C vs A+D; df 1, 16) | |
Techniques	Mean (S.D.)	Mean (S.D.)	Mean (S.D.)	Mean (S.D.)	F ratio	P
% Closed questions	45 (11)	38 (11)	13 (7)	22 (10)	8.09	< .012
Ratio open:closed questions	.38 (.10)	.43 (.13)	1.23 (.89)	1.07 (.72)	0.53	ns
% Feelings responded to	19 (15)	38 (12)	62 (15)	29 (18)	24.08	< .0002
Requests for feelings (a)	0.4 (0.5)	2.2 (2.8)	4.3 (2.9)	0.4 (0.7)	22.14	< .0003
Interpretations (b)	1.2 (1.9)	3.8 (2.4)	9.9 (3.9)	1.4 (1.6)	70.83	< .0001
Expressions of sympathy (c)	5.5 (4.6)	10.1 (6.9)	14.8 (6.8)	5.3 (3.7)	18.94	< .0005
Any of a, b or c	13 (9)	27 (20)	44 (16)	14 (9)	42.67	< .0001
Requests for self disclosure (per 60 mins)	11.6 (7.6)	15.7 (6.3)	7.4 (4.7)	5.8 (4.8)	3.29	< .09

TABLE V

Interviewer differences on feeling-oriented techniques

| | | Styles | | | | Analysis of variance | | | |
| | | A Structured | B Systematic expl. | C Act. psychoth. | D Sounding board | Between interviewers (df 1, 16) | | Within interviewers between styles (B+C vs A+D; df 1, 16) | |
Technique	Inter-viewer	Mean (S.D.)	Mean (S.D.)	Mean (S.D.)	Mean (S.D.)	F ratio	P	F ratio	P
% Open questions	A	15.2 (4.4)	11.7 (3.5)	12.2 (1.0)	16.2 (7.7)	17.46	< .0008	4.25	< .06
	B	18.5 (4.5)	22.8 (3.5)	17.2 (6.9)	21.2 (8.0)			0.03	N.S.
% Feelings responded to	A	28.5 (14.8)	39.7 (10.6)	58.3 (9.6)	32.3 (10.7)	2.68	N.S.	13.53	< .002
	B	9.0 (8.1)	36.2 (14.1)	66.2 (19.0)	25.7 (24.3)			21.30	< .0003
Requests for feelings+interpretations+expr. symp.	A	20.7 (6.5)	41.5 (20.7)	45.5 (11.7)	18.8 (7.5)	40.57	< .0001	24.08	< .0002
	B	5.8 (4.5)	13.2 (2.9)	37.3 (19.5)	9.0 (8.6)			38.01	< .0001
Requests for self-disclosures	A	6.3 (3.2)	11.8 (6.0)	8.3 (4.9)	6.0 (2.6)	12.11	< .003	5.94	< .03
	B	16.8 (7.1)	19.5 (4.0)	6.5 (4.7)	5.5 (6.7)			29.44	< .0001

The net effect of these differences was that for interviewer A the structured style included too many feeling-oriented techniques and for interviewer B the systematic exploratory style included too few. Because of unavoidable delays in data processing this was not appreciated until well into the experimental interviewing with the result that they could not be fully corrected. The difference needs to be taken into account in data analysis but in spite of some differences in threshold it is evident that both interviewers maintained fairly consistent between-style differences. However, there was a number of interviews by both interviewers in which the style actually used departed from that specified. For some analyses these interviews were excluded in order to determine if their inclusion affected the results.

Style differences on non-verbal features

Table VI summarizes the style differences on various non-verbal measures. These were not part of the definitions of style and many of the differences were non-significant. However, there was a tendency for interviewers to provide more encouragement to mothers to continue talking, by smiling, head nods and vocal listening responses, in the two active feeling-oriented techniques. The interviewers differed somewhat in their pattern of non-verbal encouragements (interviewer A used significantly more non-verbal responses but significantly less smiles while listening) but not in their overall level of encouragement. This suggests that although they changed their technique according to prescription they nevertheless retained features of their specific personal style.

Discussion

The clinical interview is the diagnostic and thera-

peutic tool-in-trade of all professionals working in the field of psychiatric disorders. Accordingly it is important to develop and test the most effective clinical interviewing techniques, yet very little systematic research has been undertaken in this area; almost all research into the effects of different interview techniques and styles has been concerned with interviews in non-clinical settings and with purposes rather different from those in clinical psychiatry (Cox and Rutter, 1977). One reason may be the fear that such research would adversely affect clinical work or that clinical necessities would make an adequate research design impractical or unethical. Our experience indicates that neither need occur.

At the time the experimental study was undertaken, the usual waiting time in the clinic was about 6 weeks for non-emergency or non-urgent referrals, from the time of initial referral to the time of the diagnostic interview which was immediately followed by whatever therapeutic intervention was required. It was the practice to offer parents the choice of an interim consultation with a social worker during this waiting period. For parents who took up this offer, there were, thus, two initial interviews—the interim consultation and the later interview with the psychiatrist. The experimental design took up the opportunities presented by this waiting period by offering the first experimental interview immediately after referral, with the second experimental interview a fortnight later leading directly into therapy.

The main difference from the clinical practice of waiting list interviews was that the research interviewers were not usually involved in the later therapeutic interviews. This meant that the family's impetus to engage therapy might have been impaired by changes in interviewer. In fact this did not seem to

■ 79

TABLE VI

Style differences on non-verbal features

	Styles					
	A Structured	B Systematic expl.	C Act. psychoth.	D Sounding board	Analysis of variance (A+D vs B+C; df 1, 16)	
Non-verbal features	Mean (S.D.)	Mean (S.D.)	Mean (S.D.)	Mean (S.D.)	t	P
Smiles while talking	0.6 (0.8)	1.8 (2.0)	1.8 (1.6)	0.3 (0.5)	3.52	< .01
Smiles while listening	5.6 (5.3)	8.1 (4.1)	8.2 (6.0)	4.2 (3.1)	2.41	< .05
Head nods while talking	15.8 (8.2)	14.1 (6.0)	17.6 (10.9)	11.1 (6.4)		N.S.
Head nods while listening	35.3 (12.1)	47.5 (10.9)	54.8 (15.7)	45.4 (16.3)	2.60	< .02
Vocal listening responses	56.6 (17.5)	64.9 (12.3)	67.6 (17.1)	51.8 (20.6)		N.S.

British Journal of Psychiatry, 1981, vol. 138, pp. 456–465

occur. We checked on the possibility by noting early lapses or drop-out from therapy. It was found that these were no more frequent in the experimental sample than in a randomly selected sample of other clinic cases; in fact they were marginally less frequent.

A further concern might be that because the research interviews were with the mother on her own, it might be more difficult to initiate therapy with conjoint marital interviews or conjoint family interviews. In practice, this did not appear to be a major obstacle and certainly a wide variety of treatments were subsequently employed. Other research (Dare *et al*, 1980) has shown that although it may be advisable to be cautious about early changes in therapeutic approach, nevertheless the form of the initial assessment need not predetermine the form of therapeutic intervention.

In undertaking an experimental study in the course of ordinary clinic practice in a busy out-patients' department, a high degree of co-operation and close liaison between researchers and clinicians was essential. If difficulties were to be avoided, attention to detail and an alertness for potential personal anxieties was crucial. Given that, it proved readily possible to integrate research and clinical needs with only occasional problems.

From the research point of view, the most fundamental concern was whether it would be possible for two experienced clinicians with well developed and rather different styles of their own to learn to use four very disparate experimental styles in a way that both felt natural to them and appeared so to the people whom they were interviewing. Our experience showed that it was possible. The research findings indicated that both interviewers were successful in adopting four styles which were measurably very different from each other. The differentiation between styles and the lack of difference between the two interviewers was most successful in the case of the fact-oriented techniques. The differentiation between styles was also good in the case of feeling-oriented techniques but the situation was complicated by some continuing differences between interviewers.

It was not that either interviewer failed to use four very different styles; to the contrary the findings showed that both succeeded well in this. Rather the problem lay in the fact that the two interviewers were not ideally calibrated with each other. Thus, although both differed between styles in their use of feeling-oriented techniques, one interviewer had a level of usage which was generally higher than the other. The main reason for this probably lay in the difficulties in providing the interviewers with feed-back on the changes in style required to ensure good comparability. Success in getting interviewers to adopt markedly contrasting styles seemed to depend on the combination of the use of role-playing, precise definition on what was required, the opportunity to view interviews on video-tape and analyse them in some detail, together with continuing feedback after each interview on how successfully styles were being followed. We are impressed by the value of both video-tapes and role-playing as a means of teaching interviewing skills.

Acknowledgements

The research reported in this series of papers was supported by a grant from the Social Science Research Council. The Papers were prepared while Michael Rutter was a Fellow at the Center for Advanced Study in the Behavioral Sciences, and financial support was provided by the William T. Grant Foundation, The Foundation for Child Development, The Spencer Foundation and The National Science Foundation (BNS 78-24671).

The study would not have been possible without the active collaboration and support of members of the Children's Department of the Maudsley Hospital. Particular thanks are due to those who took over cases for treatment during the experimental phase.

References

BALINT, M. & BALINT, E. (1961) *Psychotherapeutic Techniques in Medicine*. London: Tavistock.

BROWN, G. W. & RUTTER, M. (1966) The measurement of family activities and relationships: a methodological study. *Human Relations*, **19**, 241–63.

COX, A. & RUTTER, M. (1977) Diagnostic appraisal and interviewing. In *Child Psychiatry: Modern Approaches* (eds. M. Rutter and L. Hersov). Oxford: Blackwell Scientific.

—— HOLBROOK, D. & RUTTER, M. (1981) Psychiatric interviewing techniques: VI. Experimental study; eliciting feelings. *British Journal of Psychiatry*, (in press).

—— HOPKINSON, K. & RUTTER, M. (1981) Psychiatric interviewing techniques: II. Naturalistic study; eliciting factual information. *British Journal of Psychiatry*, **138**, 283–91.

—— RUTTER, M. & HOLBROOK, D. (1981) Psychiatric interviewing techniques: V. Experimental study; eliciting factual information. *British Journal of Psychiatry*, (in press).

—— —— YULE, B. & QUINTON, D. (1977) Bias resulting from missing information: some epidemiological findings. *British Journal of Preventive and Social Medicine*, **31**, 131–6.

DARE, J., HEMSLEY, R. & COX, A. A comparison of individual and family assessments. (In preparation).

FINESINGER, J. (1948) Psychiatric interviewing. 1. Some principles and procedures in insight therapy. *American Journal of Psychiatry*, **105,** 187–95.

GILL, M., NEWMAN, R. & REDLICH, F. C. (1954) *The Initial Interview in Psychiatric practice.* New York: International Universities Press.

HOPKINSON, K., COX, A. & RUTTER, M. (1981) Psychiatric interviewing techniques: III. Naturalistic study; eliciting feelings. *British Journal of Psychiatry*, **138,** 406–15.

QUINTON, D., RUTTER, M. & ROWLANDS, O. (1976) An evaluation of an interview assessment of marriage. *Psychological Medicine*, **6,** 577–86.

RUTTER M. & BROWN, G. W. (1966) The reliability and validity of measures of family life and relationships in families containing a psychiatric patient. *Social Psychiatry*, **1,** 38–53.

—— & COX, A. (1981) Psychiatric interviewing techniques: I. Methods and measures. *British Journal of Psychiatry*, **138,** 273–82.

WING, J. K., BIRLEY, J. L. T., COOPER, J. E., GRAHAM, P. & ISAACS, A. D. (1967) Reliability of a procedure for measuring and classifying 'present psychiatric state'. *British Journal of Psychiatry*, **113,** 499–515.

—— NIXON, J. N., MANN, S. A. & LEFF, J. P. (1977) Reliability of the PSE (ninth edition) used in a population study. *Psychological Medicine*, **7,** 505–16.

■81

Michael Rutter, M.D., F.R.C.P., F.R.C.Psych., *Professor of Child Psychiatry, Department of Child and Adolescent Psychiatry, Institute of Psychiatry, De Crespigny Park, London SE5 8AZ*

Antony Cox, M.Phil., M.R.C.P., F.R.C,Psych., *Consultant Psychiatrist, The Maudsley Hospital, Denmark Hill, London SE5 8AZ*

Stella Egert, B,A., Dip.Ment.Health, *Department of Child Psychiatry, Queen Elizabeth Hospital for Children, Hackney Road, London E2*

Daphne Holbrook, B.A. Dip.Ment.Health, *Research Worker, Department of Child and Adolescent Psychiatry, Institute of Psychiatry*

Brian Everitt, B.Sc., M.Sc., *Reader, and Head of Biometrics Unit, Institute of Psychiatry*

(*Received 11 June; revised 28 November 1980*)

Part IV
Psychiatric disorders

Handbook of Autism and Pervasive Developmental Disorders, eds D.J. Cohen & F.R. Volkmar, 1997, pp. 370–387

Genetic Influences and Autism

MICHAEL RUTTER, ANTHONY BAILEY, EMILY SIMONOFF, AND ANDREW PICKLES

In the first report that described autism, Kanner (1943) postulated that it was an inborn disorder. Yet, for many years, little attention was paid to possible genetic factors because occurrences of two autistic children in the same family were so infrequent (some 2% of cases in the literature reviewed by Smalley, Asarnow, & Spence, 1988). Early chromosome studies also failed to reveal any abnormalities.

Three developments changed the situation radically. First, aware that even a 2% rate of autism in siblings meant a huge increase in relative risk compared to the general population, Folstein and Rutter (1977a, 1977b) conducted the first systematic, general-population-based twin study and provided evidence of a strong genetic component. Second, discovery of the Fragile X anomaly led to the finding that a substantial minority of autistic individuals had this anomaly (Blomquist et al., 1985). From the early (albeit mistaken) belief that a stronger association existed between autism and the Fragile X than between mental retardation and the Fragile X, there evolved a major research interest in the associations as well as a renewal of interest in other chromosome anomalies that might be associated with autism (Gillberg & Wahlström, 1985). Third, clinical investigations encouraged a growing awareness that some cases of autism were associated with single-gene medical disorders that showed a Mendelian pattern (see Folstein & Piven, 1991; Folstein & Rutter, 1988).

Some of the claims made in these three areas of research were short-lived (see below). It is universally accepted now that genetic factors play a major role in autism even when no associated genetic disease such as Fragile X or tuberous sclerosis is evident. Indeed, autism is the most strongly genetic of all multifactorial psychiatric disorders (Rutter, Bailey, Bolton, & Le Couteur, 1993). Attention has turned, accordingly, to a more detailed consideration of specific issues relating to the role of genetic factors.

ASSOCIATIONS WITH SPECIFIC GENETIC DISORDERS

Two conditions make the strongest case for an association with autism: (a) the Fragile X anomaly (see Simonoff, Bolton, & Rutter, 1996, for an account of the several genetic abnormalities involved) and (b) tuberous sclerosis. For each condition, a detailed consideration of the evidence is informative for understanding the broad implications as well as the specific findings.

Fragile X Anomaly

The Fragile X anomaly occurs with about the same frequency as autism, is associated with mental retardation (both mild and severe), and receives its name from the appearance of a fragile site on the long arm of the X chromosome

■ 85

A major portion of this chapter is based on "Autism: Towards an Integration of Clinical, Genetic, Neuropsychological and Neurobiological Perspectives," by A.J. Bailey, W. Phillips, and M. Rutter, 1996, *Journal of Child Psychology and Psychiatry*. Reproduced with permission.

when cultured in low-folate media (Warren & Nelson, 1994). The first reports of a link between the Fragile X anomaly and autism suggested that the anomaly occurred in at least 16% of autistic persons (Gillberg & Wahlström, 1985). When a larger number of subjects were pooled a few years later, the estimate dropped to 7% (Bolton & Rutter, 1990; Brown et al., 1986). Current estimates, based on new data, put the true rate at about 2.5%, and almost certainly below 5% (Bailey et al., 1993; Piven et al., 1991). The first point to consider, therefore, is why the estimate has fallen so dramatically.

Rutter, Bailey, Bolton, and Le Couteur (1994) suggested four reasons:

1. A publishing bias exists; positive associations tend to be published and negative ones are not.
2. With a small sample size, typical of these early studies, the proportion of false positives in the findings is higher than that with large samples (see Pocock, 1983).
3. Early reports were based on inclusion of very low (1% to 3%) rates of Fragile X expression, which do not have the same significance as rates of 4% and above. This was first evident from statistical analyses using latent class methods (Bolton et al., 1992), but it is no longer necessary to rely on demonstration of a Fragile X site using low-folate media. The Fragile X anomaly originates from a trinucleotide repeat sequence in the region containing the FMR-1 gene (Davies, 1991), which means that DNA methods can be used. These methods have shown that individuals with low rates of Fragile X expression do not have this abnormality (Gurling et al., 1997, submitted).
4. The initial reports of autism in individuals who were so identified because they had the Fragile X anomaly were mainly based on clinical impression rather than systematic standardized assessment. It is now apparent that, although Fragile X individuals can show typical autism, their pattern of social and communicative abnormalities more often takes a different form (Hagerman, 1990). Marked social anxiety, gaze avoidance, and an ambivalent social approach combined with a turning away of the face seem to be particularly characteristic (Cohen, Vietze, Sudhalter, Jenkins, & Brown, 1989; Sudhalter, Cohen, Silverman, & Wolfschein, 1990; Wolff, Gardner, Paccia, & Lappen, 1989). The cognitive features associated with the social deficits that accompany the Fragile X anomaly may also be different from those found in autism (Mazzocco, Pennington, & Hagerman, 1994).

Given this evidence of a lower rate of the Fragile X anomaly in individuals with autism, it is necessary to reconsider whether there is any specific association between the two. Einfeld, Malony, and Hall (1989) compared Fragile X males with controls matched for age and IQ. When no differences in autistic symptomatology were found between the two groups, these authors argued for a lack of a meaningful causal association. On the other hand, a 2.5% rate of Fragile X in autistic persons is well above the general population figures. The alternative is that the association arises only because both autism and the Fragile X are associated with mental retardation. In other words, the suggestion is that the basic association is between mental retardation and Fragile X, and the association between autism and Fragile X is secondary. In support of that possibility is the finding that the great majority of autistic individuals with the Fragile X are mentally retarded. On the other hand, there is no direct relationship between IQ and autism. For example, trisomy 21, the most common cause of mental retardation, is only infrequently associated with autism. It seems fair to conclude that: (a) there may be some specific association between Fragile X and autism, but (b) the association does not point strongly to any genetic mechanisms that may be involved in autism. A molecular genetic study of multiplex families by Hallmayer et al. (1994) appeared to exclude linkage to the FMR-1 gene (the gene associated with Fragile X) in the sample investigated.

For many years, there have been clinical reports of autistic features in individuals with tuberous sclerosis. This single-gene, autosomal-dominant, neurocutaneous disorder occurs in about 1 per 7,000 individuals (Osborne, Fryer, & Webb, 1991). It is characterized by a combination of skin lesions and neurological features, but protean abnormalities in other organs of the body also occur. Depigmented maculas that show up best in ultraviolet light are usually the earliest and most common skin lesion (but they occur occasionally in the general population). Facial angiofibromatosis, typically in a butterfly distribution, is often striking but may not appear until adolescence or adult life. Fibrous plaques on the forehead, shagreen patches (thickened skin) on the lower back, and fibromas of the nails also occur. Retinal hamartomas (phakomas), usually near the optic disk, may be revealed in an ophthalmoscopic examination. Glial nodules along the lateral walls of the lateral ventricles are present in some four-fifths of cases. They usually calcify and are identifiable on a cranial CT scan. About two-thirds of patients develop epileptic seizures, and a general learning disability is present in about two-fifths. About three-fourths of cases derive from new mutations (i.e., there is no family history). The physical manifestations of tuberous sclerosis vary greatly from individual to individual, even within the same family. A very mild condition may be manifest only in hypomelanotic maculas (Smalley, Burger, & Smith, 1994). Gene loci have been discovered on chromosome 9 (Fryer et al., 1987) and chromosome 16 (European Chromosome 16 TS Consortium, 1993). Each accounts for about half the cases.

Hunt and Dennis (1987), who used a checklist approach, reported that 50% of children with tuberous sclerosis showed autistic behavior. A later more systematic study (Hunt & Shepherd, 1993) showed that 24% of children with tuberous sclerosis met *DSM-III-R* criteria for autism, and an additional 19% showed autistic traits. The findings of Smalley and colleagues (Smalley, Smith, & Tanguay, 1991; Smalley, Tanguay, Smith, & Gutierrez, 1992) are broadly similar and Gillberg, Gillberg, and Ahlsén (1994) reported that 61% showed autism. There are fewer data on the proportion of autistic individuals with tuberous sclerosis and it has been necessary to make various extrapolations. These have produced figures ranging from 3% (Smalley et al., 1992) to 9% (Gillberg et al., 1994). Currently available data do not provide a precise figure, although it is probably nearer the bottom than the top of the range mentioned. A low percentage would

still establish a more specific association than has been found to date with any other genetically determined medical condition.

Again, the question must be raised: What does the association mean? It is likely to be causal in some way (because of its relative strength) but it is noteworthy that the main association occurs when tuberous sclerosis is accompanied by both mental retardation and epilepsy. It has been reported in the absence of mental retardation (Gillberg, Steffenburg, & Jakobsson, 1987); nevertheless, autism seems much less common when tuberous sclerosis is associated with normal intelligence, especially if epilepsy is not found. The latter observation suggests that the risk for autism arises through the brain disorder accompanying tuberous sclerosis and not because a gene for autism is closely associated with the locus of one of the two genes known to be linked with tuberous sclerosis.

Other Genetic Conditions and Chromosome Abnormalities

The literature includes reports of autistic features in individuals with untreated phenylketonuria (see Folstein & Rutter, 1988), but because none of the reports was based on standardized assessments of autism, the strength of the association, and perhaps even its reality, must be in some doubt. Untreated phenylketonuria is now a rare occurrence; hence, it must be an even rarer cause of autism. Gillberg and Forsell (1984) published case reports of two children with autism and a third with an autistic-like condition who showed neurofibromatosis. A few similar cases have been reported, but there are no systematic studies that would allow any estimate of the validity, or strength, of the association. Possibly, the association is real, even if it does not account for many cases; as with tuberous sclerosis, a combination of skin lesions and neural tumors is involved, which may be relevant. A diverse range of other genetically determined medical conditions have been reported from time to time to be associated with autism (see the systematic review by Gillberg & Coleman, 1992) but in no case is there good evidence of a strong association.

It is quite likely that autism is associated with some increase in the rate of chromosome anomalies. Probably the rate is something of the order of 5%, in addition to the Fragile X (Gillberg & Coleman, 1992). That figure is high enough to warrant routine examination of the chromosomes in the clinical assessment of autistic individuals, but the meaning of the association remains in considerable doubt. Many of the abnormalities reported are of quite uncertain clinical significance. Thus, some are balanced translocations (i.e., they involve exchange, but not loss, of chromosomal material) and these and other anomalies are known to arise in individuals without handicap. It might have been hoped that the particular chromosome abnormalities associated with autism would provide clues to the possible locus of the gene or genes that underlie autism. Unfortunately, they do not; autism has been associated with anomalies involving almost all chromosomes. Perhaps the only chromosome in which there is any suggestion of a stronger specific association is chromosome 15. There are reports that autism is sometimes associated with an extra marker chromosome deriving from chromosome 15 (Baker, Piven, Schwartz, & Patil, 1994; Gillberg et al., 1991; Hotopf & Bolton, 1995).

QUANTIFICATION OF GENETIC RISK IN IDIOPATHIC CASES

Evidence on the strength of the genetic component in cases of autism that are unassociated with a known medical condition derives from both family and twin studies. Clinical reports initially put the rate of autism in siblings at about 2% (Smalley et al., 1988). However, this figure was not based on systematic assessment of all siblings. Bolton et al. (1994) studied the 153 siblings of 99 autistic subjects, of whom 2.9% showed autism, and a further 2.9% showed atypical autism, with a 0% rate of both in the 65 siblings in the Down syndrome comparison group. Piven et al. (1990) found a 3% rate of autism in siblings and a 4% rate of severe social impairment. Szatmari et al. (1993) found a rate of 5.3% pervasive developmental disorder (PDD) in siblings compared with 0% in controls. Jorde et al. (1991), reporting data from a large-scale Utah family study, reported a recurrence risk of 3.7% if the first autistic child was male and 7.0% if female. It may be concluded that the rate in siblings is probably in the region of 3% to 7%, which represents a

50-fold to 100-fold increase in risk. Although it does not seem likely that this could be environmentally mediated, family studies cannot separate genetic and nongenetic influences, and it is necessary to turn to twin data.

There have been three general-population-based twin studies of idiopathic autism. Folstein and Rutter (1977a, 1977b), in a British study, found a 36% pairwise concordance rate in monozygotic (MZ) twins and a 0% rate in same-sex dizygotic (DZ) twins. Steffenburg et al. (1989), in a Nordic study, reported a 91% pairwise concordance rate for autism in MZ twins and a 0% concordance rate in same sex DZ twins. In a more recent British study, Bailey et al. (1995) found an MZ pairwise concordance rate of 69%, and, again, 0% in DZ pairs. Pooling the two British studies, and using the rate of autism among the siblings of autistic singletons as the basis for the DZ rate, Bailey et al. (1995) calculated a heritability of 91% to 93% for an underlying liability to autism (the variation in estimate stemmed from different assumptions about the base rate of autism). Clearly, this represents a very strong genetic component. Several issues should be tackled before concluding that the genetic effect is as strong as these calculations seem to indicate. To begin with, the possibility that the findings could stem, at least in part, from obstetric complications needs to be considered. This possibility particularly arises because both the original Folstein and Rutter (1977a, 1977b) study, and the study by Steffenburg et al. (1989), showed that obstetric complications differentiated twins with autism from their cotwins without autism. In both studies, this was interpreted as indicating the possible role of environmentally induced brain damage. This possibility now seems unlikely for the following reasons:

1. Most of the obstetric complications were quite minor, the association with obstetric complications in singletons is weak, and it mainly applies to minor complications (Nelson, 1991; Tsai, 1987).
2. The association in singletons may be a function of maternal parity (Piven et al., 1993), although this seemed not to be so in the study by Bolton et al. (in press).
3. Within the Bailey et al. (1995) twin sample, obstetric complications were associated

with congenital anomalies, most of which were likely to derive from aberrations in early pregnancy.

4. In the Bolton et al. (1994, in press) family study, the familial loading was greater in the case of autistic subjects with obstetric complications.

Other evidence has shown that genetically abnormal fetuses (e.g., with Down syndrome) may give rise to an increased rate of obstetric and perinatal complications (Bolton & Holland, 1994). The totality of the evidence strongly suggests that the minor obstetric complications derive from a genetically abnormal fetus rather than from an environmental risk process (Bolton et al., in press). Isolated cases of autism may stem from neonatal brain damage that is associated with serious perinatal complications or very low-birth-weight, but such cases seem to be uncommon.

A further approach to the possible role of physical environmental factors is provided by a study of various specific infectious risks. Probably the best documented is a report by Chess, Korn, and Fernandez (1971) that autism is quite common in children with congenital rubella. However, the significance of this finding was modified by follow-up data (Chess, 1977) indicating that, as they grew older, many of the children with congenital rubella ceased to exhibit autism (a rare occurrence among autistic persons). In its course and, to some extent, in the details of its clinical features, the autism associated with rubella is atypical. Because congenital rubella is uncommon these days, it could constitute only a rare cause of autism. Deykin and MacMahon (1979) undertook a systematic study of possible associations with maternal infections during pregnancy, but the results were essentially negative. Several studies have reported seasonal variations in the births of children with autism and this has been taken to suggest an environmental pathogen may be operative during pregnancy (e.g., Gillberg & Coleman, 1992). Bolton et al. (1992) examined the postulated association in detail and concluded that it was far less definite than had been claimed and that it does not provide strong evidence for an environmental cause. A possible association between autism and the cytomegalovirus has been suggested, but this is, at best, a quite infrequent cause of autism (Gillberg & Coleman, 1992). Cases of autism associated with postnatal encephalitis have also been reported, but they, too, appear quite rare.

Psychosocial environmental risk factors are only rarely influential (see reviews by Cantwell, Rutter, & Baker, 1978; Koegel, Schreibman, O'Neill, & Burke, 1983). Early suggestions that autism might be an effect of parental neglect, rejection, or indifference have long since been abandoned. Numerous studies have failed to show any association between autism and qualities of upbringing or frequency of stress experiences. Accordingly, it seems most unlikely that environmentally mediated psychological experiences play any significant role in autism. An apparent exception to that widely accepted generalization is provided by a report (Rutter and the ERA team, 1997, submitted) that some children adopted from Romanian orphanages into UK families exhibited an autistic-like syndrome. Although this was very much a minority pattern, the rate was clearly raised in relation to the general population. Nevertheless, its relevance in relation to the broad run of autism is very doubtful because the clinical pattern was usually atypical in certain important features and, more especially, because the autistic features often faded as the children grew older. The children had suffered quite exceptional physical and psychological privation and it is not clear which aspect of their early experiences led to their being at risk for this atypical pattern. Grossly depriving experiences are not ordinarily found among autistic individuals. In general, psychosocial stressors and adversities play no significant role in the etiology of autism.

Another approach is provided by examination of the concordance rate in MZ pairs. The 91% pairwise concordance rate for autism in MZ twins, found by Steffenburg et al. (1989), would seem to leave little room for nongenetic influences, whereas the 69% pairwise concordance rate found by Bailey et al. (1995) allows more scope. However, as discussed below, the great majority of the non-autistic twins in discordant MZ pairs showed cognitive and social deficits of autistic quality, albeit of lesser degree. It may be concluded that, in the great majority of cases of autism, genetic influences predominate in the etiology of autism.

What Is the Phenotype?

The findings discussed so far all apply to autism as traditionally diagnosed. Folstein and Rutter (1977a, 1977b) noted, however, that most of the MZ pairs that were not concordant for autism were concordant for some type of cognitive deficit, usually involving language delay. By contrast, this applied to only 1 in 10 of the discordant DZ pairs. The implication was that it might not be autism as such that was inherited, but rather some broader type of cognitive abnormality including, but not restricted to, autism. The more recent British twin study undertaken by Bailey et al. (1995) found the same but also demonstrated that the cognitive deficits were usually associated with a persistent social impairment that continued into adult life (Le Couteur et al., 1996). Of the MZ pairs, 76% were concordant for a *combined* social and cognitive disorder, compared with 0% of the DZ pairs. Conversely, in only 8% of MZ pairs was the cotwin *without* either a social or a cognitive disorder, compared with 90% of the DZ pairs.

The family studies have also strongly suggested that the genetic liability applies to a range of social and cognitive abnormalities in individuals of normal intelligence. These abnormalities are very similar in quality to those found in autism, but they are very different in degree of handicap (for reviews, see Bolton et al., 1994; Folstein & Piven, 1991; Rutter et al., 1993). A parallel may be drawn with the association between schizophrenia and schizotypal personality disorder (Kendler, Gruenberg, & Kinney, 1994). Bolton et al. (1994) found that between 12% and 20% of the siblings of autistic probands (compared with 2% to 3% of the Down syndrome siblings) exhibited this lesser variant of autism. The exact figures were dependent on the stringency of definition. Other family studies vary in the extent to which the disorders in relatives have involved social, language, and/or cognitive deficits.

There has been some variability in whether these are mainly evident in parents or in siblings, but nearly all have shown a much

increased rate of abnormalities (Landa, Piven, Wzorek, Gayle, Chase, & Folstein, 1992; Landa, Wzorek, Piven, Folstein, & Isaacs, 1991; Murphy, Bolton, Pickles, & Rutter, 1997, submitted; Narayan, Moyes, & Wolff, 1990; Piven et al., 1994; Silliman, Campbell, & Mitchell, 1989; Wolff, Narayan, & Moyes, 1988). Thus, the social characteristics have included a lack of empathy, rapport, and emotional responsiveness; hypersensitivity; and single-minded pursuit of special interests. Communication difficulties have primarily involved pragmatic deficiencies, overcommunicativeness and undercommunicativeness, excessive guardedness and disinhibition. Language-related cognitive deficits have also been present but, strikingly, neither mental retardation nor general cognitive impairment has been evident (Fombonne, Bolton, Prior, Jordan, & Rutter, in press; Freeman et al., 1989; Szatmari, Jones, Tuff, Bartolucci, Fisman, & Mahoney, 1993). Perhaps surprisingly, the pattern of verbal and visuospatial skills is not helpful in the diagnosis of the broader phenotype of autism and, possibly, the relatives of autistic individuals may tend to have slightly superior verbal skills, rather than the verbal deficits that are characteristic of autism itself (Fombonne et al., in press).

Only two studies have yielded essentially negative findings. Gillberg, Gillberg, and Steffenburg (1992) found few differences in a rather small-scale study, but over one-third of their sample had a known medical syndrome and half were severely retarded. Szatmari et al. (1993) compared the unaffected siblings and parents of 52 probands with PDD and 33 Down's syndrome and low-birth-weight controls. No significant differences were found between the groups. It is not clear why the findings are so different from most of the other studies, but it is notable that the probands were clinically more heterogeneous, and the findings on siblings were not internally coherent. For example, speech delay was nearly three times as common in the siblings of PDD subjects (16.3% versus 6.8%), but reading problems were far less frequent (3.8% versus 20.5%). Rates of special education were also very high in both groups (10.0% in the PDD subjects and 18.2% in the controls). In addition, Spiker et al. (1994), in their study of multiplex families, argued that autism was either present or absent, and there was no need to involve the concept of a broader phenotype. However, their own data showed a substantial number of individuals who were clearly not autistic (at least as usually diagnosed) but were equally far from normal (see Le Couteur et al., 1996).

Although there are some inconsistencies, the twin and family studies, taken together, strongly suggest that the autism phenotype extends well beyond the traditional diagnosis. The extension involves characteristics that are closely similar to autism in quality but markedly different in degree, and which are found in individuals of normal intelligence. The clinical picture chiefly differs from autism (as traditionally diagnosed) in the following ways: lack of abnormal nonpragmatic language features (such as pronominal reversal and delayed echolalia); less striking stereotyped repetitive behavioral patterns; subtler social deficits; and lack of an association with epilepsy. Nevertheless, there are three main reasons for confidence in the assumption that this clinical picture is indeed part of autism: (a) the social abnormalities have been found to persist into adult life; (b) the concordance in MZ pairs for the broader phenotype, even after exclusion of autism and PDD, is much higher than in DZ pairs (Le Couteur et al., 1996); and (c) family data show a much increased loading for the broader phenotype compared with Down syndrome families (see, e.g., Bolton et al., 1994).

The boundaries of the broader phenotype remain to be determined. Questions remain on whether it may be evident in language abnormalities, social deficits, or circumscribed interest patterns in isolation, or whether its manifestation requires two or more of these. In each of this trio of abnormalities, what specific qualities are pathognomonic of autism? Even more basic, are such features categorically present or absent, or are they more appropriately considered in terms of a dimension? There is a need to differentiate the broader phenotype (or lesser variant) of autism from other forms of social abnormality and especially from schizotypal personality disorder, a quite different disorder that is associated with schizophrenia rather than with autism. (The broader phenotype of autism appears clinically different, as follows: it is first manifest in early childhood; it is associated with circumscribed interests rather than ideas of reference, magical thinking, and unusual perceptual experiences; and deficits in social reciprocity and pragmatic aspects of communication are prominent. However, systematic comparisons have yet to be undertaken.) Some means of validation of the broader phenotype of autism would be helpful. Potentially, this validation might be provided by patterns of psychological abnormality (with respect, for example, to "theory of mind," executive planning, central coherence, or pragmatic aspects of language; see Bailey, Phillips, & Rutter, 1996), but that research remains a task for the future.

More surprisingly, several studies (Bolton, Pickles, Murphy, & Rutter, 1997, submitted; DeLong, 1994; DeLong & Nohria, 1994; Murphy et al., 1997, submitted; Piven et al., 1990; Smalley, McCracken, & Tanguay, 1995) have reported an apparently increased familial loading for affective disorders and for social phobia/anxiety traits and disorders, but it is not yet clear whether this is genetically mediated. Smalley et al. (1995) compared 36 families with an autistic child with 21 families with a nonautistic child who showed either tuberous sclerosis or epilepsy. Major affective disorder was three times as common in the first-degree relatives of the autistic individuals. In nearly two-thirds of the parents with affective disorder, the onset preceded the birth of an autistic child. Social phobia was also much increased in the autism families when the autism was unaccompanied by mental retardation. Bolton et al. (1997, submitted), using both standardized interview (Schedule for Affective Disorders and Schizophrenia Lifetime Version (SADS-L) and pedigree methods, showed that the raised rate of major affective disorders in the first- and second-degree relatives of autistic individuals, compared with the relatives of individuals with Down syndrome, was not a function of the broader phenotype as defined in terms of cognitive and social abnormalities. Moreover, unlike the broader phenotype, affective disorder was more frequent in females and had a different pattern of correlates.

At first sight, it would seem unlikely that autism and affective disorders could constitute different manifestations of the same underlying genotype. Rather, the increased familial loading for depressive disorders might reflect the strains and stresses associated with rearing an autistic child and there is some evidence that, possibly, this may constitute part of the explanation (Bolton et al., 1997, submitted). Nevertheless, despite the apparent implausibility of the association, four findings suggest that it may be real: (a) the increase in affective disorders applies to second-degree, as well as first-degree, relatives; (b) the increase applies to bipolar and severe unipolar disorders as much as to milder depressive disorders; (c) the increase applies to affective disorders with an onset before the birth of the autistic individual as well as those arising afterwards; and (d) the increase has been noted in studies using quite different samples. Accordingly, although few of the investigations included adequate controls, the apparent association between autism and affective disorders clearly requires further study. One crucial test would be provided by examining the association from a different perspective. If autism and major depression are truly genetically associated, there should be an increased loading for autism in the families of individuals with major depressive disorders (although the low base rate of autism would make this difficult to detect). There are no reports that that is the case but systematic studies have yet to be undertaken. If the association between autism and affective disorders is confirmed, it will be important to examine competing hypotheses on the underlying mechanisms. Bolton et al. (1997, submitted) showed that the raised rate of affective disorders was probably not just a function of the broader phenotype as defined in terms of cognitive and social abnormalities. Nevertheless, there are many possibilities of artifact in the findings, and further research is needed both to test the reality of the association and to investigate its meaning if confirmed.

In addition, there have been suggestions that the phenotype should be extended to include Tourette's syndrome (Comings & Comings, 1991) and anorexia nervosa (Gillberg, 1992) but in neither case is the evidence particularly convincing.

Given the likelihood that the phenotype does extend beyond autism, questions must be raised about the connections between autism as traditionally diagnosed and the so-called lesser variant. The latter shares a number of features with autism proper; for example, it, too, is much more common in males than in females (although this is less true of the milder degrees of the phenotype), and the features are usually evident from early childhood onward. On the other hand, there are at least two marked differences; (a) the relatives who showed this broader phenotype in the various studies have been of normal intelligence, and (b) no association with epilepsy has been found. This could represent simply a lower "dose" of the genetic predisposition, but the possibility of some kind of "two-hit" mechanism must also be considered; that is, one set of causal factors may predispose to the broader phenotype, and a separate set of causal factors may be involved in the transition to the handicapping condition of autism proper. At one time, it was thought that this second step might involve perinatal complications (Folstein & Rutter, 1977a, 1977b; Steffenburg et al., 1989), but, for the reasons given above, that possibility now seems unlikely. The issue is unresolved, but there is an apparent paradox in the fact that most cases of autism occur in individuals who are also mentally retarded and who have a much increased rate of epilepsy, but the familial loading mainly involves qualitatively similar abnormalities in individuals without epilepsy and of normal intelligence.

GENETIC HETEROGENEITY

The history of medical genetics strongly suggests that genetic heterogeneity is to be expected in autism. There are numerous examples of different genetic abnormalities all leading to what appears to be the same clinical picture. Thus, as already noted, some cases of tuberous sclerosis are associated with a gene locus on chromosome 9, and others are associated with a locus on chromosome 16. Other neurological conditions show even greater genetic heterogeneity (see Simonoff et al., 1996). Some genetic heterogeneity has already been demonstrated insofar as autism is associated with the Fragile X anomaly, tuberous sclerosis, and various other genetic conditions. Claims have been made that more than one-third of cases of autism are associated with such known medical conditions (Gillberg, 1992) but review of the evidence suggests that the true rate of known medical conditions in autism is probably about 10% (Rutter et al., 1994). On the other hand, the rate may be higher in atypical cases of autism and in autism associated with profound mental retardation. The question then is whether there are currently any clinical indicators of heterogeneity in the remaining 90% of cases of idiopathic autism. One way to tackle this issue is to examine the variabilities in clinical expression within MZ pairs, a strategy followed by Le Couteur and colleagues (1996). In brief, they compared the variability within MZ pairs with the variability between MZ pairs. If the clinical variations index genetic heterogeneity, it would be expected that the between-pair variation should be much greater than the within-pair variation. That is because MZ cotwins will necessarily share all their genes whereas that will not be the case across pairs. The findings showed that, with respect to both autistic symptoms and verbal IQ, there was almost as much variation within pairs as there was between pairs. Differences in verbal and nonverbal IQ within concordant MZ pairs ranged up to more than 50 points. These findings strongly pointed to a wide range of phenotypic expression and provided few clinical pointers on possible clinical indicators of genetic heterogeneity. One possible exception was provided by epilepsy where there was a greater tendency for concordance within pairs. On the other hand, the presence of epilepsy was not associated with any other indications of meaningful differences, and the Bolton et al. (1994) family study showed no variation in familial loading by epilepsy. Spiker et al. (1994) used a somewhat similar strategy with respect to differences between affected family members in families that were multiplex for autism. Again, substantial variation within

pairs of affected relatives was found for both clinical features and IQ. It may be concluded that the *same* genes involved in liability to autism can give rise to a surprisingly wide range of clinical manifestations. The same evidence makes it unlikely that the several different genes involved in autism (see below) give rise to different facets of the clinical syndrome.

There is some slight suggestion that autism associated either with profound mental retardation or with a lack of useful spoken language may be different. Thus, Bolton et al. (1994) found that, although the familial loading was strongly associated with the symptom score in verbal probands, this was not so in those without useful language. August and his colleagues (August, Stewart, & Tsai, 1981; Baird & August, 1985) found a raised rate of severe mental retardation in the siblings of autistic probands who were also severely retarded, something that has not been evident in any of the studies of less retarded subjects. Their findings were based on a very small number of cases and cannot be taken as anything more than a possibility worth examining further. About one-third of autistic individuals have hyperserotoninaemia, and there is some evidence that this may be a familial trait to some extent (Cook, 1990). Although untested, this might prove to be a marker of genetic heterogeneity; but again, this is no more than a suggestion worth following up. Genetic heterogeneity is likely to be proven eventually but, so far, there are no strong leads on how this might be indexed in terms of phenotypic characteristics, and variable expression will make its identification a hard task.

ARE THE GENETIC INFLUENCES AUTISM-SPECIFIC?

A somewhat related question is whether the genetic influences are autism-specific. Clearly they are not to the extent that autism is secondary to conditions such as tuberous sclerosis or the Fragile X anomaly, but these account for only 1 in 10 cases. It has been suggested that autism is no more than a final common pathway for a heterogeneous range of etiological processes and that there is no point in searching for autism-specific causal factors (Coleman,

1990; Gillberg, 1992). The available evidence, however, suggests that this conclusion is not valid. Four key sets of data are relevant:

1. Neither brain pathology nor mental retardation carries a consistent risk for autism. Some conditions (such as cerebral palsy or Down syndrome) carry only a small additional risk (but see Howlin, Wing, & Gould, 1995); for others (such as tuberous sclerosis), the risk is much higher.
2. The twin and family studies show strong associations with a relatively specific pattern of social and cognitive deficits, but not with mental retardation or brain disease more generally.
3. The concordance for the broader phenotype of autism in MZ pairs is very high (over 90%).
4. Although there is considerable variability of phenotypic expression within MZ pairs (and within multiplex families), the variability is within the range of autistic features and does not extend to other psychiatric manifestations of brain pathology. Also, both twin and family studies have failed to find any association between autism and cognitive impairment when the latter is not accompanied by autism.

In the great majority of cases, the genetic influences are likely to prove to be autism-specific, even though it is probable that they will be multiple.

Mode of Genetic Transmission

The last issue with respect to genetics concerns the mode of genetic transmission. A segregation analysis undertaken by Ritvo et al. (1985), using families that had two or more affected siblings, suggested autosomal recessive inheritance and apparently ruled out a multifactorial model. However, the biased nature of the sample, together with a nonexclusion of cases due to known medical conditions and uncertainties about diagnosis (including a failure to take into account the possibility of a broader phenotype), calls for caution in accepting the conclusions. Also, a further study by the same research group (Jorde et al., 1990) produced a different set of conclusions. An additional complication may be the tendency of families to stop having children after an autistic child is borne (Jones & Szatmari, 1988), although this was not found by Bolton et al. (1994) in a study with limited statistical power to detect the effect. Altogether, the evidence suggests that multiple interacting genes are a much more likely cause than a single gene operating in Mendelian fashion. Two main findings point to that conclusion. First, there is a marked decline in rate, going from MZ cotwins to DZ cotwins or siblings (Bailey et al., 1995; Folstein & Rutter, 1977a, 1977b; Steffenburg et al., 1989), and a further decline occurs going from first-degree to second-degree relatives (Jorde et al., 1990; Pickles et al., 1995; Pickles, Bolton, Macdonald, Rios, Storoschuk, & Rutter, 1997, submitted). Using a development of the Risch (1990) approach based on a decline in rates, Pickles et al. (1995) estimated that a three-gene model was most likely, although the range could be anywhere between two and ten genes. The rationale for this inference is that, whereas MZ twins share all their genes and therefore all combinations of genes, DZ twins (or singleton siblings), on average share only half their genes. This necessarily means that they will share only one-quarter of any specified two-gene combinations and only one-eighth of any specified three-gene combinations. Hence, the marked decline suggests the likelihood that particular combinations of genes underlie autism, and not just one major gene. However, the estimate of approximately three genes provides only a rough guide to the likely number because the calculations are necessarily affected by the strength of effect of each gene and by the degree of genetic heterogeneity.

Second, Bolton et al. (1994) found that the familial loading increased with the severity of the autism as measured in terms of the number of autism-diagnostic interview algorithm symptoms. This, too, suggests that the severity indexes the number of genes. However, this finding does not tally well with the hypothesis that *specific combinations* of genes are required for autism to occur. The one finding that does not seem consistent with that model is that the familial loading seems only slightly greater in the families of female autistic subjects (the sex difference is nonsignificant in

94 ∎

most studies). This is apparently inconsistent because a multifactorial threshold model leads to the expectation that the loading should be higher in the less often affected sex—namely females. On the other hand, the statistical power to detect a sex difference was low in all studies, and the matter remains unresolved (see Rutter et al., 1993).

SCREENING FOR GENETIC ABNORMALITIES

A key clinical issue that derives from the genetic findings is what assessments, or investigations, should be undertaken as part of the initial diagnostic assessment. The first requirement is to combine a careful, systematic, searching of clinical history with a thorough medical examination. Particular attention needs to be paid to the possibility of tuberous sclerosis, and this requires careful examination of dermatological features. Use of Wood's light when looking for depigmented leaf-shaped maculas is essential, because differential diagnosis is often quite difficult on the basis of inspection alone. If epileptic seizures have occurred, a skull X ray or CT scan (to look for calcified lesions), as well as an EEG, may be informative, although a negative picture does not rule out tuberous sclerosis. Chromosomal examination, together with DNA study for the Fragile X anomaly, should be undertaken routinely. Although only some 5% of cases of autism are associated with Fragile X, the implications are sufficiently important to rule it out (or identify it) in all cases. As noted, some 1 in 20 other cases of autism may have associated chromosome anomalies, and this is a sufficient ratio to justify screening for them. However, in most cases, their clinical meaning is quite uncertain, and a major etiological role should not necessarily be assumed.

It has been traditional in many medical centers to screen all individuals presenting with either autism or mental retardation for metabolic abnormalities (using a range of urinary and blood tests). Clearly, screening *is* indicated if the clinical history or examination suggests the possibility of a medical condition that would be detected by these means. On the other hand, because the detection rate in the absence of clinical indications is so low as to cast doubt on the value of routine

screening (Scott, 1994), the use of such screening now needs to be re-evaluated (Bailey, 1994).

Some commentators (e.g., Gillberg, 1990) have even recommended the routine use of cerebrospinal fluid (CSF) examinations and brain scans. Although it is important not to miss etiologically relevant medical conditions, there is a lack of evidence that these more invasive or stressful investigations detect diseases that would otherwise be missed. We recommend that they should be undertaken only if there are clinical indications.

The personal history should include a detailed account of the pregnancy and neonatal period, always supplemented by the medical records made at the time. The crucial issue is not so much whether obstetric or perinatal complications occurred, as whether they were associated at the time with either brain-imaging evidence of brain damage (usually through ultrasound studies) or clinical evidence of the same (neonatal convulsions, neurological abnormalities, and so on).

GENETIC COUNSELING

Families should be given information on the role of genetic factors in autism, and genetic counseling should be made available to those who request it. Such counseling needs to start with a careful diagnostic assessment, because some individuals thought to have autism turn out to have some other disorder when a systematic evaluation is undertaken. If the autism is causally associated with some genetically determined medical condition (such as the Fragile X or tuberous sclerosis), the genetic risks should be discussed in terms of that condition. Also, when it is possible to test relatives directly (as is the case, for example, with the Fragile X anomaly), this possibility should be offered. Knowledge of patterns of Mendelian inheritance allows quantitative advice on risks when the mode of inheritance is known (see Simonoff, McGuffin, & Gottesman, 1994). However, the possibility of new mutations (common with tuberous sclerosis) and the effects of intergenerational change (as with the Fragile X, in which the risk of having an affected child seems to be related to the number of maternal trinucleatide repeats;

95

Handbook of Autism and Pervasive Developmental Disorders, eds D.J. Cohen & F.R. Volkmar, 1997, pp. 370–387

Warren & Nelson, 1994) should be carefully taken into account.

In the great majority of cases, however, autism is not associated with any known medical condition. In these circumstances, counseling is less straightforward. The first task is usually to explain that although the *relative* risk of autism in other family members is very greatly raised in relation to the general population, the *absolute* risk is rather low. Thus, if the issue is risk of recurrence with respect to future children born to the same biological parents, this can be stated as an approximate increase of 50 to 100 times overall, but still only a 1-in-20 chance. Because, at first hearing, that fact is hard to grasp, it is usually helpful to go on to explain, in simple terms, how this arises with conditions in which combinations of several genes are required. Although it is not known for certain that that is so with autism, it appears very likely, and this should be explained.

Several other issues need to be considered. Families will want to know whether the risks in their particular family are greater or less than the overall average. That question rarely has an easy answer. It seems reasonable to suppose that the risks may be lower if the autism is associated with some definite nongenetic cause, but that inference is not straightforward. In the unusual circumstance that such a definite cause can be identified (as with congenital rubella or early encephalitis), a lower risk can reasonably be assumed. More commonly, however, the story is one of obstetric complications, or an onset following immunization or some unknown fever. In this situation, the inferred causal role is usually in doubt. Unless there is contemporaneous clinical or imaging evidence of organic brain pathology, it would be unwise to assume a nongenetic etiology (Bailey, 1994). In particular, mild obstetric complications may derive from a genetically abnormal fetus (see above) and not reflect any environmental risk mechanism. Again, great caution should be exercised in making any causal inference. There is no convincing evidence that autism can be caused by any ordinarily stressful life circumstances (such as hospital admission, family discord, or loss of an attachment figure). In rare instances, an autism-like syndrome can develop as a result of unusually severe and prolonged physical and psychological privation, but, even here, the clinical picture is usually somewhat atypical. Nevertheless, in this very rare circumstance, a lower risk may be inferred.

Equally important is the need to consider whether the absence of any case of autism, including its broader phenotype, in the extended family lowers the risk, or, conversely, whether the occurrence of several such cases increases the risk. Two problems immediately arise. First, there is bound to be huge individual variation across families in the number of affected members. Accordingly, an unusually high or low familial loading does not necessarily mean anything and little weight can be attached to it. That is especially the case with respect to a lack of other affected members in the family because this will often be so simply because autism has a low base rate.

Second, given the considerable uncertainties regarding the boundaries of the broader phenotype it may be quite difficult to decide which family members are affected. Thus, there will necessarily be doubt about whether to include isolated instances of severe language delay or social oddity in the absence of a clear indication that these are autistic in type. The main situation in which the possibility of an increased risk needs to be considered is when there are definite cases of autism on both sides of the family or when one or both parents are themselves affected. Even here, empirical evidence is lacking that the risk is actually increased, although it would seem prudent to assume that it may be. The absence of a family loading, however, should not be taken to imply a reduced risk.

A further consideration is whether the risk needs to be adjusted up or down on the grounds that the autism is atypical in some respect, or that it is unusually severe or unusually mild. Bolton et al. (1994) found that, other things being equal, the risks tended to be greater if the autism was severe, although possibly not so much greater if the affected individual was nonverbal. There is also some slight suggestion (see above) that at least some cases of autism associated with profound mental retardation may be genetically different (although that does not necessarily mean that the *level* of risk is different). The point is an important one, but, in the present state of knowledge, there are no solid grounds for concluding that the risk is any different (although it may be so) when the clinical picture is atypical in some way or is unusually mild.

Queries often arise regarding four particular points. First, families want to know whether any investigations can be undertaken to measure or identify genetic risk. At the present time, regrettably, no such test is possible in idiopathic cases, although identification of the gene should make that possible, and, with the advances in molecular genetics, that is likely to happen during the next decade. Second, a frequent concern centers on possible risks to the offspring of nonaffected siblings (i.e., nephews or nieces or second-degree relatives). The few available data on second-degree relatives (Jorde et al., 1991; Pickles et al., 1997, submitted) indicate a rate of probably less than 1 in 500. However, the figure is necessarily a most uncertain one, and it is unclear how much the risk is influenced by the fact that parents are likely to have been selected on the basis of not being affected (or being less affected) themselves (see Pickles et al., 1997, submitted). The limited available evidence suggests that siblings who exhibit all but the mildest phenotypic expression are less likely than unaffected siblings to marry (or cohabit) and have children.

A third query concerns the risks in other family members for milder problems that are part of the autistic spectrum but not autism as traditionally diagnosed. The family and twin data (Bailey et al., 1995; Bolton et al., 1994) indicate that the risks are substantially greater than for autism itself, but, given the uncertainties over how far the broader phenotype extends, no precise figure is possible. Probably, however, the risk in siblings for the lesser manifestations of autism may be in the 10% to 20% range. It should be emphasized to families that most such affected individuals are *not* seriously handicapped, and the great majority go on to live fulfilling lives as independent and self-sufficient adults.

The fourth query concerns whether some *specific* family member (usually a sibling) who has been delayed in speaking, or is socially unusual, or has idiosyncratic circumscribed interests, does or does not suffer from some

variant of autism. Often, that question constitutes a quite difficult clinical decision. The only guideline is that the closer the specific social or communicative qualities of the deficit or abnormality are to those found in autism, and the greater the extent to which the abnormalities extend across all three domains of reciprocal social relationships, communication, and repetitive or stereotyped interest patterns, the greater the likelihood that the picture does represent autism. Because autism is so strongly associated with specific cognitive patterns (see Bailey et al., 1996), there is the possibility that the diagnosis of the broader phenotype could be validated through cognitive testing (see above). That is quite likely to become possible in the future, but it will require adaptation of the cognitive tests to make them suitable for nonhandicapped individuals of normal intelligence.

Three other points need to be made about genetic counseling:

1. If is often helpful to put the risks into perspective by expressing them in positive terms (i.e., a 19-out-of-20 chance that a future child will *not* be autistic).
2. It is not the job of the counselor to make decisions for the family. Rather, his/her responsibility is to provide the family with (a) the factual information that will allow them to come to their own decisions, and (b) the clinical context in which there can be a sensitive discussion of the dilemmas involved and the individual family members' own feelings about them.
3. There must be ethical concern over the inappropriateness of counseling one family member on behalf of some other member who has not asked for such information (including those who are still too young to ask for genetic counseling).

CLINICAL VALUE OF GENETIC KNOWLEDGE

At present, genetic influences are known to be strong in autism, the precise genetic mechanisms involved have yet to be determined. That situation is likely to change during the next decade as a result of advances in molecular genetics (see Bailey et al., 1996; Rutter,

1994). Accordingly, it is necessary to consider the usefulness of identifying the gene (or, more likely, several genes) involved in a liability to autism. Merely knowing where such genes are to be found (i.e., their loci on particular chromosomes) will not in itself be clinically very useful. The point, however, is that this constitutes a necessary first step in order to identify the gene itself, and the identification, in turn, constitutes a key step in the search for how the gene leads to autism. In other words, it will then be possible to determine the gene product and find out *how* that leads to autism; whether specific environmental features interact with genetic susceptibility, and why the cognitive impairment associated with autism varies from severe and general to mild and specific. An understanding of that process is likely to carry very important implications for prevention and treatment. Therein lies the enormous potential value of molecular genetics.

CONCLUSION

Our understanding of the role of genetic factors in the liability to autism has increased greatly over the last decade, although basic questions have yet to be answered. It is now clear that genetic factors play a very important role in the causation of autism; indeed, autism is probably the most strongly genetic of all non-Mendelian psychiatric disorders. Evidence has also shown that the phenotype extends beyond (perhaps quite a long way beyond) autism as traditionally diagnosed, and that several (but probably a small number of) interacting genes are responsible. In a minority of cases, however, autism arises on the basis of some single-gene medical condition. These findings already have important implications for the diagnosis of autism and for genetic counseling, and they need to be appreciated by practitioners as well as researchers. Identification of the precise genetic mechanisms will have an even greater impact on clinical practice.

Cross-References

Neurological aspects of autism and medical conditions frequently associated with autism are discussed in Chapters 16 and 18.

REFERENCES

August, G.J., Stewart, M.A., & Tsai, L. (1981). The incidence of cognitive disabilities in the siblings of autistic children. *British Journal of Psychiatry, 138,* 416–422.

Bailey, A.J. (1994). Physical examination and medical investigations. In M. Rutter, E. Taylor, & L. Hersov (Eds.), *Child and adolescent psychiatry: Modern approaches* (3rd ed., pp. 79–93). Oxford: Blackwell Scientific.

Bailey, A.J., Bolton, P., Butler, L., Le Couteur, A., Murphy, M., Scott, S., Webb, T., & Rutter, M. (1993). Prevalence of the Fragile X anomaly amongst autistic twins and singletons. *Journal of Child Psychology and Psychiatry, 34,* 673–688.

Bailey, A., Le Couteur, A., Gottesman, I., Bolton, P., Simonoff, E., Yuzda, E., & Rutter, M. (1995). Autism as a strongly genetic disorder: Evidence from a British twin study. *Psychological Medicine, 25,* 63–78.

Bailey, A., Phillips, W., & Rutter, M. (1996). Autism: Towards an integration of clinical, genetic, neuropsychological and neurobiological perspectives. *Journal of Child Psychology and Psychiatry Annual Research Review, 37,* 89–126.

Baird, T.D., & August, G.J. (1985). Familial heterogeneity in infantile autism. *Journal of Autism and Developmental Disorders, 15,* 315–321.

Baker, P., Piven, J., Schwartz, S., & Patil, S. (1994). Duplication of chromosome 15q11-13 in two individuals with autistic disorder. *Journal of Autism and Developmental Disorders, 24,* 529–535.

Blomquist, H.K., Bohman, M., Edvinsson, S.O., Gillberg, C., Gustavson, K.H., Holmgren, G., & Wahlström, J. (1985). Frequency of the Fragile X syndrome in infantile autism: A Swedish multicenter study. *Clinical Genetics, 27,* 113–117.

Bolton, P., & Holland, A. (1994). Chromosomal abnormalities. In M. Rutter, E. Taylor, & L. Hersov (Eds.), *Child and adolescent psychiatry: Modern approaches* (3rd ed., pp. 152–171). Oxford: Blackwell Scientific.

Bolton, P., MacDonald, H., Pickles, A., Rios, P., Goode, S., Crowson, M., Bailey, A., & Rutter, M. (1994). A case-control family history study of autism. *Journal of Child Psychology and Psychiatry, 35,* 877–900.

Bolton, P., Murphy, M., MacDonald, H., Whitlock, B., Pickles, A., & Rutter, M. (in press). Obstetric complications in autism: Consequences or causes of the condition. *Journal of*

98

the American Academy of Child and Adolescent Psychiatry.

Bolton, P., Pickles, A., Murphy, M., & Rutter, M. (1997, submitted). *Autism, affective and other psychiatric disorders: Patterns of familial aggregation.*

Bolton, P., Pickles, A., Rutter, M., Butler, L., Summers, S., Lord, C., & Webb, T. (1992). Fragile X in families multiplex for autism and autism-related phenotypes: Prevalence and criteria for cytogenetic diagnosis. *Psychiatric Genetics, 2,* 277–300.

Bolton, P., & Rutter, M. (1990). Genetic influences in autism. *International Review of Psychiatry, 2,* 65–78.

Brown, W.T., Jenkins, E.C., Cohen, I.L., Fisch, G.S., Wolf-Schein, E.G., Gross, A., Waterhouse, L., Fein, D., Mason-Brothers, A., Ritvo, E. et al. (1986). Fragile X and autism: A multicenter survey. *American Journal of Medical Genetics, 23,* 341–352.

Cantwell, D., Rutter, M., & Baker, L. (1978). Family factors. In M. Rutter & E. Schopler (Eds.), *Autism: A reappraisal of concepts and treatment* (pp. 269–296). New York: Plenum.

Chess, S. (1977). Follow-up report on autism in congenital rubella. *Journal of Autism and Childhood Schizophrenia, 7,* 68–81.

Chess, S., Korn, S.J., & Fernandez, P.B. (1971). *Psychiatric disorders of children with congenital rubella.* New York: Brunner/Mazel.

Cohen, I.L., Vietze, P.M., Sudhalter, V., Jenkins, E.C., & Brown, W.T. (1989). Parent-child dyadic gaze patterns in Fragile X males and in non-Fragile X males with autistic disorder. *Journal of Child Psychology and Psychiatry, 30,* 845–856.

Coleman, M. (1990). Is classical Rett Syndrome ever present in males? *Brain and Development, 12,* 31–32.

Comings, D.E., & Comings, B.G. (1991). Clinical and genetic relationships between autism-pervasive developmental disorder and Tourette Syndrome: A study of 19 cases. *American Journal of Medical Genetics, 39,* 180–191.

Cook, E.H. (1990). Autism: Review of neurochemical investigations. *Synapse, 6,* 292–308.

Davies, K. (1991). Breaking the Fragile-X. *Nature, 351,* 439–440.

DeLong, R. (1994). Children with autistic spectrum disorder and a family history of affective disorder. *Developmental Medicine & Child Neurology, 36,* 674–687.

DeLong, R., & Nohria, C. (1994). Psychiatric family history and neurological disease in autistic spectrum disorders. *Developmental Medicine & Child Neurology, 36,* 441–448.

Deykin, E.Y., & MacMahon, B. (1979). The incidence of seizures among children with autistic symptoms. *American Journal of Psychiatry, 136,* 1310–1312.

Einfeld, S., Malony, H., & Hall, W. (1989). Autism is not associated with the Fragile X syndrome. *American Journal of Medical Genetics, 34,* 187–193.

European Chromosome 16 TS Consortium. (1993). Identification and characterization of the tuberous sclerosis gene on chromosome 16. *Cell, 75,* 1305–1315.

Folstein, S., & Piven, J. (1991). Etiology of autism: Genetic influences. *Pediatrics, 87*(Suppl.5), 767–773.

Folstein, S., & Rutter, M. (1977a). Infantile autism: A genetic study of 21 twin pairs. *Journal of Child Psychology and Psychiatry, 18,* 297–321.

Folstein, S., & Rutter, M. (1977b). Genetic influences and infantile autism. *Nature, 265,* 726–728.

Folstein, S., & Rutter, M. (1988). Autism: Familial aggregation and genetic implications. *Journal of Autism and Developmental Disorders, 18,* 3–30.

Fombonne, E., Bolton, P., Prior, J., Jordan, H., & Rutter, M. (in press). Family study of autism: Cognitive patterns and levels in parents and siblings. *Journal of Child Psychology and Psychiatry.*

Freeman, B.J., Ritvo, E.R., Mason-Brothers, A., Pingree, C., Yokota, A., Jenson, W.R., McMahon, W.M., Petersen, P.B., Mo, A., & Schroth, P. (1989). Psychometric assessment of first-degree relatives of 62 autistic probands in Utah. *American Journal of Psychiatry, 146,* 361–364.

Fryer, A.E., Chalmers, A., Connor, J.M., Fraser, I., Povey, S., Yates, A.D., Yates, J.R., & Osborne, J.P. (1987). Evidence that the gene for tuberous sclerosis is on chromosome 9. *Lancet, 21,* 659–661.

Gillberg, C. (1990). Medical work-up in children with autism and Asperger Syndrome. *Brain Dysfunction, 3,* 249–260.

Gillberg, C. (1992). Autism and autism-like conditions: Sub-classes among disorders of empathy. *Journal of Child Psychology and Psychiatry, 33,* 813–842.

Gillberg, C., & Coleman, M. (1992). *The biology of autistic syndromes* (2nd ed.). London: MacKeith Press.

Gillberg, C., & Forsell, C. (1984). Childhood psychosis and neurofibromatosis—more than a coincidence? *Journal of Autism and Developmental Disorders, 14,* 1–8.

100 ∎

Gillberg, C., Gillberg, I.C., & Steffenburg, S. (1992). Siblings and parents of children with autism: A controlled population-based study. *Developmental Medicine and Child Neurology, 34,* 389–398.

Gillberg, C., Steffenburg, S., & Jakobsson, G. (1987). Neurobiological findings in 20 relatively gifted children with Kanner-type autism or Asperger Syndrome. *Developmental Medicine and Child Neurology, 29,* 641–649.

Gillberg, C., Steffenburg, S., Wahlström, J., Sjöstedt, A., Gillberg, I.C., Martinsson, T., Liedgren, S., & Eeg-Olofsson, O. (1991). Autism associated with marker chromosome. *Journal of the American Academy of Child and Adolescent Psychiatry, 30,* 489–494.

Gillberg, C., & Wahlström, J. (1985). Chromosome abnormalities in infantile autism and other childhood psychoses: A population study of 66 cases. *Developmental Medicine and Child Neurology, 27,* 293–304.

Gillberg, I.C., Gillberg, C., & Ahlsén, G. (1994). Autistic behaviour and attention deficits in tuberous sclerosis: A population-based study. *Developmental Medicine and Child Neurology, 36,* 50–56.

Gurling, H.M.G., Bolton, P.F., Vincent, J., Melmer, G., & Rutter, M. (1997, submitted). *Molecular and cytogenic investigations of the fragile X region in families multiplex for autism and related phenotypes.*

Hagerman, R.J. (1990). The association between autism and Fragile X syndrome. *Brain Dysfunction, 3,* 219–227.

Hallmayer, J., Pintado, E., Lotspeich, L., Spiker, D., McMahon, W., Petersen, P.B., Nicholas, P., Pingree, C., Kraemer, H.C., Wong, D.L., Ritvo, E., Lin, A., Hebert, J., Cavalli-Sforza, L.L., & Ciaranello, R.D. (1994). Molecular analysis and test of linkage between the FMR-1 gene and infantile autism in multiplex families. *American Journal of Human Genetics, 55,* 951–959.

Hotopf, M., & Bolton, P. (1995). A case of autism associated with partial tetrasomy 15. *Journal of Autism and Developmental Disorders, 25,* 41–49.

Howlin, P., Wing, L., & Gould, J. (1995). The recognition of autism in children with Down syndrome—implications for intervention and some speculations about pathology. *Developmental Medicine and Child Neurology, 37,* 406–414.

Hunt, A., & Dennis, J. (1987). Psychiatric disorder among children with tuberous sclerosis. *Developmental Medicine and Child Neurology, 29,* 190–198.

Hunt, A., & Shepherd, C. (1993). A prevalence study of autism in tuberous sclerosis. *Journal of Autism and Developmental Disorders, 23,* 329–339.

Jones, M.B., & Szatmari, P. (1988). Stoppage rules and genetic studies of autism. *Journal of Autism and Developmental Disorders, 18,* 31–40.

Jorde, L.B., Hasstedt, S.J., Ritvo, E.R., Mason-Brothers, A., Freeman, B.J., Pingree, C., McMahon, W.M., Peterson, B., Jenson, W.R., & Moll, A. (1991). Complex segregation analysis of autism. *American Journal of Human Genetics, 49,* 932–938.

Jorde, L.B., Mason-Brothers, A., Waldman, R., Ritvo, E.R., Freeman, B.J., Pingree, C., McMahon, M.W., Petersen, P.B., Jenson, W.R., & Mo, A. (1990). The UCLA–University of Utah epidemiologic survey of autism: Genealogical analysis of familial aggregation. *American Journal of Medical Genetics, 36,* 85–88.

Kanner, L. (1943). Autistic disturbances of affective contact. *Nervous Child, 2,* 217–250.

Kendler, K.S., Gruenberg, A.M., & Kinney, D.K. (1994). Independent diagnosis of adoptees and relatives as defined by *DSM-III* in the provincial and national samples of the Danish adoption study of schizophrenia. *Archives of General Psychiatry, 51,* 456–468.

Koegel, R., Schreibman, L., O'Neill, R.E., & Burke, J.C. (1983). The personality and family-interaction characteristics of parents of autistic children. *Journal of Consulting and Clinical Psychology, 51,* 683–692.

Landa, R., Piven, J., Wzorek, M., Gayle, J.O., Chase, G.A., & Folstein, S.E. (1992). Social language use in parents of autistic individuals. *Psychological Medicine, 22,* 245–254.

Landa, R., Wzorek, M., Piven, J., Folstein, S., & Isaacs, C. (1991). Spontaneous narrative discourse characteristics of parents of autistic individuals. *Journal of Speech and Hearing Research, 34,* 1339–1345.

Le Couteur, A., Bailey, A., Goode, S., Pickles, A., Robertson, S., Gottesman, I., & Rutter, M. (1996). A broader phenotype of autism: The clinical spectrum in twins. *Journal of Child Psychology and Psychiatry, 37,* 785–801.

Mazzocco, M.M.M., Pennington, B.F., & Hagerman, R.J. (1994). Social cognition skills among females with Fragile X. *Journal of Autism and Developmental Disorders, 24,* 473–485.

Murphy, M., Bolton, P., Pickles, A., & Rutter, M. (1997, submitted). *Personality traits of relatives of autistic probands.*

Narayan, S., Moyes, B., & Wolff, S. (1990). Family characteristics of autistic children: A further report. *Journal of Autism and Developmental Disorders, 20,* 523–536.

Nelson, K. (1991). Prenatal and perinatal factors in the etiology of autism. *Pediatrics, 87,* 761–766.

Osborne, J.P., Fryer, A.E., & Webb, D. (1991). Epidemiology of tuberous sclerosis. *Annals of the New York Academy of Sciences, 615,* 125–127.

Pickles, A., Bolton, P., MacDonald, H., Bailey, A., Le Couteur, A., Sim, C-H., & Rutter, M. (1995). Latent class analysis of recurrence risks for complex phenotypes with selection and measurement error: A twin and family history study of autism. *American Journal of Human Genetics, 57,* 717–726.

Pickles, A., Bolton, P., MacDonald, H., Rios, P., Storoschuk, S., & Rutter, M. (1997, submitted). *A case control family history study of autism: Further findings from extended pedigrees.*

Piven, J., Chase, G.A., Landa, R., Wzorek, M., Gayle, J., Cloud, D., & Folstein, S. (1991). Psychiatric disorders in the parents of autistic individuals. *Journal of the American Academy of Child and Adolescent Psychiatry, 30,* 471–478.

Piven, J., Gayle, J., Chase, J., Fink, B., Landa, R., Wzorek, M., & Folstein, S. (1990). A family history study of neuropsychiatric disorders in the adult siblings of autistic individuals. *Journal of the American Academy of Child and Adolescent Psychiatry, 29,* 177–183.

Piven, J., Simon, J., Chase, G.A., Wzorek, M., Landa, R., Gayle, J., & Folstein, S. (1993). The etiology of autism: Pre-, peri- and neonatal factors. *Journal of the American Academy of Child and Adolescent Psychiatry, 32,* 1256–1263.

Piven, J., Wzorek, M., Landa, R., Lainhart, J., Bolton, P., Chase, G.A., & Folstein, S. (1994). Personality characteristics of the parents of autistic individuals [Preliminary communication]. *Psychological Medicine, 24,* 783–795.

Pocock, S.J. (1983). *Clinical trials: A practical approach.* Chichester: John Wiley & Sons.

Risch, N. (1990). Linkage strategies for genetically complex traits. *American Journal of Human Genetics, 46,* 222–253.

Ritvo, E.R., Spence, M.A., Freeman, B.J., Mason-Brothers, A., Mo, A., & Marazita, M.L. (1985). Evidence for autosomal recessive inheritance in 46 families with multiple incidences of autism. *American Journal of Psychiatry, 142,* 187–192.

Rutter, M. (1994). Psychiatric genetics: Research challenges and pathways forward. *American Journal of Medical Genetics (Neuropsychiatric Genetics), 54,* 185–198.

Rutter, M., & the English and Romanian Adoptees (E.R.A.) Study Team. (1997, submitted). *Quasi-autistic patterns following severe privation.*

Rutter, M., Bailey, A., Bolton, P., & Le Couteur, A. (1993). Autism: Syndrome definition and possible genetic mechanisms. In R. Plomin & G.E. McClearn (Eds.), *Nature, nurture, and psychology* (pp. 269–284). Washington, DC: APA Books.

Rutter, M., Bailey, A., Bolton, P., & Le Couteur, A. (1994). Autism and known medical conditions: Myth and substance. *Journal of Child Psychology and Psychiatry, 35,* 311–322.

Scott, S. (1994). Mental retardation. In M. Rutter, E. Taylor & L. Hersov (Eds.), *Child and adolescent psychiatry: Modern approaches* (3rd ed., pp. 616–646). Oxford: Blackwell Scientific.

Silliman, E.R., Campbell, M., & Mitchell, R.S. (1989). Genetic influences in autism and assessment of metalinguistic performance in siblings of autistic children. In G. Dawson (Ed.), *Autism: Nature, diagnosis & treatment* (pp. 225–259). New York: Guilford Press.

Simonoff, E., Bolton, P., & Rutter, M. (1996). Mental retardation: Genetic findings, clinical implications, and research agenda. *Journal of Child Psychology and Psychiatry, 37,* 259–280.

Simonoff, E., McGuffin, P., & Gottesman, I.I. (1994). Genetic influences on normal and abnormal development. In M. Rutter, E. Taylor & L. Hersov (Eds.), *Child and adolescent psychiatry: Modern approaches* (3rd ed., pp. 129–151). Oxford: Blackwell Scientific.

Smalley, S., Asarnow, R., & Spence, M. (1988). Autism and genetics: A decade of research. *Archives of General Psychiatry, 45,* 953–961.

Smalley, S., McCracken, J., & Tanguay, P. (1995). Autism, affective disorders, and social phobia. *American Journal of Medical Genetics (Neuropsychiatric Genetics), 60,* 19–26.

Smalley, S., Smith, M., & Tanguay, P. (1991). Autism and psychiatric disorders in tuberous sclerosis. *Annals of New York Academy of Science, 615,* 382–383.

Smalley, S. L., Burger, F., & Smith, M. (1994). Phenotypic variation of tuberous sclerosis in a single extended kindred. *Journal of Medical Genetics, 31,* 761–765.

Smalley, S.L., Tanguay, P.E., Smith, M., & Gutierrez, G. (1992). Autism and tuberous sclerosis. *Journal of Autism and Developmental Disorders, 22,* 339–355.

Spiker, D., Lotspeich, L., Kraemer, H.C., Hallmayer, J., McMahon, W., Petersen, P.B., Nicholas, P.,

Pingree, C., Wiese-Slater, S., Chiotti, C., Wong, D.L., Dimicelli, S., Ritvo, E., Cavalli-Sforza, L.L., & Ciaranello, R.D. (1994). Genetics of autism: Characteristics of affected and unaffected children from 37 multiplex families. *American Journal of Medical Genetics, 54,* 27–35.

Steffenburg, S., Gillberg, C., Helgren, L., Anderson, L., Gillberg, L., Jakobsson, G., & Bohman, M. (1989). A twin study of autism in Denmark, Finland, Iceland, Norway, and Sweden. *Journal of Child Psychology and Psychiatry, 30,* 405–416.

Sudhalter, V., Cohen, I.L., Silverman, W., & Wolfschein, E.G. (1990). Conversational analyses of males with Fragile X, Down syndrome, and autism: Comparison of the emergence of deviant language. *American Journal on Mental Retardation, 94,* 431–441.

Szatmari, P., Jones, M.B., Tuff, L., Bartolucci, G., Fisman, S., & Mahoney, W. (1993). Lack of cognitive impairment in first-degree relatives of children with pervasive developmental disorders. *Journal of the American Academy of Child and Adolescent Psychiatry, 32,* 1264–1273.

Tsai, L. (1987). Pre-, peri-, and neonatal factors in autism. In E. Schopler & G.B. Mesibov (Eds.), *Neurobiological issues in autism* (pp. 180–189). New York: Plenum Press.

Warren, S.T., & Nelson, D.L. (1994). Advances in molecular analysis of Fragile X syndrome. *The Journal of the American Medical Association, 271,* 536–542.

Wolff, P.H., Gardner, J., Paccia, J., & Lappen, J. (1989). The greeting behavior of Fragile X males. *American Journal of Mental Retardation, 93,* 406–411.

Wolff, S., Narayan, S., & Moyes, B. (1988). Personality characteristics of parents of autistic children. *Journal of Child Psychology and Psychiatry, 29,* 143–154.

Journal of Child Psychology and Psychiatry, 1985, vol. 26, pp. 193–214

THE TREATMENT OF AUTISTIC CHILDREN

MICHAEL RUTTER

Institute of Psychiatry, London

INTRODUCTION

■103

DURING the four decades that have passed since the late Leo Kanner (1943) delineated the syndrome of infantile autism there have been important advances in our understanding of the nature of the condition. Firstly, a variety of empirical studies made it clear that autistic children suffered from a basic cognitive deficit, and that this deficit underlay many other language and behaviour problems (Hermelin and O'Connor, 1970; Rutter, 1974, 1983). Secondly, it became apparent that in many cases there was overt organic brain dysfunction. This was first evident in the observation that about a quarter of autistic children develop epileptic seizures during adolescence (Deykin and MacMahon, 1979; Rutter, 1970). However, it is also shown by the sporadic association with various diseases such as congenital rubella (Chess *et al.*, 1971) or infantile spasms (Riikonen and Amnell, 1981); by the occasional presence of metabolic, neurophysiological or neurochemical abnormalities; and by the weak association with perinatal complications (Deykin and MacMahon, 1980; DeMyer *et al.*, 1981; Rutter, 1979*a*; Rutter and Garmezy, 1983). In addition, both twin (Folstein and Rutter, 1977) and sibling studies (August *et al.*, 1981) have pointed to the importance of genetic factors.

It will be appreciated that these findings could lead in two very different therapeutic directions. On the one hand, the focus on medical causes could lead to a search for medical treatment; and on the other, the demonstration of cognitive deficits and of associated behavioural abnormalities could lead to an emphasis on psychological methods of intervention. Both have occurred. The search for possible medical treatment may pay rich dividends in the end, but so far the outcome has been generally disappointing. Drugs have a place in treatment, but the benefits are decidedly modest (Corbett, 1976; Campbell, 1978). Megavitamin therapy seems to bring about slight non-specific improvements in a few autistic children (Rimland *et al.*, 1978; Lelord *et al.*, 1981), but the gains are quite limited. A recent report (Geller *et al.*, 1982) based on just three children has suggested that there may be some behavioural improvement following pharmacological reduction of raised serotonin levels. Obviously that lead must be followed up, but evidence on the non-specific associations of rasied serotonin levels (*British Medical Journal*, 1978; Boullin *et al.*, 1982) makes it unlikely that a reduction in serotonin would affect the basis of autism.

Requests for reprints to: Department of Child and Adolescent Psychiatry, Institute of Psychiatry, De Crespigny Park, Denmark Hill, London SE5 8AF, U.K.

Accepted manuscript received 10 *June* 1983

Journal of Child Psychology and Psychiatry, 1985, vol. 26, pp. 193–214

It is important that research into possible medical treatments for autism should continue but, equally, it is clear that, for the moment, we need to look to other directions for effective ways of helping autistic children and their families.

The 'other' direction that seems most promising is the field of educational and behavioural methods of treatment. During the last 20 years these have constituted the most important therapeutic advance with respect to autism (DeMyer *et al.*, 1981). Educational and behavioural approaches seem to provide the logical way of tackling autistic children's problems if our current concepts of autism are correct (Rutter, 1979*b*) and, more importantly, both clinical experience and systematic research have shown that such approaches bring about worthwhile improvements (Bartak, 1978; Hemsley *et al.*, 1978; Schopler *et al.*, 1982). Nevertheless, many problems and many unanswered questions remain.

In order to consider how our present methods of treatment could be improved in the future it is necessary to appreciate the meaning of these problems and questions. But first, it is important to get clear the *goals* of treatment, the strategies and *principles* of treatment, and also to note what can be *achieved* by treatment today.

THE HANDICAPS ASSOCIATED WITH AUTISM

The goals of treatment need to be decided on the basis of our knowledge of the nature of autism and of autistic children's handicaps (Rutter, 1978, 1979*a*, 1983, 1984*b*). These are considered most conveniently under three main headings. Firstly, it is obvious that, more than anything else, autistic children suffer from a serious abnormality of development. This applies particularly to cognition, language and socialization. In all three of these areas it is apparent that there is both an impairment or retardation in development and deviance or abnormality. That is to say, the course of development is slowed and held back and, in addition, in some respects it follows an atypical or deviant course. Thus many autistic children have a low IQ (they are mentally retarded as well as autistic), but also their *pattern* of cognitive skills and deficits is unusual. In most cases the skills tend to apply to memory and to visuo-spatial or puzzle-type tasks; and the deficits concern processes of symbolization, abstraction and conceptual meaning.

Similarly, nearly all autistic children are delayed in learning to speak and some never acquire speech. But, also, when language does develop it is abnormal in many respects. In particular, there is a failure to *use* language for social communication, so that autistic children tend not to 'chat' in the reciprocal to-and-fro fashion that is characteristic of the conversation of even very young normal children. Also, autistic children's spoken language often shows abnormal elements such as the extensive use of stereotyped phrases and the echoing of their own as well as other people's words.

Socialization, too, shows the same combination of retardation and deviance (Lord, 1984). Autistic children are generally delayed in their early social milestones —in smiling as a social signal, in putting up their arms to be lifted up and in the emergence of selective attachments. But also, even when social relationships do develop they are not normal in form. Perhaps, more than anything else, autistic children seem to lack empathy, the ability to sense or share other people's feelings; they find it difficult to appreciate social cues and social signals (see Hobson, 1983) and, as a result, their relationships tend to lack reciprocity and responsiveness to *other* people's needs and concerns. When older, many autistic individuals *want* friendships but they just do not know how to set about making friends and, probably in many cases, they lack the emotional feeling for what true love and friendship mean.

The second set of, rather different, handicaps reflect a style of functioning characterized by rigidity, stereotypy and inflexibility. This style tends to pervade all aspects of autistic children's functioning, but some features are particularly common or noticeable. For example, autistic children can be taught new skills, but they seem unable to generalize what they have learned to new situations or new tasks. Similarly, when older they lack flexibility and initiative in the application of what they know. Often they fear and resist change and prefer a routinized, highly predictable existence.

Similarly, in normal people the most obvious feature of language is its creativity. Even young normal children use an almost infinite variety of word combinations, endlessly making up new phrases and sentences. In contrast, autistic children tend to talk in a semi-predictable series of questions and answers made up of stereotyped phrases and repetitions.

Their play shows the same characteristics. When young they may line up objects or put them into patterns, doing the same thing time and again. There is little imagination, little use of pretend or make-believe, little sequencing and even little use of toys for their appropriate purposes (spinning the wheels of toy cars or feeling their texture rather than running them along the floor making car noises as the toy cars are raced or made to go into pretend car parks). When older, autistic children's interests tend to reflect narrow preoccupations with bus routes, or numbers or time tables.

Sometimes there may be overt obsessive–compulsive rituals—especially during adolescence or early adult life. Thus autistic children may engage in checking or touching rituals, or they may insist on following certain fixed routines as they enter or leave rooms. As with rituals that form part of an obsessional disorder in normal children, they may be associated with a strongly compulsive quality and great anxiety if the rituals are interrupted or cannot be followed.

Some autistic children develop unusual attachments to particular objects—to stones, tin cans, belts or tin openers, that they insist on carrying everywhere with them. They are not interested in the function or use of the objects to which they are attached, but the attachment is to a *specific* object and there is great distress if the object is removed or lost.

Particularly when autism is accompanied by severe mental retardation, motor stereotypies are often present. The most characteristic of these are finger flapping and flicking, usually near the corner of the eyes; the twirling or whirling of bits of string or other objects; and complex whole-body movements. However, many others also occur.

These first two sets of handicaps are relatively specific to autism. In addition, many autistic children show a variety of non-specific problems in no way pathonomic of autism but, nevertheless, that provide some of the most serious difficulties in management. Some autistic children are generally overactive and problems of disruptive behaviour are common. Temper tantrums are frequent and sometimes aggression is a difficulty. There may be self-destructive behaviour—such as wrist-

■ 105

Journal of Child Psychology and Psychiatry, 1985, vol. 26, pp. 193–214

biting or head-banging. Fears and phobias are often present. In most cases these are of a type usually found in young children—such as fear of dogs. There may be difficulties in getting off to sleep or in waking in the night, so disturbing other family members. As with other developmental disorders, bedwetting or soiling are often present—especially in younger age groups and in those with severe mental retardation.

GOALS, STRATEGIES AND PRINCIPLES OF TREATMENT

Promotion of normal development

106 ▪

The goals of treatment need to be considered with these handicaps in mind. As with any developmental disorder, the first goal must be to foster normal development. In deciding how this aim is to be met it is necessary to take into account both what is known about the *normal* developmental process and about the factors that facilitate optimal development, and also what is known regarding the abnormal features that *interfere* with development in autistic children (Rutter and Sussenwein, 1971). In other words, there should be a focus on the mechanisms that underlie normal growth and maturation in order to provide what is needed to promote these mechanisms but also a recognition of the autistic features that cause interference so that means can be found to reduce or circumvent that interference.

The overall methods to be employed for that purpose are generally straightforward and well known. Thus it is a matter of creating the right sort of facilitating, of encouraging progress in the right directions through the use of differential reinforcement and of direct teaching to provide the skills needed.

However, the concern has to be with the 'effective' rather than the 'objective' environment: the environment as it *actually* impinges on the child rather than as we perceive it. The implication is that the environment that is best for a normal child may not be best of the handicapped child. For example, it seems that deaf children are more likely to develop optimally if reared by deaf parents than if brought up by normal parents (Meadow, 1975).

TABLE 1. AIM: PROMOTION OF COGNITIVE DEVELOPMENT

Need	Problem	Solution
1. Active, meaningful experiences	self-isolation	planned periods of interaction
	impaired understanding	simplified communication / individual teaching
	specific deficits	selection of learning tasks
	lack of initiative	structuring of learning / direct teaching
2. Cognitive capacity	incapacity	direct teaching / teaching at appropriate developmental level

What these issues mean in practice is best considered by taking different aspects of development in turn. For example, it is known that active, meaningful experiences are required to foster normal cognitive development (Rutter, 1984a). Note the importance of 'active'—children learn more from doing things themselves than from having things done to them (the concept of a 'stimulating' environment is seriously misleading). Also, it is necessary that the experiences be meaningful, interesting and understood by the child. Autistic children face several problems in this connection. Firstly, because they tend to isolate themselves they lack the learning experiences that stem from adult–child interaction. Thus it is necessary to structure the day so that planned periods of interaction are provided. Secondly, their defects in comprehension may mean that they cannot understand what is said to them and cannot make sense of teaching or instruction in groups. This means that, at least at first, teaching needs to be on an individual basis, and communications to the children must be kept simple with short, easily understood sentences. Thirdly, the presence of specific cognitive deficits means that learning tasks must be carefully selected to capitalize on skills that the children *do* possess and to provide help with areas of special difficulty. Fourthly, autistic children tend to lack initiative. All too often, if left to their own devices they tend to engage in solitary, stereotyped, repetitive activities. Accordingly, especially with younger and with more handicapped autistic children, there is a need for both the learning situation and teaching itself to be more structured and directive than usually needed with normal children (Schopler *et al.*, 1971).

The other requirement for cognitive development, of course, is that children have the capacities to profit from their experiences. The problem in that connection is that many autistic children suffer from quite severe and pervasive biologically determined cognitive handicaps. It is important to appreciate the limitations that that imposes. All studies have shown that IQ level is the most important single prognostic indicator (Rutter, 1970; Lotter, 1978). Moreover, it has been found that treatment makes little difference to IQ (Rutter, 1980; Howlin, 1981). Severely retarded autistic children may improve in their overall functioning as a result of treatment, but almost always they remain severely retarded. The implication is that it is necessary to provide direct teaching at an appropriate developmental level; clearly, this means that an adequate psychological assessment is crucial.

Similar issues apply with respect to language development. Normal children acquire their language skills through conversational interchange in a social context. Autistic children need the same but, because of their handicaps, it is necessary to provide planned periods of interaction in which special attempts are made to ensure that there is reciprocity and to-and-fro. Of course, opportunities of this kind should be seized whenever they occur at home or at school, but usually parents should be asked to set aside some 30 minutes a day when they can have an uninterrupted period of play and conversation with their autistic child. This period needs to be relatively short both because such structured interactions are quite hard work for parents but also because it is important for parents to be able to lead their own lives and spend time with their other non-autistic children. In addition, steps taken to promote social development are important for language because language is a social skill and because it needs to develop in a social context. If autistic children can become more social they are more likely to *have* the language learning experiences they need.

107

Journal of Child Psychology and Psychiatry, 1985, vol. 26, pp. 193–214

TABLE 2. AIM: PROMOTION OF LANGUAGE DEVELOPMENT

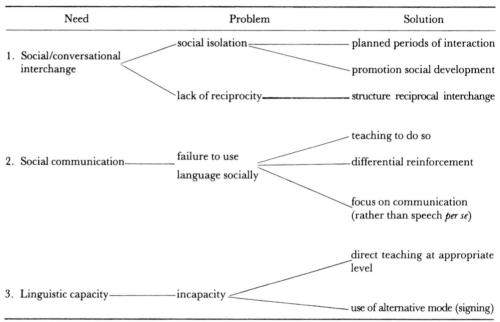

Need	Problem	Solution
1. Social/conversational interchange	social isolation	planned periods of interaction
		promotion social development
	lack of reciprocity	structure reciprocal interchange
2. Social communication	failure to use language socially	teaching to do so
		differential reinforcement
		focus on communication (rather than speech *per se*)
3. Linguistic capacity	incapacity	direct teaching at appropriate level
		use of alternative mode (signing)

108■

The main need is not to give the autistic child 'words' (although these are useful), but rather to facilitate social communication. The problem here is that autistic children tend not to use language for social communication. Moreover, unlike deaf children, if they lack speech they tend not to use gesture or mime in its place. The solutions lie in a focus on communication (encouraging any and all forms of communication and not just speech *per se*), on the differential use of praise to encourage communication and on teaching that is deliberately structured to provide an emphasis on social usage of language. Our own treatment evaluation study (Hemsley *et al.*, 1978; Howlin, 1980, 1981) showed that it is possible to increase social communication. Indeed, in the long term, treatment has a greater effect on the *usage* of language than on basic language *capacities*.

That last point emphasizes the limitations imposed by the autistic child's language handicaps. Inevitably, children's progress is determined by the severity and extensiveness of the biological incapacities. Some autistic children will never learn to speak regardless of what is done, whereas others will acquire extensive spoken language even in the absence of any form of specific treatment. All studies have demonstrated the huge individual differences in outcome and in response to language training. By and large, language training is most effective when there is evidence of some limited language skills before treatment commences—as shown by some understanding of language; by speech-like cadences in babble; by the presence of imitation and of pretend play; and by some echoed speech. Speech training has little to offer the mute child without any of these linguistic and pre-linguistic skills (Rutter, 1980; Howlin, 1980). As with cognition, direct teaching (using operant and other techniques) needs to be geared to the children's developmental language level and, again, that demands careful assessment. But also, if there is little or no progress with speech in spite of the presence of some understanding of language, it may be worthwhile introducing sign language (Carr, 1979; Bonvillian *et al.*, 1981; Kiernan, 1983). There have been few systematic evaluations of the use of signing with autistic children, but it is clear that some can learn to sign when they cannot speak, and that this is of general benefit to their communication skills. The use of signs does not impede speech development and may actually facilitate spoken language.

TABLE 3. AIM: PROMOTION OF SOCIAL DEVELOPMENT

Need	Problem	Solution
1. Intensive personal interaction that is: pleasurable, responsive, comforting	lack of social approach / lack of responsivity	structured interaction with social intrusion
2. Personalized caretaking	institutional upbringing	avoidance of residential care in early childhood
3. Social cognitive capacity	incapacity	direct teaching (social skills training)

The third area of development is that of socialization. Curiously, until very recently this has been the least investigated of all therapeutic goals, although social deficits are the symptoms that give rise to the name of autism and although they constitute both highly persistent disabilities (Lord, 1984). The evidence on the environmental qualities that promote attachment and social relationships in normal children suggests that what is needed is intense personal interaction that is pleasurable to the child, responsive to the child's needs and provides comfort and security at times of stress and distress (Bowlby, 1969; Rutter, 1981a). The sheer duration of interaction is less important than the personal qualities just mentioned. Thus normal children are more likely to become attached to their mothers than to the caretakers who look after them all day at the nursery (Rutter, 1981a). The problem for autistic children lies both in their lack of social approaches and initiatives and in their lack of responsiveness to *other* people's overtures to them. The solution lies in the parents' (or therapists') deliberate *intrusion* into the children's solitary activities so that the children need to be involved with other people in order to engage in their preferred activities (Rutter and Sussenwein, 1971). Of course, this must be done in a way that makes the social interaction pleasurable to the child. But, still, the aim is to structure interactions so that they are reciprocal and social rather than solitary.

Another consideration is that the caretaking should be personalized. It is known that children reared in institutions with a roster of multiple, ever-changing caretakers tend to show serious abnormalities in social relationships (Rutter, 1981a). The implication is that the use of prolonged institutional care for autistic children should be avoided, especially in early childhood. Also, of course, steps should be

Journal of Child Psychology and Psychiatry, 1985, vol. 26, pp. 193–214

110■

taken to provide personalized caretaking in institutions for those children who require residential care and treatment.

As with the other developmental disabilities, it is important to recognize the importance of autistic children's social incapacities: their difficulties in experiencing empathy, in recognizing socioemotional cues and in responding to others with reciprocity and responsiveness. So far, knowledge on how to remedy these deficits is quite limited. Nevertheless, there is evidence that active structuring of social experiences combined with direct teaching of social skills may lead to worthwhile improvements in autistic children's social interactions (Lord, 1984). Social responses are most likely to be elicited from autistic children when other people are directive and persistent in their play with them. On the whole, adults are more likely than other children to take the steps necessary to engage autistic children in social inter-actions. Placement in a group of non-autistic children is not likely to achieve much on its own because the autistic child's lack of responsivity discourages other children from attempting to interact. Nevertheless, it has been found that non-autistic peers can be actively encouraged to engage autistic children in play and that this leads to social gains (Lord, 1984). The use of peers to aid autistic children's social interactions warrants further exploration.

TABLE 4. AIM: PROMOTION OF LEARNING

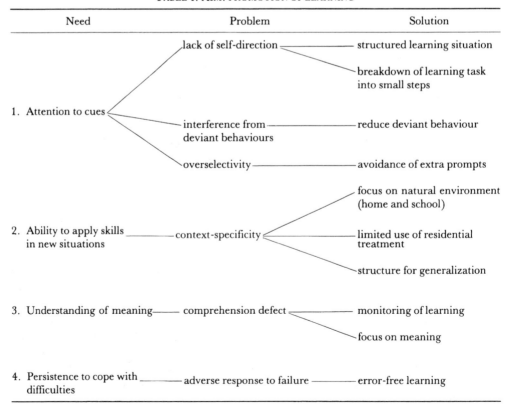

Need	Problem	Solution
1. Attention to cues	lack of self-direction	structured learning situation
		breakdown of learning task into small steps
	interference from deviant behaviours	reduce deviant behaviour
	overselectivity	avoidance of extra prompts
2. Ability to apply skills in new situations	context-specificity	focus on natural environment (home and school)
		limited use of residential treatment
		structure for generalization
3. Understanding of meaning	comprehension defect	monitoring of learning
		focus on meaning
4. Persistence to cope with difficulties	adverse response to failure	error-free learning

As well as fostering normal development, there should be a concern to promote autistic children's learning more generally. Obviously, that is the main objective of education, but also it is the goal of therapy as a whole. The first point is that numerous studies have shown that autistic children can and do profit from schooling (Bartak, 1978; Schopler *et al.,* 1982). Our own comparative study of different educational approaches (Bartak and Rutter, 1973; Rutter and Bartak, 1973) suggested that systematic teaching in an ordered environment was more effective than freer, permissive approaches.

There are several specific considerations in planning the promotion of learning by autistic children. The first problem is raised by autistic children's lack of application, or self-direction. If left to get on by themselves, all too often their interest wanders off the task. There is a need to structure the learning situation appropriately, providing guidance and supervision, not just at the beginning, but through task performance. Even more than with normal children, it is important, too, to break down the task into a series of manageable small steps. Also, it is helpful to programme the learning (through 'chaining' elements in the learning task, 'prompt-fading' and other techniques) to encourage the children to be able to work on their own (Rincover and Koegel, 1977; Koegel *et al.,* 1982). In many cases, autistic children's application to tasks is impeded by interference from deviant behaviours of one kind or another; when this is so, steps must be taken to reduce such behaviours. In common with other children suffering from a severe developmental delay, many autistic children exhibit 'overselectivity' in their response to cues—focusing on one to the neglect of others (Lovaas *et al.,* 1979). One consequence of this phenomenon is that learning tends to be *worse* if autistic children are given extra prompts or cues that are not inherent to the discriminations required for the learning task (Schreibman, 1975; Koegel and Rincover, 1976; Nelson *et al.,* 1980). It might seem that extra stimuli would guide learning but, instead, they interfere with learning and should be avoided.

If what children learn is to be of any value to them, it is necessary that they be able to apply their skills to new situations outside the classroom. One of the major difficulties with the teaching of autistic children is their tendency *not* to do so; their learning shows a handicapping context-specificity. Because of this tendency the gains following in-patient treatment often fail to generalize to the home and to school. As a result, over the last decade much less use has been made of residential treatments; of course, they have a place, and in some cases placement in hospital may be essential in order to deal with severe behavioural problems, but they do *not* provide a satisfactory general solution. Instead, therapeutic efforts have been focused on the children's natural environment, working with the parents at home and ensuring close links between programmes at home and school (Hemsley *et al.,* 1978). In addition, however, it has proved necessary to organize training in such a way as to encourage generalization of learning (Holman and Baer, 1979; Wahler *et al.,* 1979; Handleman and Harris, 1980). Such steps as training in multiple settings; ensuring that cues, stimuli and rewards are comparable across settings; the use of intermittent rather than continuous reinforcement; and an emphasis on the development of self-direction, self-monitoring and the *use* of skills may all be helpful.

A major feature of autism is the tendency to learn by rote without attention to

▪ 111

Journal of Child Psychology and Psychiatry, 1985, vol. 26, pp. 193–214

meaning or concepts. Obviously, this tendency greatly limits the usefulness of the skills acquired. Thus it is common to find that autistic children acquire quite good mechanical reading skills but yet fail to understand the *meaning* of the prose passages that they have succeeded in reading accurately. It is important to monitor the children's learning carefully so that teachers and parents are clear about what the children do and do not know, so that the teaching programme may be planned accordingly. Also, of course, it is necessary throughout all teaching, formal and informal, to focus explicitly on meaning and on understanding.

If children are to learn effectively it is necessary that they be able to persist in the face of difficulty in order to cope successfully with new learning. Autistic children are impaired in this because of their tendency to respond adversely to failure, often retreating into a stereotyped, repetitive style of response (Koegel and Egel, 1979; Clark and Rutter, 1979; Volkmar and Cohen, 1982). In order to avoid this problem it is necessary to organize the learning task to put a premium on success, with the steps in the tasks so arranged that the children make the minimum number of errors. It is especially crucial with autistic children to *start* with tasks on which they can succeed.

Reduction of rigidity/stereotypy

The second major goal of treatment is the reduction of the rigidity and stereotypy that pervades so many aspects of autistic children's functioning. The goal is 'reduction' rather than 'elimination' because this rigidity, repetitiveness and maladaptive imposition of patterns seem such an intrinsic aspect of autism (Frith, 1971) and because, in practice, it seems very difficult to eliminate the characteristic completely (although this is desirable if it can be achieved). Treatments to reduce rigidity rely on several different kinds of rationale. For example, there is the principle of 'graded change'. In essence, this means that although children may resist and reject the imposition of *major* changes in their stereotyped patterns and routines, nevertheless such major changes may be brought about if they can be introduced step by tiny step —by means of a series of separate changes so small that they are accepted by the child as not amounting to any noticeable alteration in pattern. These tiny changes may involve physical structure, timing, routine or, indeed, any aspect of the behaviour. For example, one autistic child was greatly impeded by a large blanket that he insisted on carrying everywhere he went. Because his hands were engaged in holding the blanket he could do little else. The intervention in this case consisted of getting the parents to cut off a tiny piece of blanket each night. Over the course of time, it was possible to reduce the blanket to just a few threads (Marchant *et al.*, 1974). The child accepted this reduction without upset but, interestingly, there was great distress if these few threads were taken away or mislaid. However, although the attachment remained, the object was so tiny that it provided no interference with other activities. An alternative strategy, using the same principle, is to get the child to put the object down for a few moments, then gradually increase the time it is relinquished. Or, again, children may be induced to accept tiny variations in obsessive routines and rituals: over time the variations can be gradually increased in order to break up the rigidity and the fixity of pattern.

A rather different approach is provided by attention to the environmental features that seem to elicit stereotyped behaviours or which increase the frequency of their occurrence. Of course, the determination of just which aspects of the environment serve that purpose needs to be determined by systematic observation and experimentation in the individual case. However, it has been found that, often, stereotypies tend to be at a maximum in barren, bleak, unstimulating environments (Baumeister, 1978). The implication is that it is likely to be helpful to ensure that autistic children are kept actively engaged in play or work, that there is ample provision of toys and activities and that there are plenty of structured opportunities for personal interactions. Our experimental comparisons showed that autistic children were at their best when the situation was highly structured for them and at their worst when it was left for them to take the initiative (Clark and Rutter, 1981). But it has also been found by Goodall and Corbett (1982) that the experimental provision of extrasensory stimulation may reduce stereotypies in some severely retarded children. In addition, it is apparent that the reduction of stereotyped behaviours may be aided by the introduction of alternative behaviours or activities that are incompatible with, and hence compete with, stereotypies.

■113

Elimination of non-specific maladaptive behaviours

The third goal of treatment involves the elimination of non-specific maladaptive behaviours. For the most part, behavioural approaches provide the most suitable form of intervention. These require both a functional analysis of behaviour and an application of the various principles of learning. A functional analysis simply means a careful and systematic analysis of the *preceding* circumstances that increase or decrease the likelihood of occurrence of particular maladaptive behaviours, together with a comparable analysis of the *succeeding* circumstances that seem to be associated with a prolongation or diminution of the behaviours in question. The point is that if behavioural techniques are to be employed it is essential to determine which environmental features influence the specific behaviour, *not* in children as a whole but, rather, in that particular child.

Pharmacological interventions have a place, albeit a rather limited one, in treatment. There are *no* drugs that are specific to autism. On the other hand, drugs may be useful for the control of specific behaviours. For example, the major tranquillizers may serve to reduce agitation, tension and overactivity (Corbett, 1976). Care is needed in their usage in view of the possibility of adverse effects on learning (Taylor, 1984), but they may be of value—especially, perhaps, in adolescence. Phenothiazines have the limitation of sedation as a side-effect but, on the whole, they are safer than the butyrophenones (such as haloperidol). The latter have been found to have more powerful effects on behaviour in some studies (see DeMyer *et al.*, 1981), but the side-effect of dystonic reactions make them troublesome drugs. In general, stimulants have appeared less effective in the control of overactivity in autistic children than in non-autistic hyperkinetic groups and often they seem to make retarded autistic children *worse*; hence their usage is to be avoided (Aman, 1982). Hypnotics have an occasional place in the treatment of sleep disturbance, but habituation develops rapidly, as it does in normal children. Accordingly, they are of use mainly at times of crisis or as an adjunct in the early stages of introduction of a behavioural programme.

Journal of Child Psychology and Psychiatry, 1985, vol. 26, pp. 193–214

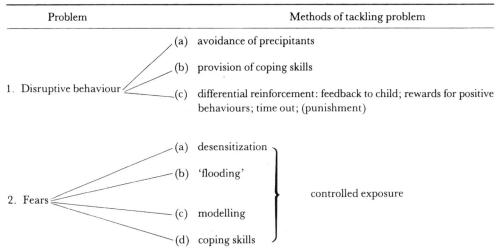

TABLE 5. EXAMPLES OF BEHAVIOURAL TECHNIQUES

Problem	Methods of tackling problem
1. Disruptive behaviour	(a) avoidance of precipitants
	(b) provision of coping skills
	(c) differential reinforcement: feedback to child; rewards for positive behaviours; time out; (punishment)
2. Fears	(a) desensitization
	(b) 'flooding' } controlled exposure
	(c) modelling
	(d) coping skills

114■

The principles of learning that may be used in behavioural treatments are many. Perhaps they may be illustrated most easily through a consideration of two key problem behaviours. For example, Table 5 shows a few approaches that may be adopted in the treatment of disruptive behaviour. In the first place, it is necessary to consider what steps may be taken to *avoid* its onset. A functional analysis should be undertaken to identify possible precipitants in order that they may be circumvented or overcome. Similarly, it may be helpful to teach autistic children coping skills to enable them to deal better with the situations that provoke emotional upset and behavioural disruption. For example, one mute autistic boy in a long-stay hospital caused considerable difficulties through his tendency to have outbursts at meal-times, during which he both threw food and hit out at staff and fellow patients. Careful observation indicated that these outbursts occurred only when he was given certain foods. The behavioural programme designed to deal with the problem involved three elements: (1) the provision of alternative foods to those to which he took exception; (2) the teaching of a means of indicating 'yes' and 'no', so that he could convey his wishes; and (3) the use of graded change to widen the range of foods that were acceptable to him.

Operant techniques are those that have been most widely employed as a means of controlling disruptive behaviour. Essentially, the approach involves no more than the breakdown of complex behaviours into smaller, more manageable elements which may be encouraged or discouraged through the use of differential reinforcement. The first essential is the provision of accurate feedback to the child regarding which behaviours are, and which are not, acceptable. This procedure must include feedback on (and, if necessary, teaching of) *alternative* responses to those that are to be eliminated. Then it is necessary to identify those elements in the child's behavioural pattern that are adaptive and positive in their effects. There need not be many of these, so long as there are some. The objective then is to use some form of *immediate* positive reinforcement or reward to encourage the child in the use of these behaviours, the aim being to extend and develop such acceptable behaviours by a process of differential *shaping*. At one time material rewards, such as sweets, were widely used in the belief that autistic children would not be responsive to praise and social reinforcement. However, it has become clear that most autistic children *are* responsive to social rewards and, moreover, that there are considerable disadvantages to the use of material rewards. Accordingly, although in some circumstances with some children they are necessary, the aim should always be to move to social rewards as soon as possible. Praise and encouragement are readily available in the natural environment whereas material rewards are not. Also, it should be appreciated that the objective is *not* to bring children's behaviour under the complete control of external reinforcement—that would be extremely limiting. Rather, the aim must be to seem for internal, self-directed controls. With this in mind, reinforcement should be intermittent and steps should be taken to make acceptable behaviour enjoyable and rewarding in its own right. It should be added that not only is there no point in the introduction of external rewards for behaviour inherently pleasurable and spontaneously engaged in by the child, but also the use of rewards in these circumstances may actually *reduce* such behaviour (Lepper, 1981).

■ 115

Often, whatever its origin, disruptive behaviour may come to serve as an attention-gaining device. The general upset and attention provoked by the disruption may be rewarding to the child and hence may act to prolong the disruption. In these circumstances the procedure of 'time-out' may be useful. The term simply means a period of withdrawal from positive reinforcement (or rewarding attention). In practice, this means ignoring disruptive behaviour, withdrawing attention from the child or unemotionally removing him without fuss from the situation to be on his own until he calms down. If this procedure is to be effective it is essential that the response be *swift*, that there is an immediate return or provision of attention *as soon as the disruption stops* and that there is ample attention given to the child at *other* times when he is behaving appropriately.

There has been some controversy in the literature over the use of punishment for disruptive behaviours. Of course, it is accepted that immediate disapproval and other forms of punishment as ordinarily used in normal families may be appropriate for autistic children. However, it is important that such disapproval be immediate and readily understood. Delayed punishments are not likely to be understood and hence are not likely to be effective. What is more controversial is the use of *physical* punishments of various kinds. They may be effective in the control of unacceptable behaviours (Corbett, 1975; Foxx *et al.*, 1979) and, on occasions, they may be both justified and necessary when it is essential to control dangerous behaviour, such as serious self-injury (Romanczyk *et al.*, 1982). Nevertheless, such extreme measures are *not* often needed, they have considerable disadvantages and they should be avoided whenever possible. They are a *last* resort and should *not* be employed as a first recourse.

Fears and phobias constitute a common but quite different form of maladaptive behaviour. The techniques to be employed are the same as those used with fears in non-autistic children. Thus desensitization may be effective. This involves the establishment of a hierarchy ranging from the least feared stimulus to the most feared. In effect, the procedure involves the gradual introduction of the fear stimuli,

Journal of Child Psychology and Psychiatry, 1985, vol. 26, pp. 193–214

116■

starting with those bottom of the hierarchy (i.e. least feared) so that the autistic child 'gets used to' the feared object. This process may be helped by a linkage of the fear stimuli with a pleasurable stimulus that provides an emotional and autonomic response that is incompatible with fear. 'Flooding', the rapid introduction of a massive exposure to the fear stimuli, seems to work on the opposite principle but may also be effective (provided the child is cooperative, willing and understands what is involved). Modelling, i.e. enabling the child to watch someone else cope successfully with the feared object, may be helpful in some cases (but usually only with older, less handicapped autistic individuals). Alternatively, the child may be helped by gaining coping skills: learning to swim as a way of overcoming a fear of water constitutes an example. Whereas we do not fully understand all the mechanisms involved, it seems that controlled exposure to the feared object constitutes an essential element, probably together with some means by which the child can learn to cope with the fear stimulus and to appreciate that when he does so no harm befalls him.

These constitute no more than a few examples of the very wide range of behavioural techniques that may be employed in the treatment of autistic children. The art, as well as the science, of successful therapy lies in the accurate identification of the environmental features that influence the child's behaviour (the purpose of functional analysis), together with the application of ingenuity and imagination in the construction of behavioural methods that will be effective in altering such environmental features in a direction that alters the child's behaviour in the desired fashion.

Alleviation of family distress

The fourth major goal of treatment concerns the alleviation of family distress. The parents and siblings of handicapped children face many difficulties and carry many burdens, and this is especially the case with autistic children, many of whom are unresponsive and unrewarding to be with, difficult to play and talk with and demanding in their needs for supervision, structuring and control. Often, the parents are very puzzled by their child's abnormal behaviour and hence worried and uncertain regarding what they should do. It is important that they be helped to gain an understanding of the child's problems. But it is also necessary that they learn *what* to do—that is, that they be helped to gain effective problem-solving skills. Often, they have worries, anxieties and guilt that are, in part, irrational as well as rational. Many parents of handicapped children worry at some time that they have caused their children's disability by what they did or did not do. The therapeutic approach must provide an opportunity to deal with such concerns if they are present. In addition, it is likely that there will be many practical burdens on the family and ways must be sought to reduce them so far as possible.

A variety of methods may be employed for these purposes; thus it is important for families to have full feedback on the results of the diagnostic appraisal (see Rutter, 1984a). This may take more than one session, and the feedback should include an understanding of the nature and patterning of the child's problems; his developmental level with respect to the key areas of functioning, and educational and other needs; and as much information as it is possible to give on the probabilities of the child's later development and outcome in late childhood and adult life. The parents (and, in appropriate cases, the siblings as well) should be engaged as co-therapists

(Schopler and Reichler, 1971; Hemsley *et al.,* 1978). After all, it is they who have to deal with their autistic child day in and day out; and it is necessary that they acquire the requisite skills to do so. In this connection, it is desirable that the parents do more than just learn how to deal with the immediate problems of the moment. If they are not to be forever dependent on professional help, they must go on to gain coping skills so that they can know how to decide what to do with the *next* set of problems to arise. That constitutes a more difficult goal, and the extent to which it is generally attainable remains uncertain.

The engagement of parents as co-therapists may raise concerns and conflicts. The focus on the autistic child is likely to have implications for the balance of relationships and for the pattern of life in the family as a whole. It is important to be sensitive to the needs of each parent as an individual, to needs with respect to their marital relationships and to the needs of other children in the family. *What* parents are expected to do for their autistic child and *how* they are expected to do it must be adapted to the personal situation and characteristics of each family. But, also, the therapist must be alert to irrational guilt felt by many parents, to despair and depression when their child seems to make so little progress, and to anger and frustration aroused by the parents' difficulty in dealing with resistent problems, by disappointment or hostility at the child's relative lack of affection and social response and by resentment over having a handicapped child at all. Of course, these are normal and understandable reactions experienced at some time by most parents of seriously handicapped children. Counselling and case work are needed to help parents to realize that they are not alone in these feelings; that love and anger can co-exist; and that there are ways of coming to terms with these troubling feelings and of channelling them in positive directions. Often, too, advice and guidance may enable parents to deal with these family matters in a more constructive and adaptive fashion. One specific concern that should not be overlooked is the need for genetic counselling on the risks that any further children may be autistic or show other handicaps. This requires both the provision of information and the opportunity to discuss the implications that follow from it (Rutter, 1981*b*). Lastly, families require practical help with regard to such matters as baby-sitting arrangements so that they can go out in the evenings without the autistic child, holiday provisions for handicapped children, financial allowances to which they may be eligible, dental care and special educational provision.

■117

OVERALL TREATMENT PROGRAMME

So far, treatment has been considered in terms of the multitude of separate elements required to deal with particular problems. Those need to be brought together to construct an overall treatment programme. Such a programme should have at least three key features: a full diagnostic appraisal, special educational provision and a home-based programme for the family.

The diagnostic appraisal is required for many different purposes, including the accurate delineation of the children's assets and deficits, together with a functional analysis of the behaviours to be treated at home or at school. In addition, it must include an adequate screening for possible underlying medical conditions. When

Journal of Child Psychology and Psychiatry, 1985, vol. 26, pp. 193–214

118■

these are present (which they are in only a small minority of cases), appropriate treatment should be provided. However, also, it is necessary to identify possible medical complications (such as the development of epileptic seizures during adolescence), to investigate them appropriately and to provide suitable treatment. It is always essential to undertake the necessary skilled investigations to identify any defects or abnormalities in hearing or vision, so that these may be corrected. Dental care, too, must not be overlooked. Because of their behavioural difficulties, many autistic children do not receive the dental care they need and, if necessary, referral should be made to one of the dental centres specializing in the treatment of handicapped children. It is obvious from these requirements that there can never be any 'once and for all time' diagnostic appraisal, In all cases the child's needs must be reassessed from time to time as required by changing problems or changing circumstances, or simply in order to ensure that important matters are not being overlooked.

For autistic children of school age, and for those requiring preschool education, there must be a careful analysis of their educational requirements so that a suitable class, unit or school may be found. In many cases a unit specially designed for autistic children may be best, but it should *not* be assumed that this is necessarily preferable. Often, facilities for mentally retarded or for language-impaired children may be equally (or more) appropriate, especially if there can be flexibility in the provision of speical help of one kind or another. Units that are exclusively for autistic children have the advantage of a concentration of the skills involved in the teaching of children with that particular constellation of handicaps; however, they have the disadvantage of a lack of peer interactions. Units that cater for children with more varied handicaps have the potential for better use of the peer group, but considerable efforts are required for that potential to be realized. Moreover, it may be more difficult in mixed units to develop the expertise required to cope with the most disturbed or most handicapped autistic children. Probably, both sorts of units have a place. A few of the more intellectually able, and more mildly handicapped, may even be most suitably placed in an ordinary school if means can be found to adapt the school situation to cater for any special individual needs of the autistic child. In most circumstances day schooling is preferable for younger autistic children, but it is necessary that residential schooling be available for those young people that require it for reasons associated with their own handicaps, family needs or geography. Whatever the schooling decided upon, there should be consideration of whether or not any extra facilities (such as speech therapy) are needed.

Finally, there must be a therapeutic programme for the family. This is termed a 'home-based' programme in order to emphasize that it must be planned in such a way that it tackles problems as and how they arise in the home environment. Almost always this need means that there must be at least one prolonged home visit to observe the child, to appraise parent–child interaction and to note any particular features of the house of neighbourhood that have implications for treatment. We have found it advantageous to undertake most of the treatment in the home itself, but practical considerations may impose limits on how far that is possible. The elements that should be included in such a home-based approach to treatment have been discussed at length already, but they include: the use of behavioural/developmental methods, drugs where appropriate, counselling, practical help and the availability of in-patient care for the very few occasions when it is necessary.

EVALUATION OF TREATMENT

The crucial issue with respect to treatment, of course, is the extent to which it is successful in the achievement of its aims. There are numerous studies to show that treatment can bring about behavioural gains in the short-term. But autism is a chronic disorder and the more important question is whether treatment can improve the *long-term* outcome of autistic children. The evidence on this point is limited, but our own findings show that it can.

Thus the educational progress of autistic children in three very different types of unit (Bartak and Rutter, 1973; Rutter and Bartak, 1973) showed that: ''an autistic unit with large amounts of specific teaching in a well-controlled classroom situation is likely to bring the greatest benefits in terms of scholastic progress'' (Rutter and Bartak, 1973).

In a more recent evaluation study (Rutter *et al.*, 1977; Hemsley *et al.*, 1978; Rutter, 1980; Howlin, 1980, 1981) the long-term benefits of an intensive home-based behaviourally oriented treatment programme were compared with those of a more traditional out-patient approach. The findings showed that the results of the home-based programme were significantly superior on almost all behavioural measures. The differences were less marked on the language measures. Indeed, there were no significant differences between the groups on the tests of language *skills*, although the home-based group tended to perform slightly better. However, the home-based group showed better *social usage* of language. There was no evidence that treatment made any differences to IQ. It was also apparent that there was huge individual variation in outcome. The most handicapped children made the least progress, in spite of a comparable investment of therapists' time and energy in treatment. The outlook was especially poor for mentally retarded mute school age children without babble, imaginative play or understanding of language. Such children cannot be expected to gain useful language or acquire self-reliance, even with the best treatment. Nevertheless, appropriate treatment can substantially reduce behavioural disturbance and, in so doing, improve social functioning.

The last point in terms of the evaluation of treatment concerns parental satisfaction. In order to assess this aspect of the therapeutic programme an independent investigator was asked to follow up both the home-based treatment group and their controls to determine their reactions to the treatment programme a year or so later. The findings (Holmes *et al.*, 1982) confirmed the value of the therapeutic programme, although it was also apparent that many parents had experienced difficulties in applying what they had learned when the children developed new and different problems.

In summary, then, we may conclude that the benefits of treatment in both the short and long term are real and worthwhile. This applies to both special schooling and work with parents. However, it is also clear that there is an immense variation in outcome, with some autistic children remaining very severely handicapped.

Journal of Child Psychology and Psychiatry, 1985, vol. 26, pp. 193–214

CONCLUSIONS ON TREATMENT: LESSONS AND QUESTIONS

In conclusion, the research findings may be drawn together in order to make some inferences on the lessons that stem from what has been found out and on the questions that remain to be answered. The lessons may perhaps be summarized in terms of the broad terms that have taken place in treatment approaches.

Thus behavioural and educational techniques have largely replaced insight-oriented psychotherapy. But, within behavioural approaches, there is less use of material rewards and greater use of social rewards and social cues. Also, it has become generally appreciated that the treatment programme must be planned in order to be appropriate to the developmental level of the individual child.

Most especially, the main centre of treatment has moved from the hospital and the laboratory to the school and the home; and parents have been involved as co-therapists in treatment programmes. The therapeutic aims have broadened considerably. The early focus on speech has been extended to social communication and that on the suppression of deviant behaviours has been widened to include efforts to aid the more normal development of social relationships. In the same kind of way, the range of therapeutic techniques has been increased to provide effective combinations of behavioural, developmental and counselling approaches.

Four caveats or cautions need to be emphasized regarding the results of treatment. Firstly, there are huge individual differences in response to treatment; no therapy overrides the importance of the severity of the initial handicaps, especially in intelligence and language. Secondly, treatment makes most difference to the *non*-specific problems of autistic children. It makes only a slight difference to language competence (although slightly more to language usage) and no difference at all to general intelligence. Thirdly, unless particular steps are taken to avoid the problem, the gains following treatment tend to be situation-specific. That is, unless specifically taught to do so, autistic children tend not to generalize their behaviour and, especially, do not spontaneously apply what they have learned to new situations and new circumstances. Fourthly, the claims of the therapeutic enthusiasts far exceed what can in fact be accomplished, although a lot of useful and worthwhile things *can* be achieved through appropriate treatment.

It is also necessary to consider some of the many remaining questions on treatment. To begin with, it is apparent that there is much to learn on how best to facilitate normal social development. Although, on general grounds, it would seem likely that more could be achieved if treatment was started early in the infancy period, it is not known whether early treatment is more effective.

Although language training can do much in the short term and a little (albeit much less) in the long term, very little is known about *how* it works or *which* are the essential elements in the treatment programme. It is not even known whether it is important to teach language directly or whether more can be achieved by establishing the appropriate social interactions for autistic children to learn by themselves (Rutter, 1980).

Our work (Hemsley *et al.,* 1978) and that of Eric Schopler and his colleagues (Schopler and Reichler, 1971) both emphasize the importance of helping parents acquire coping skills so that they can decide for themselves what to do with the next problem or crisis when it occurs. However, the extent to which treatment

120 ■

programmes can succeed in that aim remains uncertain, and it is unclear which elements in the therapeutic approach are crucial for that purpose.

Most therapeutic experience and research has been with younger autistic children and less is known on how to help adolescent and adult autistic individuals. Many of the more mildly handicapped autistic persons become unhappy and concerned over their difficulties as they become older and more self-aware. Probably, counselling and psychotherapy may be of value at this stage, although they are of little use with younger children. However, the benefits of counselling have not yet been assessed. Some autistic people experience quite marked depression in late adolescence and early adult life and it may be that antidepressants are indicated then.

■ 121

The transition from school to work is a difficult one for many autistic individuals and it seems important that they have help at that stage. Unfortunately, there is a paucity of systematic data on just what is needed or how much can be achieved.

There is some suggestion that social skills training may be helpful in the teenage period, but we lack knowledge both on the best approaches to follow and on their efficacy.

Various small-scale studies suggest that, in some cases, training in sign language or gesture may be more useful than efforts to teach speech and spoken language. However, we lack knowledge on *which* autistic children most need signing and we do not know how much can be attained through the use of this modality of communication. Moreover, there is a lack of evidence on the extent to which the autistic child's use of gesture manifests the same problems as those shown in speech (stereotyped utterances, lack of spontaneity, etc.). Preliminary evidence suggests that there may be comparable abnormalities in their use of gesture.

To date there has been little indication that drugs make any decisive difference, although they are of some value in the treatment of overactivity, sleep disturbance and aggression. Clinical experience suggests that the phenothiazines may have a greater place in the treatment of severe tension in adolescence and adult life, and anti-depressant medication, too, may sometimes be useful. Furthermore, the possibility that drugs to reduce serotonin levels may bring benefits should be explored further. The field of pharmacotherapy as a whole needs greater development.

Some people have suggested that vitamins and diet may aid the treatment of autism. So far, that remains a highly speculative suggestion that has not been adequately substantiated by research. Nevertheless, it is possible that vitamins or diets may be of *some* benefit in a few autistic children; another area warranting study.

Finally, there have been competing claims regarding what sort of social milieu is best for autistic children. The findings so far indicate that a substantial degree of structure and organization is important, but the last word has not yet been said on this topic and the needs may well vary according to the autistic child's age and development level.

It is apparent that an enormous amount has been learned over the last 20 years and that we are now in a position where therapeutic interventions can do some good. Nevertheless, much remains to be learned, both about the nature and causes of autism and about its treatment.

Journal of Child Psychology and Psychiatry, 1985, vol. 26, pp. 193–214

SUMMARY

The goals of treatment need to be decided on the basis of knowledge on the nature of autism. As with any developmental disorder, the first goal must be to foster normal development; with autistic children this involves a focus on intellectual, language and social development. The further goals include: the reduction of rigidity/stereotypy; the elimination of non-specific maladaptive behaviours; and alleviation of family distress. Research findings are used to translate these goals into a practical overall therapeutic programme with three main elements: a full diagnostic appraisal, special educational provision and a home-based programme for the family. Finally, the research findings are drawn together to derive inferences on the lessons to be learned and the questions that remain to be answered.

122 ∎

REFERENCES

AMAN, M. C. (1982) Stimulant drug effects in developmental disorders and hyperactivity: toward a resolution of disparate findings. *J. Aut. devl Disord.* **12**, 385–398.

AUGUST, G. J., STEWART, M. A. and TSAI, L. (1981) The incidence of cognitive disabilities in the siblings of autistic children. *Br. J. Psychiat.* **138**, 416–422.

BARTAK, L. (1978) Educational approach. In *Autism: a Reappraisal of Concepts and Treatment* (Edited by RUTTER, M. and SCHOPLER, E.), pp. 423–438. Plenum, New York.

BARTAK, L. and RUTTER, M. (1973) Special educational treatment of autistic children—I. Design of study and characteristics of units. *J. Child Psychol. Psychiat.* **14**, 161–179.

BAUMEISTER, A. A. (1978) Origins and controls of stereotyped movements. In *Quality of Life for Severely and Profoundly Retarded People* (Edited by MEYERS, C. E.), American Association on Mental Deficiency Series 3, pp. 353–384. Research Foundations for Improvement, Washington, DC.

BONVILLIAN, J. D., NELSON, K. E. and RHYNE, J. M. (1981) Sign language and autism. *J. Aut. devl Disord.* **11**, 125–138.

BOULLIN, D., FREEMAN, B. J., GELLER, E., RITVO, E., RUTTER, M. and YUWILER, A. (1982) Toward the resolution of conflicting findings. *J. Aut. devl Disord.* **12**, 97–98.

BOWLBY, J. (1969) *Attachment and Loss—I. Attachment.* Hogarth, London.

BRITISH MEDICAL JOURNAL (1978) Editorial: Serotonin, platelets and autism. *Br. med. J.* **1**, 1651–1652.

CAMPBELL, M. (1978) Pharmacotherapy. In *Autism: a Reappraisal of Concepts and Treatment* (Edited by RUTTER, M. and SCHOPLER, E.), pp. 337–355. Plenum, New York.

CARR, E. G. (1979) Teaching autistic children to use sign language: some research issues. *J. Aut. devl Disord.* **9**, 345–360.

CHESS, S., KORN, S. J. and FERNANDEZ, P. B. (1971) *Psychiatric Disorders of Children with Congenital Rubella.* Brunner/Mazel, New York.

CLARK, P. and RUTTER, M. (1979) Task difficulty and task performance in autistic children. *J. Child Psychol. Psychiat.* **20**, 271–285.

CLARK, P. and RUTTER, M. (1981) Autistic children's responses to structure and interpersonal demands. *J. Aut. devl Disord.* **11**, 201–217.

CORBETT, J. (1975) Aversion for the tratment of self-injurious behaviour. *J. ment. Defic. Res.* **19**, 79–95.

CORBETT, J. (1976) Medical management. In *Early Childhood Autism* (2nd Edn.) (Edited by WING, L.), pp. 271–286. Pergamon, Oxford.

DEMYER, M. K., HINGTGEN, J. N. and JACKSON, R. K. (1981) Infantile autism reviewed: a decade of research. *Schizophr. Bull.* **7**, 388–451.

DEYKIN, E. Y. and MACMAHON, B. (1979) The incidence of seizures among children with autistic symptoms. *Am. J. Psychiat.* **136**, 1310–1312.

DEYKIN, E. Y. and MACMAHON, B. (1980) Pregnancy, delivery, and neonatal complications among autistic children. *Am. J. Dis. Child.* **134**, 860–864.

FOLSTEIN, S. and RUTTER, M. (1977) Infantile autism: a genetic study of 21 twin pairs. *J. Child Psychol. Psychiat.* **18**, 297–321.

FOXX, R. M., SNYDER, M. S. and SCHROEDER, F. (1979) A food satiation and oral hygiene punishment program to suppress chronic rumination by retarded persons. *J. Aut. devl Disord.* **9**, 399–412.

FRITH, U. (1971) Spontaneous patterns produced by autistic, normal and subnormal children. In *Infantile Autism: Concepts, Characteristics and Treatment* (Edited by RUTTER, M.), pp. 113–131. Churchill Livingstone, Edinburgh.

GELLER, E., RITVO, E. R., FREEMAN, B. J. and YUWILER, A. (1982) Preliminary observations on the effect of fenfluramine on blood serotonin and symptoms in three autistic boys. *New Engl. J. Med.* **307**, 165–169.

GOODALL, E. and CORBETT, J. A. (1982) Relationships between sensory stimulation and stereotyped behaviour in severely mentally retarded and autistic children. *J. ment. Defic. Res.* **26**, 163–175.

HANDLEMAN, J. S. and HARRIS, S. L. (1980) Generalization from school to home with autistic children. *J. Aut. devl Disord.* **10**, 323–324.

HEMSLEY, R., HOWLIN, P., BERGER, M., HERSOV, L., HOLBROOK, D., RUTTER, M. and YULE, W. (1978) Training autistic children in a family context. In *Autism: a Reappraisal of Concepts and Treatment* (Edited by RUTTER, M. and SCHOPLER, E), pp. 379–411. Plenum, New York.

HERMELIN, B. and O'CONNOR, N. (1970) *Psychological Experiments with Autistic Children.* Pergamon, Oxford.

HOBSON, R. P. (1983) Origins of the personal relation, and the unique case of autism. Paper presented to the Association for Child Psychology and Psychiatry, London, May 1983.

HOLMAN, J. and BAER, D. M. (1979) Facilitating generalization of on-task behavior through self-monitoring of academic tasks. *J. Aut. devl Disord.* **9**, 429–446.

HOLMES, N., HEMSLEY, R., RICKETT, J. and LIKIERMAN, H. (1982) Parents as co-therapists: their perceptions of a home-based behavioral treatment for autistic children. *J. Aut. devl Disord.* **12**, 331–342.

HOWLIN, P. (1980) The home treatment of autistic children. In *Language and Language Disorders in Childhood* (Edited by HERSOV, L. A. and BERGER, M.), pp. 115–145. Pergamon, Oxford.

HOWLIN, P. (1981) The effectiveness of operant language training with autistic children. *J. Aut. devl Disord.* **11**, 89–106.

KANNER, L. (1943) Autistic disturbances of affective contact. *Nerv. Child* **2**, 217–250.

KIERNAN, C. (1983) The use of nonsocial communication techniques with autistic individuals. *J. Child Psychol. Psychiat.* **24**, 339–376.

KOEGEL, R. L. and EGEL, A. L. (1979) Motivating autistic children. *J. abnorm. Psychol.* **85**, 418–426.

KOEGEL, R. L., RINCOVER, A. and EGEL, AL.L. (1982) *Educating and Understanding Autistic Children.* College Hill, San Diego, CA.

KOEGEL, R. L., RINCOVER, A. and EGEL, AL.L. (1981) *Educating and Understanding Autistic Children.* Colley Hill, San Diego, CA.

LELORD, G., MUH, J. P., BARTHELEMY, C., MARTINEAU, J., GARREAU, B. and CALLAWAY, E. (1981) Effects of pyridoxine and magnesium on autistic symtoms: initial observations. *J. Aut. devl Disord.* **11**, 219–229.

LEPPER, M. R. (1981) Intrinsic and extrinsic motivation in children: detrimental effects of superfluous social controls. In *Aspects of the Development of Competence* (Edited by COLLINS, W. A.), pp. 155–214. Erlbaum, Hillsdale, NJ.

LORD, C. (1983) The development of peer relations in children with autism. In *Applied Developmental Psychology* (Edited by MORRISON, F. J., LORD, C. and KEATING, D. P.). Academic, New York.

LOTTER, V. (1978) Follow-up studies. In *Autism: a Reappraisal of Concepts and Treatment* (Edited by RUTTER, M. and SCHOPLER, E.), pp. 475–495. Plenum, New York.

LOVAAS, O. I., KOEGEL, R. L. and SCHREIBMAN, L. (1979) Stimulus overselectivity in autism: a review of research. *Psychol. Bull.* **86**, 1236–1254.

MARCHANT, R., HOWLIN, P., YULE, W. and RUTTER, M. (1974) Graded change in the treatment of the behaviour of autistic children. *J. Child Psychol Psychiat.* **15**, 221–227.

MEADOW, K. P. (1975) The development of deaf children. In *Review of Child Development Research* (Edited by HETHERINGTON, E. M.), Vol. 5, pp. 441–508. University of Chicago Press, Chicago, IL.

NELSON, D. L., GERGENTI, E. and HOLLANDER, A. C. (1980) Extra prompts versus no extra prompts in self-care training of autistic children and adolescents. *J. Aut. devl Disord.* **10**, 311–322.

Journal of Child Psychology and Psychiatry, 1985, vol. 26, pp. 193–214

RIIKONEN, R. and AMNELL, G. (1981) Psychiatric disorders in children with earlier infantile spasms. *Devl Med. Child Neurol.* **23**, 747–760.

RIMLAND, B., CALLAWAY, E. and DREYFUS, P. (1978) The effects of high doses of vitamin B$_6$ on autistic children: a double-blind crossover study. *Am. J. Psychiat.* **135**, 472–475.

RINCOVER, A. and KOEGEL, R. L. (1977) Classroom treatment of autistic children—II. Individualized instruction in a group. *J. abnorm. Child Psychol.* **5**, 113–126.

ROMANCZYK, R. G., KISTNER, J. A. and PLIENIS, A. (1982) Self-stimulating and self-injurious behaviour: etiology and treatment. In *Advances in Child Behavioral Analysis and Therapy*, Vol. 2. *Autism and Severe Psychopathology* (Edited by STEFFEN, J. J. and KAROLY, P.), pp. 189–254. Lexington Books, D. C. Heath, Lexington, MA.

RUTTER, M. (1970) Autistic children: infant to adulthood. *Semin. Psychiat.* **2**, 435–450.

RUTTER, M. (1974) The development of infantile autism. *Psychol. Bull.* **4**, 147–163.

RUTTER, M. (1978) Diagnosis and definition. In *Autism: a Reappraisal of Concepts and Treatment* (Edited by RUTTER, M. and SCHOPLER, E.), pp. 1–25. Plenum, New York.

RUTTER, M. (1979a) Language, cognition and autism. In *Congenital and Acquired Cognitive Disorders* (Edited by KATZMAN, R.), pp. 247–264. Raven, New York.

RUTTER, M. (1979b) Autism: psychopathological mechanisms and therapeutic approaches. In *Cognitive Growth and Development: Essays in Memory of Herbert G. Birch* (Edited by BORTNER, M.), pp. 273–299. Brunner/Mazel, New York.

RUTTER, M. (1980) Language training with autistic children: how does it work and what does it achieve? In *Language and Language Disorders in Childhood* (Edited by HERSOV, L. A. and BERGER, M.), pp. 147–172. Pergamon, Oxford.

RUTTER, M. (1981a) *Maternal Deprivation Reassessed* (2nd Edn). Penguin Books, Harmondsworth.

RUTTER, M. (1981b) *Hereditary Factors and Autism.* National Society for Autistic Children, London.

RUTTER, M. (1983) Cognitive deficits in the pathogenesis of autism. The Kenneth Cameron Memorial Lecture. *J. Child Psychol. Psychiat.* **24**, 513–531.

RUTTER, M. (1984a) Family and school influences: meanings, mechanisms and implications. In *Practical Lessons from Longitudinal Studies* (Edited by NICOL, A. R.). Wiley, Chichester. In press.

RUTTER, M. (1984b) Infantile autism: assessment, differential diagnosis and treatment. In *Diagnosis and Treatment in Pediatric Psychiatry* (Edited by SHAFFER, D., ERHARDT, A. and GREENHILL, L.). Free Press, New York. In press.

RUTTER, M. and BARTAK, L. (1973) Special educational treatment of autistic children: a comparative study—II. Follow-up findings and implications for services. *J. Child Psychol. Psychiat.* **14**, 241–270.

RUTTER, M. and GARMEZY, N. (1983) Developmental psychopathology. In *Social and Personality Development.* Vol. 4. *Handbook of Child Psychology* (Edited by HETHERINGTON, E. M.), pp. 775–911. Wiley, New York.

RUTTER, M and SUSSENWEIN, F. (1971) A developmental and behavioral approach to the treatment of pre-school autistic children. *J. Aut. Childh. Schizophr.* **1**, 376–397.

RUTTER, M., YULE, W., BERGER, M. and HERSOV, L. *An Evaluation of a Behavioural Approach to the Treatment of Autistic Children.* Final Report to the Department of Health and Social Security, London, 1977.

SCHOPLER, E., BREHM, S., KINSBOURNE, M. and REICHLER, R. J. (1971) Effect of treatment structure on development in autistic children. *Archs gen. Psychiat.* **24**, 415–421.

SCHOPLER, E., MESIBOV, G. and BAKER, A. (1982) Evaluation of treatment for autistic children and their parents. *J. Am. Acad. Child Psychiat.* **21**, 262–267.

SCHOPLER, E. and REICHLER, R. J. (1971) Parents as cotherapists in the treatment of psychotic children. *J. Aut. Childh. Schizophr.* **1**, 87–102.

SCHREIBMAN, L. (1975) Effects of within-stimulus and extra-stimulus prompting on discrimination learning in autistic children. *J. appl. Behav. Anal.* **8**, 91–112.

TAYLOR, E. (1984) Drug treatment. In *Child Psychiatry: Modern Approaches* (2nd Edn) (Edited by RUTTER, M. and HERSOV, L.). Blackwell Scientific, Oxford. In press.

VOLKMAR, F. R. and COHEN, D. J. (1982) A hierarchical analysis of patterns of non-compliance in autistic and behavior-disturbed children. *J. Aut. devl Disord.* **12**, 35–42.

WAHLER, R. G., BERLAND, R. M. and COE, T. D. (1979) Generalization processes in child behavior change. In *Advances in Clinical Child Psychol* (Edited by LAHEY, B. B. and KAZDIN, A. E.), Vol. 2, pp. 36–69. Plenum, New York.

Motivation and Delinquency. Vol. 44 of the Nebraska Symposium on Motivation, ed. D. W. Osgood, 1997, pp. 44–118

Heterogeneity of Antisocial Behavior: Causes, Continuities, and Consequences

Michael Rutter
MRC *Child Psychiatry Unit and Social, Genetic & Developmental Psychiatry Research Centre, Institute of Psychiatry, London*

Barbara Maughan
Joanne Meyer
Andrew Pickles
Judy Silberg
Emily Simonoff
Eric Taylor

Any consideration of the reasons why people engage in antisocial behavior must be based on a recognition of the heterogeneity of antisocial behavior (Rutter, in press-a). At one extreme, isolated acts that could have led to prosecution are committed at some time by the majority of young people. The extremely high base rate means that the great majority grow up to be ordinary, reasonably well func-

Particular thanks are due to Deborah Jones for her help in preparing this chapter and especially for her production of the figures used. The research reported here owes much to the contribution of many colleagues; we are particularly indebted to Lindon Eaves, Richard Harrington, John Hewitt, David Quinton, Lucinda Shillady, David Smith, and William Yule. Further details on the individual programs of research are given in the notes.

126 ∎

tioning adults. At the other extreme, some young people who show persistent and widespread antisocial behavior in childhood go on to exhibit antisocial personality disorders in adult life that are accompanied by pervasive and persistent social malfunction across a wide spread of life's domains. Such disorders are found in some 1 in 30 males in the general population (Robins, Tipp, & Przybeck, 1991). Between these two extremes are the third or more of boys living in cities who have an official court record (Rutter & Giller, 1983); about half of these have only one conviction, but the remainder have varying degrees of recidivism. In addition, a small proportion of criminal acts are associated with major mental disease or disorder.

Although there is a general recognition that antisocial behavior is heterogeneous, doubts and uncertainties remain on how best to subdivide this overall behavioral grouping. Indeed, there is not agreement as yet on whether the heterogeneity reflects qualitatively distinct subcategories or whether it is a consequence of varying admixtures of dimensional traits and risk factors. In this chapter, we focus on possible meaningful heterogeneity as reflected in the overlap between conduct disorder in childhood and three other broad groupings: emotional disorder (especially depression), hyperactivity, and reading difficulties. Data from studies over the last 30 years employing a range of epidemiological, longitudinal, clinical, and genetic research strategies are used to consider the possible implications for causal mechanisms, continuities and discontinuities between childhood and adult life, and consequences for adult functioning and psychopathology.

The questions to be addressed were laid out in the findings of the Isle of Wight surveys undertaken in the mid-1960s (Rutter, Tizard, & Whitmore, 1970). Findings for the children at age 10 emphasized the high frequency with which conduct disorders were accompanied by symptoms of overactivity, restlessness, fidgetiness, and inattention. The importance of the association was indicated by the results of the follow-up study at age 14–15 years (Schachar, Rutter, & Smith, 1981). The persistence of conduct disturbance across the time period extending from middle childhood into mid-adolescence was much higher in the children whose conduct disturbance was accompanied by hyperactivity, especially where this was evident both at home and at school. Follow-up findings were also informative in indicating the different course shown by emotional disorders and conduct disorders, with the latter more likely to persist (Graham & Rutter, 1973). But, the findings at both age periods emphasized the high frequency with which emotional and conduct disorders co-occurred. The epidemiological correlates suggested that, on the whole, these mixed disorders had more in common with "pure" conduct disorders than with "pure" emotional disorders, but the data on this point were necessarily limited. Severe reading difficulties were also extremely common in children showing conduct disorders. Over 40% of boys with conduct disorders showed severe reading difficulties, as did nearly a third of girls with conduct disorders. Co-occurrence of reading difficulties and emotional disorder was very much less frequent. The other finding from the Isle of Wight studies to which we draw attention is that reading difficulties were far more frequently found accompanying disorders that were already evident at age 10 than accompanying those disorders arising *de novo* at some point between 10 and 14 years. It appeared that age of onset might be an important source of meaningful heterogeneity. Persistence of disorder was also relevant; family risk factors were much more strongly associated with disorders that were evident at *both* age 10 and age 14 than with those manifest at only one of the two age periods.

■127

Some Causal Considerations

Before considering how far research findings are informative on the meaning of this heterogeneity in antisocial behavior, we need to address the question of what is meant by *motivation*. The term is often used in the sense of the emotion or cognition that leads to a conscious choice or decision or will to behave in a particular way. That is to say, the focus is on what was in a person's mind that caused him or her to commit some act. Alternatively, the term *motivation* is used to refer to the underlying causes of a behavior, and that is the sense in which we primarily use it here. In order to understand why a person engages in some behavior, it is necessary to determine how genetic factors and prior experiences create a predisposition to act in that way—a predisposition that may operate through behavioral styles (e.g., impulsivity or sensation seeking), or patterns of attribution (e.g., assumptions of hostile intent), or thinking patterns (e.g.,

128 ∎

acting without thought for the future). The predisposition may, in addition, come about through the situations in which people find themselves. A teenager's decision to leave a hostile, rejecting home environment through the route of early marriage and pregnancy may involve no unusual motivational process, but, nevertheless, it is likely to place the teenager at an increased risk for a range of social outcomes involving risk circumstances. The factors involved in a decision to commit an antisocial act need to be considered as the end result of direct and indirect causal chains and not as a process that is independent of the past. Longitudinal research strategies are essential if there is to be an adequate understanding of how internal psychological processes serve to influence later environments, and vice versa. It is also necessary to appreciate that the motivational factors will include those that concern individual differences in liability to engage in antisocial behavior and the factors that concern the translation of that liability into the commission of antisocial acts. There can be no assumption that deliberate decisions are required. Clearly, conscious choices are involved, but they constitute only part of the story. This approach to motivation also differs from the former in its focus on both distal and proximal processes.

It is important to recognize that causal processes involve, not one causal question, but many (Rutter, in press-b; Rutter, 1994). With respect to antisocial behavior, there is the question of individual differences; why "X" is criminal whereas "Y" is not. There is also the quite different question of the causes of differences in level either over time or place (Rutter & Smith, 1995). Thus, one may ask why the crime rate has risen so greatly in most Western countries over the last 50 years or why the murder rate in the United States is 15 times that in Europe. A third causal question refers to differences in actualization. We need to consider why this person with a predisposition to antisocial behavior actually commits a crime now in this particular circumstance (Tonry & Farrington, 1995). This distinction is one that applies widely in psychopathology, and not just antisocial behavior. Whether someone attempts suicide will be influenced, not just by their suicidal tendencies, but by the availability of means of self-destruction and whether, at the relevant time, their inhibitions are reduced by drugs or alcohol. Similarly, severely stressful life events play a major role in the precipitation of onset of episodes of depression (Brown & Harris, 1978), but it is quite likely that such events are less important with respect to individual differences in the overall liability to depression when considered over time (Kendler, Neale, Kessler, Heath, & Eaves, 1993). A fourth question concerns changes over time within the individual. Thus, it is well documented that criminal behavior falls off markedly during early adult life (Farrington, 1986). The factors involved in desistance from crime may or may not be the same as those involved in the initiation of antisocial activities at a much earlier age (Sampson & Laub, 1993).

A rather different sort of distinction among causal explanations concerns the different levels to which they refer. To begin with, there are the features that concern neural structure and function. Thus, research has focused on the possible importance of serotonin levels and of neurotransmitter functions. Alternatively, research may focus on susceptibility traits such as novelty seeking (Cloninger, Adolfsson, & Svrakic, 1996). Recent research linking the D4 dopamine receptor gene with novelty seeking has indicated a potential bridge between these first two levels in causal explanation. However, susceptibility traits may involve not only temperamental characteristics but also styles of cognitive processing (Dodge, 1986; Dodge, Pettit, McClaskey, & Brown, 1986), and such traits are likely to be influenced, not only by genetic factors, but also by parenting and other experiences during the early years (Dodge, Pettit, Bates, & Valente, 1995). A third level of causal explanation might concern the route by which such susceptibility traits lead on in some individuals either to a disorder (for example, conduct disorder) or the manifestation of a tendency to engage in antisocial behavior. A fourth level of explanation might address the question of individual differences (among those with that disorder or propensity) with respect to the frequency and/or severity of their antisocial behavior. One might ask why this individual has only 1 criminal conviction whereas that one has 10. A fifth level concerns the factors involved in why an individual act is committed at the time and in the particular circumstances in which it took place. Thus, there is a sizeable literature on situational factors that influence delinquent and criminal activities (Tonry & Farrington, 1995).

Along with these approaches to causal explanation, it is necessary to adopt a developmental perspective (Loeber & Hay, 1994). That is, one also needs to consider how behavior may change in form over the course of lifespan development. For example, one

■ 129

Motivation and Delinquency. Vol. 44 of the Nebraska Symposium on Motivation, ed. D. W. Osgood, 1997, pp. 44–118

may ask why and how hyperactivity in the preschool years leads to an oppositional/defiant disorder in early or middle childhood, why some cases of oppositional/defiant disorder become conduct disorders in adolescence, and why some cases of conduct disorder lead to personality disorders of various types in adult life.

130 ∎

Some Epidemiological Findings on Risk Factors

During the 1970s and early 1980s, epidemiological methods were used to examine quite a wide range of risk factors for antisocial behavior at individual, family, school, and community levels. In each of these studies, we sought to determine how the risk might be mediated. For example, following the Isle of Wight surveys (which concerned an area mainly made up of small towns), it was necessary to consider the extent to which the findings would be the same in the very different circumstances of socially disadvantaged inner London (Rutter, 1973; Rutter, Cox, Tupling, Berger, & Yule, 1975; Rutter, Yule, et al., 1975; Berger, Yule, & Rutter, 1975). A survey in London, using exactly the same methods as those employed in the Isle of Wight, was undertaken with a focus on 10-year-olds. The findings were clear-cut in showing that the rate of psychopathology in inner London was twice that on the Isle of Wight.[1] The difference was evident on both questionnaire and interview measures; moreover, it was found not to be an artifact of selective in- or out-migration. The twofold increase in disorder applied to children born and bred in the two areas.

The study included a detailed examination of a range of possible risk factors, and the findings showed that all these factors were considerably more prevalent in inner London than on the Isle of Wight (see Figure 1). About half the child population in inner London came from families exhibiting some form of psychosocial adversity, whereas this applied to only about 1 in 5 of the children living on the Isle of Wight (Rutter & Quinton, 1977). Multivariate analyses showed that almost the whole of the difference in rates of psychopathology between the two areas was explicable in terms of the area differences in family adversity. In other words, it seemed that the causal route was likely to involve some mechanism by which living in a socially disadvantaged inner-city area increased family adver-

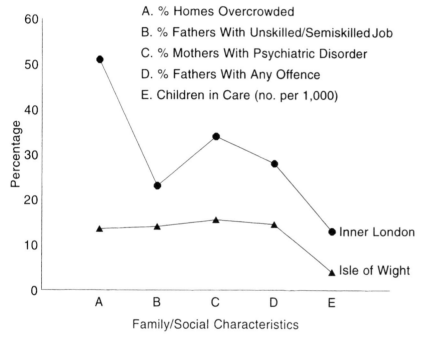

A. % Homes Overcrowded
B. % Fathers With Unskilled/Semiskilled Job
C. % Mothers With Psychiatric Disorder
D. % Fathers With Any Offence
E. Children in Care (no. per 1,000)

Figure 1. Psychosocial features in inner London and on the Isle of Wight (adapted from Rutter & Quinton, 1977).

sity rather than any direct effect on the child that was independent of the family. Follow-up data were informative, too, in showing that (at least as measured by teacher questionnaires) the main effect of the area in which children grow up applied to disorders that persisted to age 14–15 years but that were already manifest at age 10, and not to those developing *de novo* in adolescence without behavioral disturbance at age 10 (Rutter, 1980).

The Isle of Wight–London comparison also suggested that a contributory factor to the area difference was to be found in school adversity. Thus, indices such as high pupil turnover, high rates of absenteeism, and a high pupil-teacher ratio were more frequent in inner London than on the Island. These school characteristics were associated with disorder, with the main effect apparently being on children from nondisadvantaged families. This led to a more systematic study of possible school influences on children's behavior and scholastic attainments.[2] Our starting point lay in the epidemiological study of 10-year-olds in an inner London borough. We followed the children across their transfer into secondary school at age

132 ▪

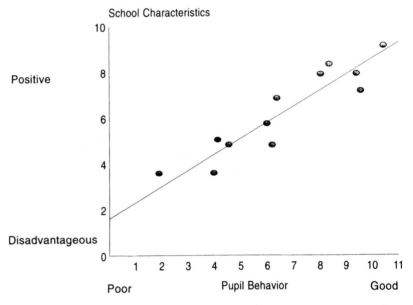

Figure 2. School characteristics and pupil behavior. From *Fifteen Thousand Hours: Secondary Schools and Their Effects on Children* (p. 142), by M. Rutter, B. Maughan, P. Mortimore, & J. Ouston, 1979, London: Paul Chapman Publishing Ltd. Copyright 1979 by Paul Chapman Publishing Ltd. Reprinted with permission.

11–12, focusing on the progress of those children who attended the 12 secondary schools taking the bulk of the children from the borough that we had studied (Rutter, Maughan, Mortimore, Ouston, & Smith, 1979). These children were followed throughout their secondary schooling and into their first year of employment (Gray, Smith, & Rutter, 1980). In parallel with studying the children's progress, we made a detailed study of the characteristics of the schools.

The findings were striking, not just in their demonstration of huge variations among the schools on all indices of pupil progress, but more particularly in showing that these variations were systematically associated with characteristics of the schools as social institutions. Because we had systematic longitudinal data extending from the period before the children entered secondary school, we were able to take account of variations among the schools in the characteristics of their pupil intake. The findings were clear-cut in showing major school effects on pupil behavior such as truancy, fighting, breaking school rules, and classroom disruption (see Figure 2). The causal inference that the associations represented effects of the school on the children, rather than the effects of the children on the school, was supported by the finding that the correlation between school characteristics and children's behavior during the later years of their secondary schooling (0.92) was considerably greater than the correlation between school characteristics and the children's behavior at the time of school entry (0.39). The school characteristics associated with better pupil behavior included good classroom management, appropriately high expectations of the pupils, good models of teacher behavior, positive feedback to the children, consistency of school values, pleasant working conditions and good teacher-child relationships, shared activities between staff and pupils, and opportunities for the children to exercise responsibility.

Although pupil misbehavior at school is associated with delinquency, the two are far from synonymous, and the role of the school was not quite the same for both. School effects on delinquency were quite strong, but the details differed from effects on misbehavior in that the composition of the school intake played a rather greater role than the characteristics of the school ethos. The implication was that peer group pressures might well be playing a larger role in relation to delinquency than with other aspects of the pupils' behavior. Causal inferences are, of course, always stronger when one can demonstrate effects following a change in the putative causal factor. We were able to use this strategy to a limited extent in a study of three schools that had been in considerable difficulties and that then experienced a change in school principal (Maughan, Pickles, Rutter, & Ouston, 1991; Ouston, Maughan, & Rutter, 1991). The results showed a dramatic effect on absenteeism and scholastic attainments in one of the schools and worthwhile benefits in a second school. The findings again support the inference that schools can and do influence children. Our findings on the importance of the school environment were initially greeted with some skepticism among academics, but subsequent studies by other research groups have broadly confirmed our findings and have shown that, if anything, we underestimated the importance of school effects (see Maughan, 1994; Mortimore, 1995).

Risk factors relating to the children's upbringing were examined in two main high-risk groups: those who were reared in residential Group Homes as a result of parenting breakdown (Quinton & Rutter, 1988) and those reared by mentally ill parents (Rutter & Quinton,

134 ∎

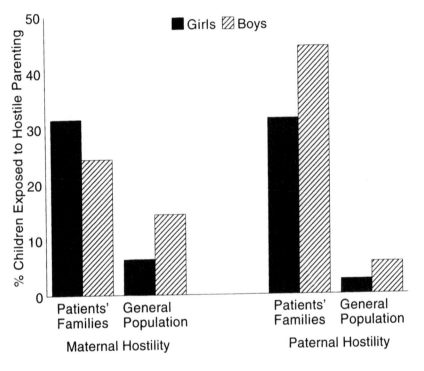

Figure 3. Frequency of hostile parenting in families with a mentally ill parent (high-risk group) and a general population community sample (adapted from Maughan et al., 1995).

1984). Both studies were based on epidemiological samples and both involved longitudinal study, as well as comparisons with the general population sample. The children taken into care by local authorities as a result of parenting breakdown showed a greatly increased rate of antisocial behavior, however measured, in both childhood and adult life. We consider the findings from that study in greater detail when looking at adult outcome later in this chapter.

The original focus on parental mental disorder, in the other study, derived from the expectation that this would constitute a major risk factor in its own right. Our comparison between the sample of families with a mentally ill parent and a general population community sample showed that the two groups differed greatly in marital discord and in adverse relationships between parents and children.[3] Children in families with a mentally ill parent (patients'

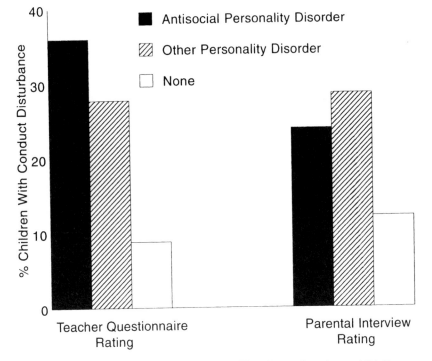

Figure 4. Parental personality disorder, parental hostility, and persistent child disturbance on teacher questionnaires (adapted from Rutter & Quinton, 1984).

families) were much more likely to be exposed to hostile parenting than were those in the general population (see Figure 3).

This led us to look in greater detail at the relative contributions from parental mental disorder and from parent-child relationships. The parental diagnosis that was associated with the highest psychopathological risk for the children was antisocial personality disorder, the main risk being for conduct disturbance in the offspring. Accordingly, we examined the relative strength of effect of parental personality disorder and the child's exposure to hostile behavior by the parents (see Figure 4). The findings were striking in showing that the main effect derived from hostile parenting, rather than from parental personality disorder. In the absence of hostile parenting, there was no increase in risk associated with parental personality disorder. However, within the group of children exposed to hostile behavior, the risk was greater when this was combined with paren-

136 ■

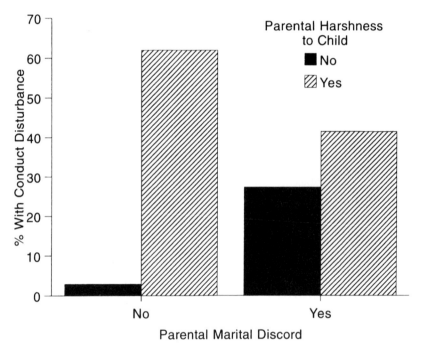

Figure 5. Parental harshness and marital discord in relation to conduct disorder in boys (adapted from Maughan et al., 1995).

tal personality disorder. These findings were evident in both questionnaire and detailed interview assessments.

At the time that this study was undertaken, the main focus in the research literature was on family-wide marital discord. Our research was unusual in measuring how the family environment impinged on each child at an individual level. Accordingly, we were able to determine the extent to which the risk for the children derived from child-specific risk experiences within the family rather than overall family circumstances. The analyses showed that, although both had some effect, the predominant impact came from individualized experiences of hostile parental behavior (see Figure 5). The finding is in line with comparable investigations by other research groups (see Reiss et al., 1995) and with the evidence from genetic research showing that child-specific environmental effects tend to be greater than family-wide shared environmental effects (Plomin & Daniels, 1987). In part, this difference is likely to stem from children's differential involvement in family-wide adverse experiences. For example, the same study showed that when mentally ill parents were feeling stressed and irritable, their hostility was not evenly distributed among the children in the family. The negative focus tended to be particularly on children with adverse temperamental characteristics (Rutter, 1978).

■ 137

Time Trends in Crime

At the same time as these epidemiological/longitudinal studies were being undertaken, there was a growing awareness on both sides of the Atlantic that levels of crime were rising greatly. This led Academia Europaea to set up a study group to examine the phenomenon, not just in relation to crime, but with respect to a broader range of psychosocial disorders in young people (Rutter & Smith, 1995).[4] Detailed attention was paid to a range of methodological considerations that could have led to an artifactual impression of a rise in crime. The evidence from a wide range of European countries and from North America showed that during the period since World War II there had been a very considerable rise in crime (Smith, 1995). The trend was shown, not only by official crime statistics, but also by victim survey data and interview studies. Unfortunately, the available crime data refer to crimes, rather than individuals, and do not differentiate between isolated offences and recidivist crime. The interview data from the U.S. Epidemiological Catchment Area study, however, suggest that the rise does include antisocial behavior persisting from childhood into adult life (Robins et al., 1991). The implication is that there has probably been some increase in the proportion of the population with a liability to antisocial behavior, and not just in the actualization of that liability (i.e., the tendency of delinquency-prone individuals to engage in delinquent activities). Clearly, a rise as rapid and as marked as this had to be the result of some change in environmental circumstances, rather than the result of any change in the gene pool. The evidence on comparable rises in other psychosocial disorders was informative in bringing in the additional consideration that the rise applied to disorders in youths and young adults but not in older age groups. Accordingly, the explanation had to be found in terms of some environmental change

Motivation and Delinquency. Vol. 44 of the Nebraska Symposium on Motivation, ed. D. W. Osgood, 1997, pp. 44–118

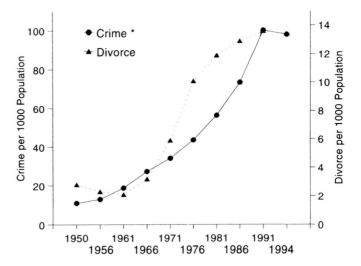

* Excluding offences of 'other criminal damage' value £20 & under

Figure 6. Changes in crime and divorce rates, 1950–1994 (data from Farrington, 1992; Home Office, 1994; OPCS, 1994).

that particularly impinged on younger age groups (Rutter, in press-b).

Social scientists have often been inclined to attribute changes in the level of crime to society-wide factors such as unemployment or income level. These probably are important at an individual level, but the evidence was clear that they could not be invoked as a main explanation for the rise in crime over time. The rise in antisocial activities began during the 1950s and accelerated during the 1960s and early 1970s at a time when unemployment rates were very low and when levels of affluence were increasing, together with an accompanying reduction in social inequalities. The parallel between the rise in crime and the rise in divorce was much closer; it is certainly possible that a rise in family breakdown has played a part in leading to a rise in crime (see Figure 6). However, quite a range of other possible explanations also need to be considered. In part, it may be that crimes have increased because opportunities for crime have risen. The rise in affluence has meant that there are more goods to steal, and changes in housing conditions (particularly the widespread introduction of high-rise housing) have meant that community surveillance is weaker. The growth of large self-service stores has meant that shopping has become less personalized; perhaps, too, this has made stealing less easy to control because the shopkeepers are less likely to know the customers and because there are far more customers milling around the shelves of goods on sale. In addition, it may be that levels of stress experienced by young people have gone up because of diminished job opportunities for unskilled workers, because of rising educational expectations, and because the extension of education has meant a prolonged period of dependence on parents. A third set of factors may involve a potentiation of antisocial activities through the greater availability and misuse of drugs and alcohol and perhaps by a focus on crime in the media, especially films and television. Public concerns about the adverse effects stemming from the media have often been in terms of people copying what they see on film. This may occasionally take place, but it is likely that the greater effect derives from creating an impression that "everyone does it" (solve problems by violence, take drugs, or steal things), and hence that such behavior is acceptable. As well as the increased liability to antisocial behavior that may have derived from the increasingly high rate of family breakdown, the parallel increase in mental disorders (such as depression, alcoholism, and drug problems) in young parents is likely to have had consequent risk effects on the children. Inevitably, there are difficulties in investigating causal factors for trends over time, and there are necessary uncertainties that apply to reliance on aggregated group data. Nevertheless, the phenomenon of change over time in rates of crime has been important in drawing attention to a range of possible causal influences that differ somewhat from those that are most striking in relation to the rather different causal question of individual differences in antisocial behavior.

Antisocial Behavior and Depression

We have already noted the evidence, from the Isle of Wight surveys onward, that there are many children who show an admixture of both emotional and conduct disturbance. Longitudinal data may help in sorting out the possible meaning of this comorbidity (see Caron & Rutter, 1991). One key question is whether conduct disturbance in childhood predisposes to emotional disturbance in adult

140■

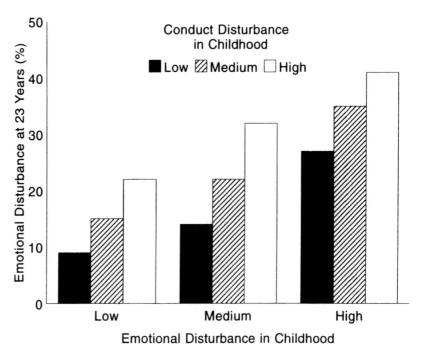

Figure 7. Emotional/Conduct disturbance in childhood and probability of high "malaise" score in females at 23 years (adapted from Rutter, 1991).

life among individuals who did *not* show emotional disturbance in childhood. The British National Child Development study of some 17,000 children followed from birth into adult life provided the necessary sample to examine this question. The childhood measures were derived from a combination of parent and teacher questionnaires given at 7, 11, and 16 years. The use of six data sources enables one to be reasonably sure that most important emotional difficulties will have been detected. As might be expected, emotional difficulties in childhood were associated with a two- to threefold increase in the rate of emotional disturbance at 23 years of age, as assessed on the Malaise Inventory (Rutter, 1991). However, what was very striking, and perhaps surprising, is that, within all levels of emotional disturbance in childhood, conduct disturbance was also associated with a doubling of the risk of emotional disturbance in adulthood. The report in 1991 provided the findings for males; Figure 7 gives the comparable data for females, which show exactly the same pattern. It is evident that conduct problems in childhood predict emotional disturbance in adult life even in the absence of emotional difficulties in childhood and adolescence. More detailed multivariate analyses, using logistic regression methods based on latent variables that account for measurement error and that focus on persistent emotional or conduct disturbance in childhood, confirmed this predictive relationship (Pickles & Clayton, 1996).

Leverage on the same issue was provided by a longitudinal study of child patients undertaken by Harrington and his colleagues (1991).[5] The main focus of that investigation was the adult outcome (at a mean age in the early 30s) for children who had shown a depressive disorder (as operationally defined on the basis of symptomatology) below 16 years of age. This depressive group was compared with a closely matched group of child patients showing some nondepressive form of psychopathology. In order to focus on the specific importance of depression, the two groups (both of which involved patients at the Maudsley Hospital) were matched on all symptoms other than that of depression itself. This design had the additional advantage of allowing us to examine the outcome for both depressive disorders and conduct disorders in childhood according to whether or not they co-occurred. The findings were surprisingly clear-cut. Conduct disturbances in childhood were powerfully predictive of a criminal conviction in adult life, and the presence or absence of depression in childhood made no difference to this adult outcome. The findings for the outcome of major depressive disorder in adult life were quite different. Depression in childhood proved to be a powerful, and diagnosis-specific, predictor, and to that extent, the findings were similar to those for conduct disorder. The key difference lay in the effect of comorbidity. Children with both depression and conduct disorder showed no increase in major depressive disorders in adult life. Together with other findings, the implication was that these comorbid depressive disorders were probably secondary to conduct disturbance and, hence, had a somewhat different meaning from "pure" depressive disorders in childhood (see also Harrington, Rutter, & Fombonne, 1996). On the other hand, the prognostic importance of conduct disturbances in childhood were completely unaffected by the co-occurrence of depression.

It is necessary to ask how this finding tallied with the earlier finding that conduct disturbances in childhood predicted emotional

142 ■

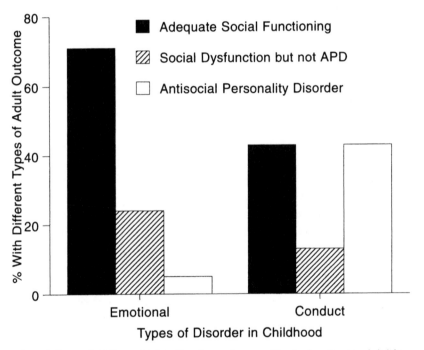

Figure 8. Type of child psychiatric disorder and personality dysfunction in adult life (adapted from Rutter et al., 1994).

disturbance in adult life. To answer that question, we focused on the difference in adult life between major and minor depressive disorders within the subgroup of child patients who showed pervasive social dysfunction of one sort or another in adult life (see Figure 8). The results showed that antisocial personality disorder was accompanied by minor depression in nearly a quarter of the individuals, but that major depressive disorders were strikingly uncommon, occurring in only 6% (Rutter, Harrington, Quinton, & Pickles, 1994). The implication was that although the co-occurrence of emotional difficulties did not seem to alter the course of antisocial behavior between childhood and adult life, nevertheless, antisocial behavior appeared to generate an increased tendency to minor depressive problems (minor, that is to say, in the pattern of symptomatology but often associated with substantial chronicity and social impairment). How might that come about?

To answer that question, we used our longitudinal study of school children in inner London followed from the age of 10 over the

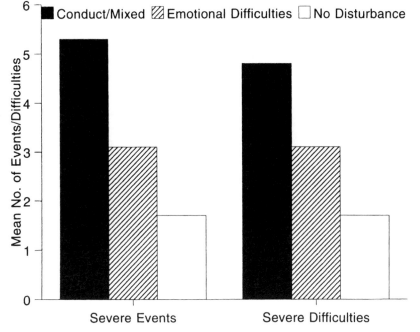

Figure 9. Severe events and difficulties in early adult life and type of disturbance at 10 years, in females (adapted from Champion et al., 1995).

next two decades (Champion, Goodall, & Rutter, 1995). The focus of this study was on whether children's behavior at age 10 predicted their environment as experienced during their late 20s (see Figure 9). The answer was that it did. Conduct disturbance as measured on a teacher questionnaire at age 10 was associated with a threefold increase in the mean number of severely negative acute life events (such as parental loss) and severely negative long-term difficulties (such as chronic family discord) experienced over a five-year period in the late 20s. There was also some increase in negative life experiences in adulthood for children who showed emotional disturbance in childhood, but the effect was much more marked in relation to conduct problems. It seems likely that part of the explanation for the association between antisocial behavior and minor depression is that people with conduct problems act in ways that predispose them to interpersonal tensions and other stressful situations. These stresses, in turn, then tend to provoke affective disturbance.

Motivation and Delinquency. Vol. 44 of the Nebraska Symposium on Motivation, ed. D. W. Osgood, 1997, pp. 44–118

Reading Difficulties and Antisocial Behavior

The same longitudinal study of London children was used to examine the interconnections between reading difficulties and antisocial behavior in greater detail.[6] Our earlier findings had suggested that some kind of two-way interplay was likely. Thus, the association between a somewhat lower IQ and an increased risk of antisocial behavior held right across the IQ range and applied within social class groupings (Rutter, Tizard, & Whitmore, 1970). Data from other studies have been consistent in confirming this association (Goodman, 1995; Goodman, Simonoff, & Stevenson, 1995). Also there was a trend (albeit a statistically nonsignificant one) for developmental delays to be more frequent in children with antisocial problems than in the remainder of the general population—a mean score of 1.5 versus 0.9 (the scores reflecting the number of delays across a range of different developmental functions such as speech or motor control).

The follow-up into the adult life of the 10-year-old children as part of the epidemiological study of an inner London borough provided the opportunity to look at effects over time. First, the effect of disruptive behavior on progress in reading was examined. As might be expected, children with disruptive behavior (who had a much increased rate of truancy and unauthorized absenteeism from school) made slightly less progress in reading during secondary school (Maughan, Rutter, & Yule, 1996).

We then looked at the association the other way round, in terms of the effect of reading difficulties on the course of antisocial behavior over time (Maughan, Dunn, & Rutter, 1985; Maughan & Hagell, 1996; Maughan, Hagell, Rutter, & Yule, 1994; Maughan, Pickles, Hagell, Rutter, & Yule, 1996). As all studies have shown, there was quite a strong association between antisocial behavior and reading difficulties in childhood. Thus, even in a high delinquency area like inner London, the rate of delinquency was some 50% higher among boys who showed severe reading difficulties. The follow-up of the children who had shown severe reading difficulties had indicated a very high degree of persistence into adult life (Maughan et al., 1994), and it might be supposed that this would be accompanied by an equally persistent association with antisocial behavior. Thus, Moffitt (1993a) has argued that neuropsychological deficits may play a key

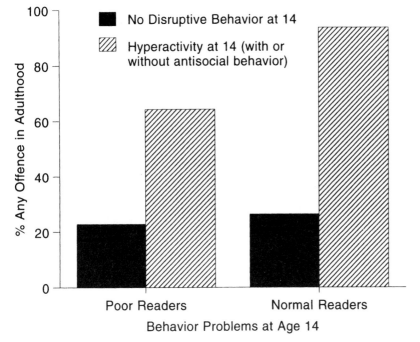

Figure 10. Hyperactivity and adult crime in individuals with and without severe reading difficulties at age 14 (adapted from Maughan et al., 1996).

role in the genesis of antisocial behavior. If that were the case, it might be supposed that this would be particularly true in relation to antisocial behavior persisting into adult life. In the event, the follow-up findings showed the opposite.

The rate of adult crime was actually slightly lower among the boys who had been poor readers than it was in the general population comparison group. Of course, this finding must be interpreted within the context of an inner London general population sample with a particularly high base rate of crime. Nevertheless, even when the adult outcome was considered in relation to broader aspects of psychopathology or social functioning, it was evident that the poor readers did *not* have any substantial increase in adult mental disorder. Multivariate analyses showed that reading difficulties were associated with disruptive behavior at age 10, that the latter predisposed children to poor school attendance at age 13, and that poor school attendance, in conjunction with some independent effect from disruptive behavior, led to juvenile delinquency. Juvenile de-

Motivation and Delinquency. Vol. 44 of the Nebraska Symposium on Motivation, ed. D. W. Osgood, 1997, pp. 44–118

146 ∎

linquency, and conduct disturbances at 14, were associated with a much increased risk of adult crime, but there was no route to adult crime that did not come through earlier antisocial behavior. A more detailed study of the data showed that antisocial behavior was somewhat less likely to persist into adult life when it was accompanied by reading difficulties (see Figure 10).

There was one particularly puzzling aspect of these findings. In childhood, as other studies have also found (Hinshaw, 1992), the association between reading difficulties and antisocial behavior in childhood was particularly evident when the antisocial behavior was accompanied by hyperactivity. As hyperactivity has been found to be a predictor of greater persistence of antisocial behavior (Schachar et al., 1981), it would seem to follow that antisocial behavior would be particularly persistent when there were reading difficulties. To look at that matter more closely, we looked at the effect of hyperactivity at age 14 on the later course of antisocial behavior according to the presence or absence of reading difficulties. In both groups, the presence of hyperactivity was associated with a greater likelihood of adult crime, but this effect was more marked in those *without* reading difficulties (see Figure 10). The implication is that at least some forms of hyperactivity associated with reading difficulty may have a somewhat different meaning than that which applies in the absence of reading problems. It might also have been expected that hyperactivity as measured at age 10 would be particularly influential, as that had been found in the Isle of Wight sample (Schachar et al., 1981), but this was not the case. It is difficult to be sure exactly why there was no effect in this sample, but perhaps the reason lies in the high level of inattentive, restless behavior among children in socially disadvantaged inner-city schools, including overactivity that derives from sources quite different from those found in hyperkinetic disorders. Unfortunately, in this sample we did not have parental interview or questionnaire measures, as these might have resolved the issue.

Adult Experiences and Course of Antisocial Behavior

Attention has already been drawn to the association between behavior in childhood and adult experiences. One particularly important aspect of that effect concerns the choice of spouse or partner. Our follow-up of children who had spent much of their years of upbringing in group foster homes showed that, compared with the general population sample, they were much more likely to have a partner with deviant behavior involving antisocial activities, drug taking, or alcohol problems (Quinton & Rutter, 1988; Quinton, Pickles, Maughan, & Rutter, 1993; Zoccolillo, Pickles, Quinton, & Rutter, 1992).[7] This tendency was much stronger in females than males. Not surprisingly, these marriages, or cohabiting partnerships, with antisocial individuals were often characterized by marked marital discord and a high rate of marital breakdown. What was particularly striking, however, was the observation that when these women from high-risk backgrounds did happen to have a nondeviant supportive partner, their adult functioning was very much better.

The key question was whether those who married nondeviant men were less antisocial themselves in childhood. There was also the query whether this might represent some peculiarity of the circumstances of young people who had experienced an institutional rearing. To tackle both these questions, the institutional sample was combined with a general population sample also followed into adult life (already described above). Latent class methods, together with other statistical approaches, were used to ensure that the apparent protective effect of a supportive marital partner was not simply a consequence of measurement error (Pickles & Rutter, 1991; Quinton et al., 1993). The results were clear-cut in indicating that there was a true turning-point effect by which the presence of support from a nondeviant partner was associated with a much better adult outcome among girls who had shown conduct disturbance in childhood (see Figure 11). In the absence of such support, antisocial behavior showed a strong likelihood of leading to pervasive social malfunction in adult life. By sharp contrast, women who were equally antisocial as children (actually marginally more antisocial) tended to go on to show *adaptive* social functioning in adult life when they had support from a nondeviant partner. A closely comparable finding was evident in the re-analysis of the Gluecks' (1950) follow-up study data by Sampson and Laub (1993). The findings are important in indicating that adult experiences can play a crucial role in influencing the social outcome (including, but not confined to, criminal activities) of young people who have shown conduct problems

• 147

148▪

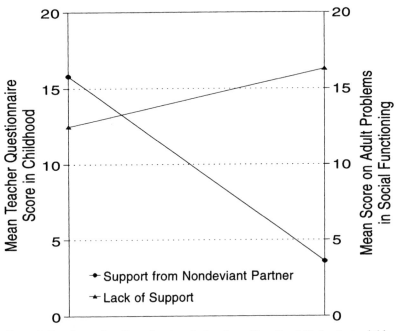

Figure 11. Turning-point effect of partner in females with antisocial behavior in childhood (analysis by Pickles from data set reported in Quinton et al., 1993).

in childhood. This protective effect in our sample was substantially greater in females than males.

In order to understand how this protective effect came about, we needed to examine the intervening years in greater detail. The question was why some young people with antisocial behavior succeeded in making a harmonious marriage with a nondeviant partner whereas many did not. Both the age at which girls married and had their first child and (for any given age) the likelihood of the partner being antisocial were important (Pickles & Rutter, 1991). Girls showing antisocial behavior in childhood were much more likely to become a teenage parent and to have a deviant partner. A range of possible influences was examined. It was found that being part of a deviant peer group and having had an institutional rearing were associated with an increased risk of cohabitation with a deviant partner by age 20 and that a tendency to show planning (meaning the taking of deliberate decisions about key life choices) and the presence of a harmonious family environment were associated with a decreased risk. Early cohabitation with a deviant partner was associated with a markedly decreased likelihood of the individual being

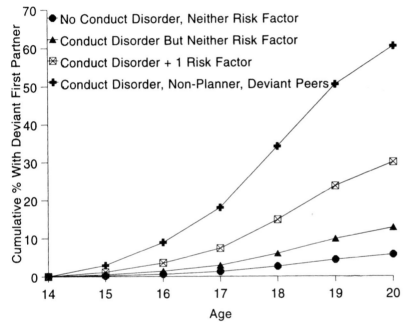

■ 149

Figure 12. Childhood conduct disturbance, planning, and deviant peers, as risk factors for deviant first partners by age 20 years (analysis by Pickles from data set reported in Quinton et al., 1993).

with a current nondeviant supportive partner at the time of follow-up in the mid-20s.

The overall effect is most easily seen when the pathways are expressed in diagrammatic form. Thus, Figure 12 shows the cumulative probability over time of living with a deviant man according to the presence of conduct disorder, a lack of a tendency to plan, and participation in a deviant peer group. The probabilities concern estimated rates derived from a survival analysis using Cox regression; this assumes a multiplicative effect of risk factors on the hazard (although not on the probability itself). The proportion of women, without conduct disorder and without either of the two risk factors of nonplanning and deviant peers, who had a deviant first partner by the age of 20 years was very low (5.7%). The presence of conduct disorder, in the absence of the two risk factors, doubled the proportion, but the main effect came from the combination of conduct disturbance with the two risk factors. The proportion with a deviant partner at age 20 was 30% when there was one risk factor; when both

150 ■

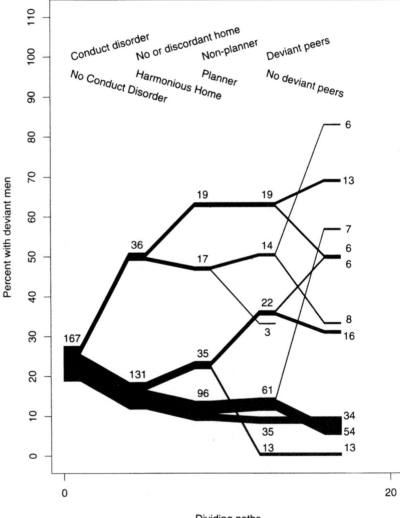

Dividing paths
Frequencies given by numbers and line width

Figure 13. Paths of women to deviant men. From "Partners, Peers and Pathways: Assortative Pairing and Continuities in Conduct Disorder," by D. Quinton, A. Pickles, B. Maughan & M. Rutter, 1993, *Development and Psychopathology, 5*, p. 778. Copyright 1993 by Cambridge University Press. Reprinted with the permission of Cambridge University Press.

risk factors were present, the proportion rose to 60%—a more than tenfold increase in risk over the base rate.

Figure 13 (based on raw data rather than estimates) shows the overall indirect pathway by examining the routes to first cohabitation with a deviant man according to risk and protective factors laid out in time sequence. The overall tendency for partnership with a deviant man was greater for those showing conduct disorder in childhood, but the likelihood went up or down in a consistent way according to the presence or absence of the protective effect of a harmonious home in the teenage years, a tendency to plan, and a nondeviant peer group. At each point, the person's life situation made a substantial difference to the ultimate likelihood of partnership with a nondeviant spouse at follow-up. In each instance, of course, the prior risk factor made it less likely that the person would *have* the protective experience, but if they did, the beneficial effect was evident. The implication is that, although undoubtedly part of the persistence of antisocial behavior needs to be seen in terms of trait or disorder persistence, much of the continuity comes indirectly from the cumulative effect of life experiences. As Caspi and Moffitt (1993) have pointed out, stressful experiences on the whole accentuate, rather than change, prior psychological characteristics. On the other hand, major turning-point effects, with a redirection of life trajectory, can occur when individuals from a high-risk background encounter a very positive life experience that is out of synchrony with their previous chain of adversities and disadvantage (Pickles & Rutter, 1991; Quinton et al., 1993; Rutter, 1996d). These effects of positive life experiences in adulthood do not stand out as major influences in outcome when considered in population variance terms simply because it is unusual for high-risk individuals to have such protective experiences. Nevertheless, when they do, the benefits can be substantial with respect to their own functioning in adult life. We have studied this issue in relation to long-term effects, but the same considerations apply to shorter-term fluctuations in antisocial behavior (Horney, Osgood, & Marshall, 1995).

Studies of Hyperactivity and Hyperkinetic Disorder

The next set of studies to consider came from the program of research undertaken into hyperactivity and hyperkinetic disorders. In

■151

152 ∎

order to investigate the question of whether there was a meaningful distinction to be drawn between hyperkinetic and conduct disorders, Taylor and colleagues (Taylor, Sandberg, Thorley, & Giles, 1991) undertook a systematic epidemiological study of 7-year-olds living in inner London.[8] Initially, the groups were divided up on the basis of the screening questionnaire findings. Whereas the children with pure conduct disturbance did not differ from general population controls with respect to objectively measured activity (using actometers) or attentional performance (as measured by a range of tests) or IQ, the group with mixed hyperactivity and conduct disturbance did differ on all three counts. They were much more active, showed much worse attention, and had a mean IQ some 6 points below the mean for the general population. The next step in the research involved the more detailed, standardized, individual study and the redefinition of diagnostic groups defined in terms of this much more detailed information. Thus, for example, hyperactivity and inattention were measured on the basis of detailed descriptions of the children's behavior across a range of situations, using operationalized criteria, rather than in terms of questionnaire scores. The contrast between diagnostic groups became much sharper at this point. The hyperkinetic 7-year-olds in the disorder group had a mean IQ some 17 points below controls, their attentional performance was much worse, they were more likely to show neurodevelopmental impairment, and they were somewhat more likely to have experienced obstetric suboptimality (meaning an increase of minor complications during the pregnancy). The hyperkinetic disorder group was very much more likely to have shown language impairment and poor coordination, and the children were several times more likely to have shown early behavior problems. By contrast, the conduct disorder group was much more likely to have a family history of conduct problems, and the children were more likely to come from families exhibiting marked marital discord. It may be concluded that hyperkinetic disorder was particularly associated with cognitive impairment and neurodevelopmental difficulties, whereas conduct disturbance was not, but such disturbance *was* associated with family adversity and a family history of antisocial behavior. The findings were very much in line with those of other investigators (see Fergusson, Horwood, & Lloyd, 1991; Fergusson, Horwood, & Lynskey, 1993). The diagnosis of hyperkinetic disorder as used in this study was substantially narrower (and in some key respects different from) that associated with the North American concept of attention deficit disorder with hyperactivity (ADHD). Accordingly, the next step was to compare the findings for hyperkinetic disorder and ADHD. The results showed that, whereas hyperkinetic disorder contrasted sharply with both pure conduct disorder and general population controls, this contrast did not apply to ADHD. In some respects children with ADHD were intermediate, but on the whole they were closer to the conduct disorder group than to the hyperkinetic disorder group (particularly with respect to their IQ level).

These data all used clinical or epidemiological correlates to investigate possible heterogeneity, but response to treatment constitutes another, complementary, approach. A double-blind, cross-over trial of stimulant medication was used to explore whether drug response (defined in terms of a benefit in relation to the active drug as compared with the placebo as used in the same child) helped with diagnostic distinctions (Taylor et al., 1987). It did not in any clear-cut way, although the overall hyperactivity level and degree of inattention did predict a positive drug response. A beneficial reaction to stimulant drugs was also more likely when the children showed low levels of anxiety and depression, and there was some tendency for neurodevelopmental impairment to predict a good drug response, although this effect disappeared when the other variables were taken into account. The degree of oppositional/conduct disturbance and the degree of family dysfunction had no effect on drug response.

A key issue in all studies examining relationships between family dysfunction and antisocial behavior of the children concerns the question of the direction of the causal arrow. To what extent has the family dysfunction predisposed children to antisocial behavior and to what extent did the antisocial behavior predispose the family to difficulties (Bell, 1968; Lytton, 1990)? The drug study provided one means of tackling this issue. The question was whether there was a change in parental behavior that accompanied the pharmacologically induced alteration in the child's behavior. Schachar and colleagues (Schachar, Taylor, Wieselberg, Thorley, & Rutter, 1987) found that, among drug responders, the use of methylphenidate was significantly associated with a rise in maternal warmth and

■ 153

154 ▪

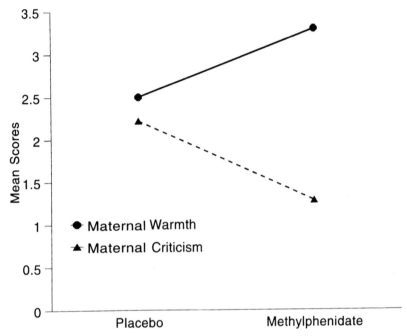

Figure 14. Effects of stimulants given to children on parental expressed emotions (adapted from Schachar et al., 1987).

a fall in maternal criticism (see Figure 14). The implication was that the child had an effect on parental behavior, although, of course, the finding did not rule out an additional effect the other way around. Indeed, other research has provided evidence of effects both ways (see Anderson, Lytton, & Romney, 1986).

Although our findings, like those of others, indicated the strength of differences between hyperkinetic disorder and conduct disorder, the fact remained that there was considerable overlap between these two patterns of psychopathology. We needed to address the question of how this came about and also what the implications were for the course of antisocial behavior over time. A follow-up study at the age of 17 years was undertaken for the groups first studied at age 7 (Taylor, Chadwick, Heptinstall, & Danckaerts, 1996) in order to tackle the question. Four main groups were compared: those showing hyperactivity (but not oppositional/conduct disturbance); those showing oppositional/conduct disturbance (but not hyperactivity); those with both types of psychopathology; and those

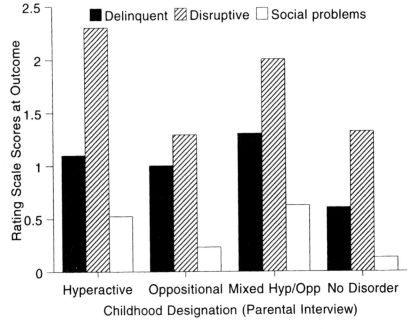

Boys in London originally studied at age 7

Figure 15. Hyperactivity and oppositional/conduct disturbance as predictors of out-come at 17 years for boys (adapted from Taylor et al., 1996).

with neither. All three psychopathological groups showed an in-creased level (relative to the general population) of antisocial behav-ior at age 17, the level being greatest in those with both hyperactivity and disruptive behavior at age 7. Hyperactivity at 7 predicted antiso-cial behavior at 17, but the reverse did not apply (i.e., antisocial be-havior at 7 did not predict hyperactivity at 17). The effects of early hy-peractivity were somewhat different, however, according to the type of outcome being considered. Hyperactivity was associated with some increase in delinquent behavior at outcome, but the main effect was most obvious with respect to other forms of disruptive be-havior and social problems more generally (see Figure 15). The group with pure hyperactivity showed much the same level of anti-social behavior at age 17 as did the pure oppositional/conduct disor-der group, and the outcome for both antisocial behavior and other forms of psychopathology was much worse in the group with the comorbid pattern. It seems that the presence of hyperactivity in

156 ■

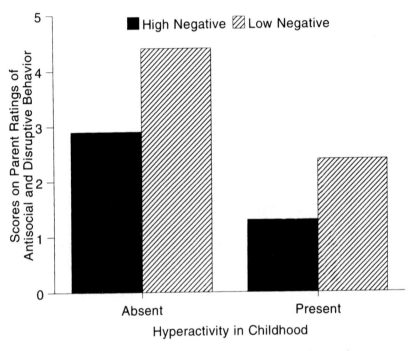

Figure 16. Negative expressed emotion with hyperactivity as predictors of outcome at 17 years for boys with antisocial problems at 7 years (adapted from Taylor et al., 1996).

early childhood is an important prognostic factor, that it does indeed predispose a child to antisocial behavior, but probably that the increased liability applies more to social malfunction that includes antisocial behavior rather than having any direct effect on delinquent activities as such.

We have already noted that hyperactivity is associated with negative parent-child relationships, so it is necessary to consider whether the effect on outcome derived from the hyperactivity in the child or rather from the negative parent-child relationships. The follow-up findings showed that both were important (see Figure 16). For children with both high- and low-negative expressed parental emotion, the outcome was worse for those with hyperactivity in childhood. Equally, however, for children who did and those who did not show hyperactivity in childhood, the outcome was worse for those experiencing parental criticism and hostility. In other words, the prognostic effect derived from *both* child characteristics and parent-child relationships. Research needs to focus on the interplay between risk factors in the child and risk factors in the environment (Rutter et al., in press).

Any research into individual risk factors has to contend with the fact that the putative individual risk factors for antisocial behavior cover quite a broad range, even when confined to those for which there is reasonably good empirical support (Farrington, 1995a, 1995b; Lahey, McBurnett, Loeber, & Hart, 1995). Thus, there are those factors that concern behavioral tendencies such as novelty seeking, impulsiveness, hyperactivity, aggressivity, and low autonomic reactivity. It is obvious that these concepts overlap to an important extent, and it is not as yet clear which concept incorporates the main risk effect. There is a second set of risk factors associated with cognitive limitation of one kind or another—including inattention, verbal impairment, and an executive planning deficit (Moffitt, 1993a). Thirdly, there are atypical thought processes as represented by a hostile attributional style (Dodge et al., 1995) or an internalized model of insecure attachment (Greenberg, Speltz, & DeKlyen, 1993). Although the behavioral tendencies, cognitive limitations, and atypical thought processes sound as if they refer to quite different risk factors, it is likely that they overlap; we do not know their relative importance or indeed what sort of underlying liability they reflect.

The issues are well illustrated by the behavioral phenomenon of impulsiveness. At a descriptive level, this is usually indexed by features such as children not being able to wait for their turn, or blurting out answers in class before they are asked, or interrupting other people's conversations. The problem here is that this could reflect a cognitive tendency, a behavioral characteristic associated with oppositional behavior, or both. The epidemiological findings from the study undertaken by Taylor et al. (1996) indicated that these behaviors increased in both the hyperactive group and the conduct disorder group. A program of experimental studies is being undertaken in order to determine more precisely what is involved in the apparently impulsive behavior that is specifically associated with hyperactivity. The study by Sonuga-Barke and his colleagues (Sonuga-Barke, Taylor, Sembi, & Smith, 1992) illustrates the approach. An experimental design was used in which children could choose either an immediate reward or a delayed reward and in which the experimental setup could be manipulated to ensure that the economic ben-

■ 157

158 ▪

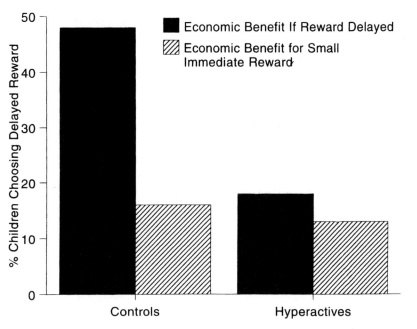

Figure 17. Reward-delay benefits and responses of hyperactive and control children (adapted from Sonuga-Barke at al., 1992).

efit to the child favored either a delayed reward or a smaller, but immediate, reward. Hyperactive children did not differ at all from controls in the experimental conditions in which the benefits were associated with a small immediate reward. By sharp contrast, however, the groups differed markedly when the economic benefit derived from a delayed reward (see Figure 17). This change in reward made virtually no difference in the hyperactive group, but in the control group, the children were much more likely to choose a delayed reward when it was beneficial for them to do so. On the other hand, when the experimental conditions were altered so that the children had to wait before they could proceed, regardless of which reward they chose, the hyperkinetic children tended to choose the delayed reward. It seemed that they had an aversion to delay that was not responsive to economic benefits, but they could wait if they had to. It may be concluded from the findings of Taylor's research program and the results of research undertaken by other investigators (Schachar, 1991; Schachar, Tannock & Logan, 1993) that the behavioral feature of impulsiveness in hyperkinetic children has several different bases when analysed at the level of neuropsychological process. First, the children show a lack of preparedness so that in circumstances when children can anticipate having to react in a particular way, hyperkinetic children show a prolonged reaction time. Second, they have difficulty suppressing or delaying a response (often called "inhibition") and hence tend to show unduly hasty responses when they would do better to take a little more time over their reactions. In different circumstances their reactions could therefore be either too quick or too slow. Third, there is a range of behavioral features for which further research is necessary to determine whether they can be explained in terms of these two processes. The tendency of hyperactive children to give inaccurate, careless responses could be due to hastiness; disorganized exploration of new situations could also be due to a premature and disinhibited response to most salient stimulus features. It remains to be seen whether these explanations will in fact hold.

Many of the earlier notions that a general deficit in attention constituted the basis of hyperactivity have had to be abandoned. Thus, children with a hyperkinetic disorder do not show impaired selective attention as was once thought to be the case. On the other hand, there is no doubt that cognitive limitations are a prominent part of what is involved in the hyperkinetic syndrome, and it remains quite possible that the key to the psychopathology will be found in some form of abnormality in cognitive processing. With respect to antisocial behavior, however, there is the additional question of whether the risk derives from some type of cognitive limitation or, rather, from the behavioral tendencies with which such cognitive features tend to be associated. The answer to that question will have to await further research.

Follow-up of Twins with Conduct Disorder

One possibly important aspect of heterogeneity in antisocial behavior concerns the persistence, or nonpersistence, from childhood into adult life. The pooled twin data from several studies of juvenile delinquency and adult crime showed that the genetic component in adult crime was substantially greater than that for juvenile delinquency (DiLalla & Gottesman, 1989). The finding is potentially im-

Motivation and Delinquency. Vol. 44 of the Nebraska Symposium on Motivation, ed. D. W. Osgood, 1997, pp. 44–118

portant, but it is constrained by three pertinent limitations: the data were based on samples that were not entirely satisfactory; the results applied strictly to official crime records and not to antisocial behavior generally; the age difference derived from quite different samples, and there was uncertainty whether the difference was a consequence of the samples or the age. In order to examine possible age changes in heritability more directly, Simonoff and her colleagues undertook a systematic study of all twins with an IQ in the normal range who attended London's Maudsley Hospital when under the age of 16 years and who displayed an emotional or conduct disorder or some admixture of the two. Subjects with developmental disorders or psychoses were excluded.[9] The follow-up was confined to the twins who would be at least 25 years of age at the time of follow-up. All sets of twins were followed into adult life and were interviewed about their lifetime psychopathology and their life experiences, using systematic standardized investigator-based interview methods. At the time of writing, a few remaining twins have yet to be seen; the results are reported on the subsample of 15 monozygotic (MZ) pairs and 40 same-sex dizygotic (DZ) pairs, in both cases the sample being restricted to those where the designation of zygosity is definite. For present purposes, the 33 opposite-sexed dizygotic pairs are excluded, as are the pairs for whom complete data are available on only one member of the pair.

In keeping with the results from studies of singletons, conduct disorder in childhood proved to be a powerful predictor of antisocial personality disorder in adult life (the adult diagnosis being made without the requirement of childhood psychopathology). Nearly half of the individuals with conduct disorder in childhood showed antisocial personality disorder compared with only about 1 in 15 of those without conduct disorder. The within-pair correlations, treating antisocial behavior as a continuous dimension (rather than a present/absent category) at both age periods, showed a marked difference between childhood and adult life (see Figure 18). In childhood, the within-pair correlations for both MZ and DZ twins were moderately high, being just below the 0.5 level, but with no appreciable difference between the two types of twins. The implication is that shared environmental influences predominate. The finding is striking because the child patients with conduct disorder showed a good deal of psychopathology; by no stretch of the imagination did

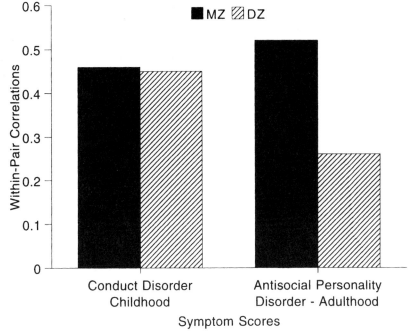

Figure 18. Within-pair correlations for MZ and DZ pairs on conduct problems in childhood and antisocial personality in adulthood (adapted from Simonoff et al., in press).

they fit the picture of relatively normal youngsters who happened to
have committed a few delinquent acts. On the other hand, previous
research had shown that family characteristics play a substantial
role in children's referral to psychiatric clinics (Shepherd, Oppenheim, & Mitchell, 1971), and it was clear from both the contemporaneous case notes and the follow-up data that the majority of the
young people came from extremely troubled families. Be that as it
may, it was clear that environmental influences accounted for most
of the variation and that a substantial proportion of the environmental effects were common to the two twins. The findings for adulthood were quite different. The within-pair MZ correlation was much
the same, but slightly higher at just over 0.5, but the within-pair DZ
correlation was just half the MZ correlation. The implication is that,
within the same group of individuals, genetic factors play a greater
role with respect to antisocial personality disorder in adulthood
than with conduct disorder in childhood. Antisocial personality disorder, of course, applies to a much lower proportion of the general

Motivation and Delinquency. Vol. 44 of the Nebraska Symposium on Motivation, ed. D. W. Osgood, 1997, pp. 44–118

162 ▪

population than does conduct disorder in childhood. Further analyses to quantify findings more precisely will be undertaken when the sample is complete, but in the meanwhile it is clear that persistence or nonpersistence of antisocial behavior into adult life constitutes an important source of heterogeneity that needs to be taken into account.

Virginia Twin Study of Adolescent Behavioral Development

Genetic research strategies were applied to the study of antisocial behavior in the very much larger (some 1,400 twin pairs) general population sample of 8- to 16-year-olds in the Virginia Twin Study of Adolescent Behavioral Development (Eaves et al., in press; Hewitt et al., in press; Silberg, Meyer, et al., 1996; Silberg, Rutter, et al., 1996; Simonoff et al., in press).[10] This is a longitudinal study in which there will be at least three waves of data collection, but the present set of analyses is based on just the first wave. A wide range of both questionnaire and investigator-based standardized interviews were used.

So far, attention has focused mainly on the co-occurrence of hyperactivity and conduct disturbance. The first approach used maternal ratings exclusively and focused on the possible difference between the younger boys and the adolescents. In both age groups, the correlation between hyperactivity and conduct disturbance was substantial (a correlation of circa 0.4 to 0.5). However, the partitioning of the variance showed a contrast between the younger and older age groups. In the children, the overlap between hyperactivity and conduct disturbance was largely explicable in terms of the same genetic factors underlying both forms of psychopathology. By contrast, although that applied to a limited extent in the adolescent age period, the genetic components of hyperactivity and of conduct disturbance were largely separate and distinct (see Figure 19). Also, conduct disturbance differed from hyperactivity in showing a substantial effect from the shared environment in the adolescent age period.

A more detailed consideration of the possible mechanisms involved is provided by expansion of the data set to include both sexes and a wider range of measures from mothers, fathers, teachers, and

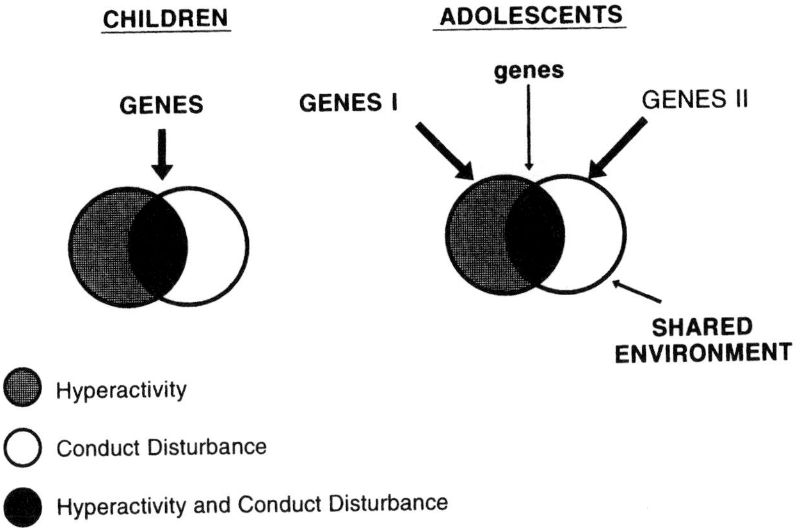

CHILDREN   **ADOLESCENTS**

GENES   **GENES I**   genes   **GENES II**

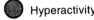

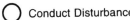

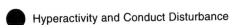

**SHARED
ENVIRONMENT**

⬤ Hyperactivity

◯ Conduct Disturbance

⚫ Hyperactivity and Conduct Disturbance

Figure 19. Genetic influences on the co-occurrence of hyperactivity and conduct disturbance in children and adolescents (adapted from Silberg et al., 1996).

the young people themselves. The first striking finding is the near-zero within-pair correlation for hyperactivity on maternal ratings for DZ pairs, as contrasted with within-pair correlations of 0.5 or above for maternal ratings of antisocial behavior in MZ pairs (Eaves et al., in press; Silberg, Rutter, et al., 1996). There are three main possible explanations for the near-zero within-pair correlations in DZ pairs for hyperactive behavior: the genetic component involves several interacting genes (i.e., epistasis); the interaction between the DZ twins serves to emphasize and exaggerate the difference between them; and when parents rate their twins they do so in ways that build on the contrast between them rather than in terms of comparison with children of the same age more generally. Both of the contrast explanations expect a greater variance in DZ pairs than MZ pairs whereas the gene-interaction hypothesis does not. The fact that, on the whole, we found greater variance in DZ pairs argues in favor of one or another of the contrast explanations.

Further light is shed by the introduction of data from the teacher questionnaires (see Figure 20). These showed a within-pair correlation for hyperactivity in DZ pairs of about 0.25—that is, substantially above zero. The difference from the maternal ratings strongly suggests a rating bias that derives from contrast effects. Statistical mod-

164 ■

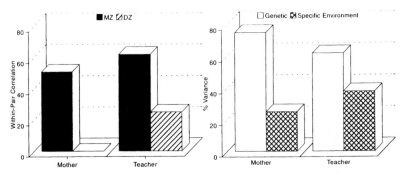

Figure 20. Within-pair correlations and genetic/environmental effects on hyperactivity as measured by mother and teacher questionnaires (adapted from Eaves et al., in press).

eling is in line with this inference and indicates that the genetic component for hyperactivity, once contrast effects have been taken into account, is somewhere in the region of 70% (Eaves et al., in press).

The findings for antisocial behavior, whether assessed by questionnaire or interview, were quite different. Both mother and child questionnaires for boys and girls showed a substantial environmental component that included both specific and shared elements. However, there was also a difference in findings that stemmed from whether the informant was the mother or the child and also whether the measurement was by questionnaire or standardized interview (see Simonoff et al., 1995). On the interview data, the environmental component was almost entirely child specific, whereas on the questionnaire measures there was also a substantial effect from the shared environment, especially in girls. The difference between mother and child reports (which applied to both interview and questionnaire measures) was that the genetic effect was at least twice as great on the mothers' reports as on the children's reports (see Figure 21 for findings on interview measures). Further analyses are required in order to determine exactly what these rater and instrument differences mean, although multivariate analyses indicate that rater bias is not likely to provide the main explanation (Simonoff et al., 1995). These differences have been found in other studies that have looked for them, so they clearly reflect nothing that is specific to the particular instruments that we used. The issue is not just that parents and children show relatively weak agreement in their reporting, but, rather, that the correlates of psychopathology differ ac-

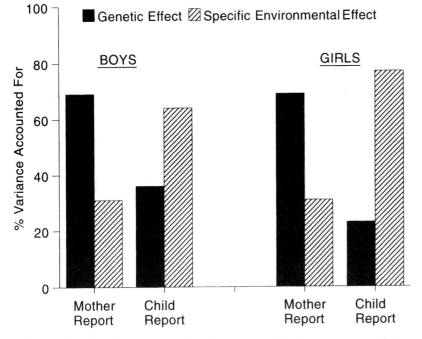

Figure 21. Genetic and environmental effects on conduct disturbance as assessed from interview with mothers and with children (adapted from Eaves et al., in press).

cording to who is reporting symptoms. A satisfactory solution to this problem has yet to be obtained because it is not known how this comes about.

Silberg, Meyer, et al. (1996) used latent class analyses in male adolescent twins, putting together data from all sources, in order to determine whether the findings could be used to infer different varieties of antisocial behavior. Using a conventional latent class analysis based on phenotypic data, four classes were derived: 1) a class of unaffected individuals with a generally low rate of psychopathology, with an estimated population prevalence of 72%; 2) a comorbid class with an estimated frequency of 14%, based upon moderately high endorsements of both hyperactivity and conduct disturbance from both mother and teacher questionnaires and, to a lesser extent, reading difficulties; 3) a class of children with conduct disturbance only, with an estimated prevalence of 8%, in which there were zero probabilities of endorsing hyperactivity items but a high probability of conduct problems, as shown on the modified version of the

Motivation and Delinquency. Vol. 44 of the Nebraska Symposium on Motivation, ed. D. W. Osgood, 1997, pp. 44–118

166 ■

Variations within Normal Range
(72% of population)

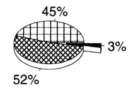

Pure Conduct Disturbance
(8% of population)

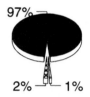

Hyperactive - Conduct Disturbance
(14% of population)

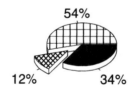

Multisymptomatic Class
(6% of population)

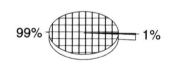

⊞ Additive Genes ⊠ Shared Environment ■ Unique Environment
■ Contrast Effect or Gene Interaction

Figure 22. Genetic evidence on heterogeneity of antisocial behavior (based on Silberg, Meyer et al., 1996).

Olweus scale, self-report ratings of oppositional and conduct problems from the child interview on the Child and Adolescent Psychiatric Assessment (CAPA) (Angold et al., 1995), reading difficulties, and, to a lesser extent, generalized anxiety; and 4) a multisymptomatic comorbid class consisting of individuals with a high probability of showing all the problem behaviors referred to above, with an estimated probability of about 6%.

As illustrated in the pie chart (Figure 22), these four classes differed dramatically in their partitioning of the variance within each class attributable to genetic and environmental effects. The multisymptomatic class showed variance that was almost entirely accounted for by genetic factors, whereas the pure conduct disturbance class showed variance that was almost entirely due to environmental factors of a shared kind. The hyperactive–conduct disturbance class was different yet again in that, although genetic factors predominated, rating contrast effects or dominant (interacting) genes were also important. The first class of relatively un-affected individuals showed additive genetic and shared environmental effects of roughly equal strength. For a variety of methodological reasons, it is likely that the true differences between these classes are not as great as these particular findings suggested (e.g., the differences between classes are as much a function of instruments as of types of psychopathology). But the genetic findings do suggest that there are both strongly genetic and strongly environmental varieties of antisocial behavior. The strongly genetic variety is one that involves a major admixture with hyperactive problems. The largely environmental variety is unassociated with hyperactivity; it particularly refers to antisocial behavior as reported by the adolescents themselves rather than their parents (and, therefore, is perhaps less likely to be accompanied by overt social malfunction) and probably is more likely to develop at a somewhat later age. Longitudinal data will be needed to resolve some of these issues, but the genetic findings are at least consistent with the distinction drawn by Moffitt (1993b; Moffitt, Caspi, Dickson, Silva, & Stanton, 1996) between the highly persistent, early-onset antisocial behavior and the transient adolescent-onset antisocial behavior.

All studies of antisocial behavior have noted the high frequency with which it is associated with mental disorder in parents. Probably the association is strongest with parental criminality, but it is also found with a wide range of other types of psychopathology (Farrington, 1995a, 1995b; Rutter & Quinton, 1984). We sought to tackle this issue by using a latent class analysis, pooling the data for mothers and fathers, to derive composite classes of parental mental disorder (Shillady et al., 1996). The first class was made up of just over half the sample and included families in which neither parent had any appreciable psychopathology. The next two classes, pooled for present purposes and accounting for just over a third of the sample, applied to families in which one or both parents had anxiety or depressive disorders. The last three classes, comprising some 13% of the overall sample, were made up of varied mixes of multiple parental disorders including alcoholism and antisocial personality disorder. The odds ratios for psychiatric disturbance in the children were determined for a range of disorders. For present purposes, the child diagnoses have been combined into broad groups of emotional disorders on the one hand and disruptive disorders on the other. There

Motivation and Delinquency. Vol. 44 of the Nebraska Symposium on Motivation, ed. D. W. Osgood, 1997, pp. 44–118

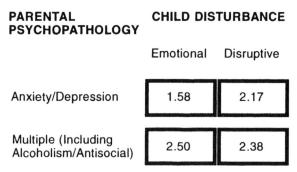

BOYS

PARENTAL PSYCHOPATHOLOGY	CHILD DISTURBANCE	
	Emotional	Disruptive
Anxiety/Depression	1.99	2.22
Multiple (Including Alcoholism/Antisocial)	1.16	2.12

GIRLS

PARENTAL PSYCHOPATHOLOGY	CHILD DISTURBANCE	
	Emotional	Disruptive
Anxiety/Depression	1.58	2.17
Multiple (Including Alcoholism/Antisocial)	2.50	2.38

Figure 23. Odds ratios for psychiatric disturbance according to parental psychopathology (adapted from Meyer et al., 1996).

was little association between multiple parental disorders and emotional disturbance in the sons, but otherwise both the main classes of parental psychopathology were associated with an increased risk of both emotional disorders and disruptive disorders in both boys and girls (see Figure 23). With the possible exception of the association between parental affective disorder and persistent emotional disturbance in sons, the latter having a substantial genetic component (Shillady et al., 1996), this relative nonspecificity of risks for psychopathology in the children is similarly evident in other research (see Rutter, 1989). As already noted, mental disorder in parents is associated with a much increased risk of family dysfunction of various kinds and likely represents both a genetic risk factor and an environmental risk factor. Further analyses will be required to gain an understanding of how these different risk routes operate.

Finally, we have used the extended twin-family design provided by the Virginia Twin Study of Behavioral Development to test for environmentally mediated risks associated with measured environmental features and operating in a fashion that is shared across twin pairs. Although there is a vast literature on the associations between various forms of family dysfunction and antisocial behavior in the children, scarcely any of the research has utilized genetically sensitive designs. This is a crucial lack because of the consistent finding that parental criminality is one of the strongest predictors of antisocial behavior in the children and because parental criminality includes a substantial genetic component. The key consideration here, of course, is that parental criminality is itself associated with disorganized and discordant family functioning in many instances. Family dysfunction was assessed using maternal reports on Olsson's Family Adaptability and Togetherness Questionnaire (Olsson, Sprenkle, & Russel, 1979) and the Dyadic Adjustment Scale (Spanier, 1976), data on the childhood symptoms of conduct disorder shown by the parents were obtained using a standardized interview, and conduct disorder in the children was assessed using the CAPA interview (Angold et al., 1995). A path-analytic model was used to test hypotheses regarding the determinants of parent-offspring similarities for conduct disorder symptomatology (Eaves, Last, Young, & Martin, 1978). A series of submodels in which parameters were dropped from the full model, or constrained to equal other parameters, were also fitted to the data in order to determine which effects were significant.

As would be expected, there was substantial covariance between marital discord (as measured on the Spanier scale) and family dysfunction (as measured by the Olsson scale). However, the pattern of significant paths was somewhat different for these two putative environmental risk factors. Figure 24 provides a simplified model for the family origins of conduct disorder, concentrating on the paths that apply to family dysfunction. It should be noted, however, that the coefficients apply to the findings from the full model

170 ■

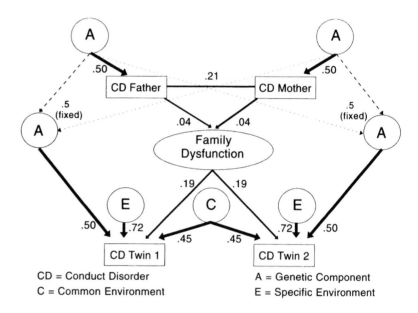

CD = Conduct Disorder   A = Genetic Component
C = Common Environment   E = Specific Environment

Figure 24. Simplified model for family origins of conduct disorder (adapted from Meyer et al., 1996).

Note: The figures in the body of the table all refer to path coefficients. Thus, .21 refers to the extent to which conduct disorder in the father is associated with the same feature in the mother. The coefficient of .50 on the path from A to CD Twin 1 and 2 refers to the genetic component; that of .72 to specific environmental effects; and that of .45 to shared environmental effects. The path coefficient of .19 from family dysfunction to CD Twin 1 and 2 refers to the shared environmental effect of this feature, after taking account of the other paths in the model.

and make mathematical sense only when the omitted coefficients are included. The main story, however, is evident in the figure shown. Having taken account of the rather weak association between the parental and child phenotypes, and the assortative mating between the parents, a significant environmentally mediated effect of family dysfunction was found. It accounts for only a rather small proportion of the shared environmental effect, and clearly other environmental factors will need to be examined. Nevertheless, these results provide a rigorously tested demonstration of the reality of an environmentally mediated risk for antisocial behavior that stems from family dysfunction.

Conclusions

Pulling together the findings from this program of research extending over the last 30 years demonstrates that the findings are as important in setting the agenda for the next 30 years as they are in showing what has been demonstrated in the past. Nevertheless, certain reasonably firm conclusions are possible.

When we initiated the research into antisocial behavior in the mid-1960s, little attention was being paid to the role of factors in the individual, and almost none to possible genetic factors. The main focus was on the supposed importance of broader social influences (such as poverty and social disadvantage) and of family breakdown and children's separations from their parents (see Rutter, 1972; Rutter & Madge, 1976; Rutter & Giller, 1983). School influences were regarded as unimportant, and there was a disregard of the extent to which children living in the same family differed in their experiences. There was also an almost complete neglect of the effects of children's behavior on their parents. All of that has changed as the result of research findings from many groups of investigators. Our own research has contributed to eight substantive conclusions on the causal factors involved in antisocial behavior.

First, it is clear that genetic factors play an important role in determining individual differences in at least some forms of antisocial behavior. The evidence indicates that this is most strikingly so in the case of antisocial behavior that is accompanied by hyperactivity. This subgroup tends to have an unusually early onset of antisocial behavior that also frequently leads to personality disorder in adult life. Perhaps it would not be much of a surprise if this finding of a strong genetic effect applied only to the severe, and uncommon, syndrome of hyperkinetic disorder, which affects perhaps some 2% of the population (Taylor, 1986; Taylor et al., 1991). After all, many clinicians have tended to view this disorder as representing some form of "organic" condition. But it is apparent that the genetic effect extends much more widely than that. The latent class analyses by Silberg, Meyer, et al. (1996) showed a predominant genetic effect in the two multisymptomatic classes that made up some 20% of the population. This also means that the findings cannot be restricted to the early-onset life course antisocial behavior that Moffitt (1993b) postulated to constitute a meaningful separate group (comprising

172 ▪

some 5% of the general population) that differed from the much commoner transient adolescent-onset delinquent pattern. It seems likely, therefore, that the genetically influenced individual risk characteristics operate more widely (probably as a risk dimension) and that the degree to which these lead to persistent antisocial behavior that in turn leads to a personality disorder in adult life depends on the co-occurrence of other risk factors (see Moffitt et al., 1996).

Three main questions derive from this finding: What is the relationship between this common feature of hyperactivity and the rarer hyperkinetic disorder syndrome? What constitute the genetically influenced susceptibility traits for antisocial behavior? Does the risk for antisocial behavior that derives from hyperactivity require any kind of interplay with environmental risk factors? Taylor's research (1986; Taylor et al., 1991) has consistently shown very important differences between the hyperkinetic disorder and the other more common varieties of overactivity/inattention. In particular, the rarer syndrome includes a much stronger component of cognitive and neurodevelopmental impairment. The possibility that this syndrome is genetically, as well as clinically, distinct requires investigation (Eaves et al., 1993). Although the genetic component in antisocial behavior is particularly associated with hyperactivity, that does not necessarily mean that excess movement (or inattention) constitutes the key susceptibility trait. We have noted the heterogeneous range of behavioral and cognitive features that need to be considered.

The possibility of gene-environment interplay might, at first sight, seem a curious consideration to raise when the evidence suggests such a strong genetic effect for antisocial behavior associated with hyperactivity. It needs raising, nevertheless, for three different reasons: this broader class of hyperactivity–conduct disorder is associated with an increased rate of features thought to represent environmental risk factors; these risk factors have been shown to predict the longitudinal course of antisocial behavior; and the findings from adoptee studies suggest that gene-environment interactions apply with respect to antisocial behavior (Bohman, 1996; Cadoret, Yates, Troughton, Woodworth, & Stewart, 1995). Thus, Silberg, Meyer, et al. (1996) found that the multisymptomatic classes were associated with high rates of parental emotional disorder that, in turn, were accompanied by increased family discord and negative parent-child relationships, which predispose to a continuation of antisocial behavior (Rutter & Quinton, 1984). Also, the Taylor et al. (1996) follow-up study of children from 7 to 17 years of age showed that parental negatively experienced emotion predicted the persistence of psychopathology. Three possibilities need to be examined: the supposed environmental risk factors are epiphenomena that are genetically determined and unimportant in risk mediation; these factors stem from the effects of children's behavior on their families rather than the other way around (i.e., active or evocative person-environment correlations); and there is a crucial gene-environment interaction that is not detected in the usual twin analyses and that particularly concerns the *persistence* of antisocial behavior over the course of development (so requiring longitudinal data for their study). The specific study of the proximal processes involved in the interplay between nature and nurture in the genesis of antisocial behavior constitutes a major research priority (Rutter et al., in press).

■ 173

The second conclusion concerns the role of environmental risk factors. Our genetic analyses demonstrate that they are very important in some forms of antisocial behavior—particularly variations within the normal range and antisocial behavior that is *not* accompanied by hyperactivity and that is reported by the adolescents themselves, rather than by their parents and teachers (Eaves et al., in press; Silberg, Meyer, et al., 1996). The question is what the environmental risk factors might be. The usual assumption is that family dysfunction and maladaptive parenting of one sort or another constitute the main causal factors. There is much evidence from other research that these are associated with early-onset antisocial behavior (Patterson, 1996). However, the epidemiological, longitudinal, and genetic findings all suggest that, on the whole, child-specific relationship features are more important than overall family characteristics. The crucial negative parenting features focused on individual children often derive from general family circumstances (such as discord), but the point is that they impinge differentially on individual children. It is these child-specific relationship problems (and other features such as surveillance, supervision, and effective feedback) that particularly require study.

However, our data, together with those of other researchers, emphasize that antisocial behavior tends to differ from other forms of psychopathology (and from most personality characteristics) in

174 ■

having a relatively strong shared environmental component. Because the "sharing" means that it affects all children in the same family to much the same degree, it is usually assumed that the risk stems from some family feature. Our findings suggest that this may not always be the case. The schools study findings point strongly to the importance of the school environment and of peer group influences. The time-trends data also suggest that population-wide factors (such as the changed meaning of adolescence and media influences) may be relevant. The crucial consideration is that because twins are of the same age, almost always attend the same school, and usually are in the same grade in school, they are much more likely than singleton siblings to share the same school and peer group influences. Insofar as they do, much of the school and peer group effects will appear as shared. The consequence is that a focus on subgroups of antisocial children in which shared environmental effects are strong may not be optimal for identifying family influences. The study of putative psychosocial causal factors needs to include school and peer group, as well as family, characteristics.

It is necessary, however, to go on to ask whether the pattern of environmental effects is likely to be the same in the more severe and pervasive forms of conduct disorder in the children who get referred to psychiatric clinics. Simonoff's twin study of this group (Simonoff, 1996), albeit based on a small sample, which calls for caution in generalizing findings, was striking in its evidence of a strong shared environmental effect. Because manifold chronic family problems were usual in this patient sample, it is most unlikely that they did not play some kind of key causal role. The results serve as a reminder that twin and adoptee studies both tend to include rather few severely disorganized families and, hence, may not be best placed to investigate the effects on children of those more extreme family environments. In general, epidemiologically based general population twin samples are to be preferred over clinic ones, but this is an instance in which a much enlarged clinic sample would be most informative.

The third conclusion concerns the important role of adult experiences in modifying the course of antisocial behavior. There are two features of our findings on this issue that stand out. First, there is the importance of investigating the course of antisocial behavior over long periods of time, with a recognition that major changes take place during the transition from adolescence to adult life, and that these changes are often systematically associated with current life circumstances in adulthood. This is an age period that particularly warrants further study for three main reasons. First, it is in the early and mid-20s that antisocial behavior decreases markedly in the general population. Second, this is a time when most young people leave school and have an increasingly wide range of activities outside the confines of the family. This means that there is a greater chance of *dis*continuity in environmental circumstances (and hence a greater opportunity for turning-point effects to occur). Third, early adult life is a time when people tend to have a much greater scope for selecting and shaping their environments. The last point leads to the second key feature of our findings; namely, that environments brought about as a result of the actions or behavior of the individuals themselves may nevertheless make a major impact on their subsequent functioning. The appreciation that the *origin* of a risk (or protective) factor has no necessary connection with its mode of risk (or protective) mediation has important research, as well as practical, implications (Rutter, Silberg, & Simonoff, 1993).

To date, there are no good longer-term published follow-up studies of individuals who have experienced an apparent change from a risk path to a more adaptive life trajectory (although we have such a data set that is now being analysed). The question to explore is whether the beneficial adult experiences bring out a lasting change in the liability to antisocial behavior or whether they are associated only with context-dependent changes in the actualization of a preexisting propensity.

The fourth conclusion is a development of the same point about adult experiences; namely, that the *course* of antisocial behavior is, to a considerable extent, dependent on indirect chain reactions. In the past, there has often been a tendency to assume that it was only *changes* in behavior that required explanation because trait persistence is the "norm." That represents a misunderstanding of what happens in development; growth (psychological and physical) involves both change and consistency (Rutter, 1996d; Rutter & Rutter, 1993). Our findings, together with those from other longitudinal studies (e.g., Caspi, Elder, & Bem, 1987, 1988), suggest a developmental process that reflects a series of interconnected probabilistic links in which continuity is influenced by the effects of people's be-

Motivation and Delinquency. Vol. 44 of the Nebraska Symposium on Motivation, ed. D. W. Osgood, 1997, pp. 44–118

havior in selecting their environments and in shaping other people's responses to them.

The fifth conclusion is that it is highly likely that cognitive factors play two rather different roles in their influence on the origins and course of antisocial behavior. On the one hand, the findings on young children with the hyperkinetic disorder strongly point to fairly direct risk effects. Although long dismissed by criminologists, neuropsychological deficits may well be involved in the causal processes underlying that disorder and, therefore, in the antisocial behavior with which it is associated (Moffitt, 1993a). The follow-up data of Taylor et al. (1996) suggest that the antisocial consequences mainly come about as part of a pattern of more widespread social malfunction, rather than as an effect on lawbreaking as such. Nevertheless, the associations are quite strong, and there is a strong need for neuropsychological research (which will need to use experimental designs) to determine which cognitive processes are involved.

On the other hand, in a follow-up of children with severe reading difficulties, Maughan, Pickles, et al. (1996) suggested that the antisocial behavior shown by the children is likely to involve more indirect effects. The antisocial behavior was *less*, not more, likely to persist into adult life in young people with severe reading problems, and the predictive power of hyperactivity was less. The finding of the antisocial tendency was *not* a consequence of the individuals' acquiring good reading skills, because the reading difficulties were remarkably likely to persist into adult life (Maughan, Hagell, et al., 1994). Rather, the general improvement in social functioning and loss of psychopathology (in many, but not all, of the poor readers) seemed to stem from moving out of the educational environment in which they were failing and from gaining alternative sources of satisfaction and reward. It should be added, however, that this relatively good outcome applied to a group of young people who left school to seek jobs at a time of very low unemployment. Whether the same would apply in the much less favorable conditions operating today in the United Kingdom is another matter.

The sixth conclusion we draw is that any consideration of the course of antisocial behavior needs to examine its consequences, as well as its causes. Up to now, researchers have tended to pay most attention to alcohol abuse and drug use, which are quite strongly associated with antisocial behavior. That constitutes one focus of our own research (not reported here), but it is equally necessary to pay attention to the association with depression and other forms of emotional disturbance. Although little recognized in the past, the data indicate that conduct problems in childhood, even when they are *not* associated with emotional difficulties in that age period, constitute quite an important precursor of emotional disturbance in early adult life (as well as predisposing to suicidal behavior—Harrington et al., 1994). Our findings suggest that this important effect may derive, in part, from the tendency of antisocial individuals to act in ways that generate stressful interpersonal interactions and life circumstances for themselves. More generally, however, the results raise the crucial question of the role of personality disturbances in predisposition to depression. To what extent, for example, is poor parenting in early childhood a risk factor for depression (Harris, Brown, & Bifulco, 1990), not because it predisposes to depression as such, but because it predisposes to personality disorder? Similarly, does part of the genetic liability to depression reflect a liability to personality disturbance?

■ 177

Although not a main focus in our own research, clearly the consequences of antisocial behavior include societal responses, the possible effects of labeling and the results of court decisions. As shown, for example, by the Sampson and Laub (1993) findings on the negative impact of incarceration (i.e., people who had been in prison found it more difficult to get jobs, and those out of work were more likely to return to crime), these consequences may well affect the likelihood that antisocial behavior persists.

A seventh conclusion from our research concerns the connections between distal and proximal risk processes. Thus, the comparative study of children in London and the Isle of Wight showed that child rearing in an inner-city area was associated with a doubling of the risk for conduct disorder—a geographical effect reflecting a distal risk. The finding that the effect was largely mediated through family discord, disorganization, and disadvantage indicated that the proximal process lay within the home and not in the children's interactions in the community. However, our more detailed studies of high-risk families went further in their demonstration that the main risk actually lay in child-specific adverse parent-child relationships rather than family-wide features. Thus, it was possible (indeed, necessary) to move from a very broad social risk indicator (i.e., child rearing in inner London) to a specific dyadic nonshared environmental risk process. The finding that the geographical area effect especially applied to early-onset chronic disorders strongly suggests that the risk processes apply to a basic liability to antisocial behavior. By contrast, this may well not be the case with either school influences or some of the societal factors that underlie the rise in crime over the last half-century. It has not been possible as yet, however, to determine the proximal processes involved.

An eighth conclusion is that study of the risk processes for antisocial behavior needs to include biological factors, but that the most profitable group to investigate in that connection is the small subgroup with hyperkinetic disorder. The particular need here is to focus on the cognitive processing abnormalities and to use functional imaging methods to determine their neural basis.

Finally, the whole body of research strongly underlines the need for both longitudinal data and genetically sensitive designs; for high-risk as well as general population samples; for a combination of dimensional and categorical measurement; for discriminating measures of environmental risk factors that operate in both a shared and nonshared fashion; and for a choice of well-designed measures and samples to test competing hypotheses on the varied range of causal questions that need to be tackled.

Model of Motivational Influences

Finally, we need to return to our starting point: the motivation of antisocial behavior. In doing so, we seek to integrate our findings with those of other research (see Cornish & Clarke, 1986; Farrington, 1995a; Felson & Tedeschi, 1993a, 1993b; Gottfredson & Hirschi, 1990; Heimer & Matsueda, 1994; Jessor, Donovan, & Costa, 1991; Loeber & Hay, 1994; Osgood, Wilson, O'Malley, Bachman, & Johnston, 1996; Patterson, 1982; Patterson, Reid, & Dishion, 1992; Rutter & Giller, 1983; Sampson & Laub, 1993; Tedeschi & Felson, 1994). The concepts and explanatory terms used by different commentators, reviewers, and theorists vary greatly, but there has been an increasing recognition that no single theory provides an adequate explanation. That is scarcely surprising because, as we noted at the outset, antisocial behavior includes a wide range of acts spanning status violations (such as truancy), illegal pleasures (e.g., drug use, joyriding, and other activities involving the thrills of risk taking and power assertion), acquisitive acts such as theft (with or without instrumental aggression), and hostile aggression both against property (e.g., vandalism) and persons (e.g., assault or homicide). The continuity between antisocial behavior in childhood and personality disorder in adult life also raises the query on the extent to which the defining criterion concerns *anti*social behavior or social *incompetence*.

Moreover, there is a growing body of evidence on the heterogeneity of antisocial patterns (Rutter, in press-a). Possibly the best validated (although even here the evidence is sparse) are the distinctions between conduct disorder associated with hyperactivity and "pure" conduct disorder (Taylor et al., 1991), and between early-onset, life-course-persistent antisocial behavior and late-onset, adolescence-limited delinquency (Moffitt, 1993b; Moffitt et al., 1996; Patterson, 1996). It appears that early-onset, life-course delinquency is associated with hyperactivity/inattention, poor social skills, varied and pervasive antisocial behaviors, associated family disorganization and coercive cycles of interpersonal interaction, and a strong genetic component. By contrast, adolescent-onset delinquency involves a lesser (but still increased) antisocial propensity accompanied by relative social competence and a lack of hyperactivity (see Patterson & Yoerger, this volume). It has to be added that, because oppositional/defiant disorders are so common in early childhood, there must also be an early-onset transient variety, about which we have fewer data. Equally, it is known that some late-onset varieties of delinquencies persist into adult life.

In addition, there may be a valid distinction between violent and nonviolent crime in adult life (see Bock & Goode, 1996); some antisocial behavior stems from mental illness; rare cases derive from medical conditions; and some cases represent highly principled moral acts (e.g., some aspects of the civil rights movement or the fight against apartheid). Is an entirely different motivational explanation needed for each of these varieties? We suggest not (at least for antisocial behavior not due to some overt illness). However, in putting forward a general model it is essential to note that very few data are available on antisocial behavior in females or in middle-class groups. Accordingly, although the explanations for these groups are

180 ∎

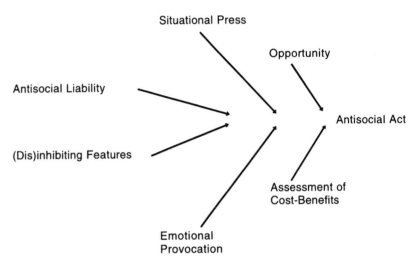

Figure 25. Schematic model of proximal motivational influences.

likely to include similar components, there may well be important differences. Nevertheless, the overall model of possibly operative causal factors is probably broadly similar across a range of antisocial behavior despite the critical fact that their relative importance, and the specifics of their operation, are likely to vary substantially both according to act (e.g., theft vs. violence vs. vandalism vs. sex offences) and person (male vs. female; white collar vs. blue collar; or differences among ethnic groups). That variation is crucially important, as we have emphasized here, but now we need to place the heterogeneity within a broader framework.

Figure 25 sets out the six broad groups of factors that may play a part in the causal processes leading to the commission of some antisocial act. That labeled *Antisocial Liability* recognizes the importance of individual differences in people's propensity to engage in antisocial behavior. That labeled *(Dis)inhibiting Features* reflects the fact that, despite individual differences, everyone has some potential for antisocial behavior; whether or not individuals engage in delinquent acts will be influenced by the strength of inhibitory controls. The other four factors serve as a reminder that a propensity to act antisocially is one thing, but the commission of a particular delinquent act is another. It will be dependent on available *Opportunities, Situational Presses* that foster antisocial activities, *Emotional Provocation,* and the individual's personal *Assessment of Cost-Benefits* of commit-

ANTISOCIAL LIABILITY	(DIS)INHIBITING FEATURES
Values	Values
Indirect Susceptibility Traits (e.g., impulsivity or novelty-seeking)	(Lack of) Anxiety
Learned Behavioral Patterns (e.g., aggression, self-seeking acquisition)	(Lack of) Empathy for Others
Cognitive Processing of Experiences (e.g., tendency to attribute hostile intent)	(Lack of) Internal Controls/Inhibitions
Reactivity to Environmental Adversities	(Lack of) Long-term Planning/Foresight
Lack of Status Attributes (e.g., high IQ, educational attainments social position, admired social qualities)	(Lack of) Surveillance/ External Controls
Previous Experiences	
"Permission" for Antisocial Behaviors (e.g., Cultural, contextual, media influences)	Alcohol / Drugs

Figure 26. Antisocial liability and (dis)inhibiting features.

ting the delinquent act (note the actual cost-benefits are not what matters; rather, it is the person's own assessment, however inaccurate and misguided, that will influence action).

The summary of some of the key aspects of an antisocial liability provided in Figure 26 emphasizes its multifaceted nature. Values favoring antisocial activities include an acceptance of the use of illegal drugs for their pleasurable effects as normal and desirable; the acceptability to many people of fiddling with income tax or expense returns or using a work telephone for private calls; and the perceived appropriateness in some groups of assaulting someone who insults you. The research findings on hyperactivity underline the importance of behavioral traits such as impulsivity or sensation seeking that do not in themselves concern antisocial features but that nevertheless, in some circumstances, create a susceptibility, or increased risk, for antisocial behavior. In addition, of course, there are learned antisocial behaviors (but subject to genetic influences) that lead more directly to delinquent activities (see Patterson, 1982, 1996; Patterson & Yoerger, this volume). The likelihood that someone will respond with violence to a negative interpersonal interaction will be

Motivation and Delinquency. Vol. 44 of the Nebraska Symposium on Motivation, ed. D. W. Osgood, 1997, pp. 44–118

182∎

influenced by their inference of the person's intent; the work of Dodge (1986; Dodge et al., 1986) has shown that aggressive boys show an increased liability to attribute hostile intent. All research into the effects of psychosocial stresses and adversities has indicated the importance of individual differences in vulnerability, and adoptee studies have suggested that part of the effects of genetic predisposition may lie in a greater susceptibility to environmental hazards (Bohman, 1996; Cadoret, Cain, & Crowe, 1983; Cadoret et al., 1995).

Our own research, like that of others, has shown that low educational attainment predisposes to antisocial behavior in childhood. The finding that it does not do so in adult life suggests that the connection is likely to be indirect, and perhaps reflects the many disadvantages experienced at school by children who fail educationally. As Tedeschi (this volume) notes, the social strain theory of delinquency has only rather modest empirical support, but it is likely that a lack of status attributes may predispose to antisocial behavior to some extent. Thus, unpopularity among peers is a risk factor (Parker & Asher, 1987), and a range of other personal qualities appear to have effects mediated through their impact on interpersonal interactions and attitudes (Engfer, Walper, & Rutter, 1994).

Labeling theorists have argued that judicial processing increases the likelihood that someone will continue his or her delinquent activities, and there is some evidence that this effect does operate to a limited extent on the first occasion, although probably not with subsequent offences (see Rutter & Giller, 1983). The precise mechanisms are ill-understood, but probably part of the explanation lies in the fact that, with most risky behaviors, there seems to be a diminishing resistance once there has been the first crossing of the prohibited threshold (whether the behavior is sexual activity, smoking, violence, or theft). Probably the process is enhanced by the person coming to accept, through public labeling, that he or she is someone who behaves in that way.

In addition, both at the individual and community-wide levels, a liability to engage in antisocial behavior will be influenced by the "permission" afforded by the impression that "everyone does it," especially admired role models, and that it brings rewards. There is evidence that portrayals of violence in the media operate in this way (Wartella, 1995), and, more arguably, it is possible that an awareness that some politicians get away with lying and cheating (over financial matters, arms deals, and other issues) and that some leaders of commerce can and do award themselves huge increases in salary while keeping down the wages of employees and making workers redundant creates an image that personal greed at the expense of others is both acceptable and rewarding.

Figure 26 summarizes some of the key facets of inhibiting or disinhibiting influences. Values are again influential in terms of an acceptance or lack of acceptance of qualities such as honesty, respect for others, and nonviolent solutions to problems. Empirical findings have shown that delinquents tend to have a diminished autonomic reactivity (Lahey et al., 1995; Raine, in press; Raine, Venables, & Williams, 1996), and it would seem that a low anxiety is likely to make it easier to engage in high-risk activities.

A lack of empathy for others has been one of the features most emphasized in writings on psychopathy and antisocial personality disorder (Hare, 1986), and possibly an awareness of the feelings of victims to some extent may inhibit person-directed criminal acts. Delinquents often define their crimes as ones that have no victim (because the theft is from an organization or because the person's loss will be covered by insurance). It is striking, however, that the population subgroups most likely to commit crimes are also the ones most likely to be victims (Rutter & Giller, 1983). Either delinquents do not feel a strong group identity, or if they do, they are not inhibited by a shared group identity with their victims.

Developmental studies have shown that the acquisition of sets of standards is a universal milestone in early childhood that probably derives from the growing cognitive capacity to appreciate other people's expectations and to recognize how things should be (Kagan, 1981). Although this acquisition is universal, the specifics of the standards that become internalized are more variable, are influenced by upbringing at home and at school, and are likely to create a greater or lesser tendency to inhibit antisocial inclinations.

Our studies, like those of others (Clausen, 1993) have shown the importance of a tendency to plan ahead with respect to key life choices and transitions. Planners tend to show better social functioning in adult life and are less likely to engage in antisocial activities. Probably, it is not so much that planning inhibits antisocial behavior directly, but rather that it enhances positive behavior and

■ 183

184 ■

creates life situations that make crime a less necessary, and a less desirable, solution to life problems.

The control of delinquent activities brought about both by monitoring and supervision within the family (Patterson, 1982, 1996; Patterson & Yoerger, this volume) and by external surveillance in public places (Clarke, 1985, 1992) is well documented.

Finally the role of drugs and alcohol in reducing inhibitions is well established. There is some limited evidence that their use makes recourse to violence (to persons and property) more likely (Fergusson, Lynskey, & Horwood, 1996; Rutter, 1996a; Sumner & Parker, 1995), although there is probably less effect on theft.

This general model of antisocial liability and disinhibitory features is similar to that put forward by many other writers. What our own research has emphasized, however, is that community, school, and peer group characteristics, as well as family upbringing, are important; that hyperactivity constitutes an important individual risk factor; that genetic factors are more important for some forms of antisocial behavior than often appreciated; that both genetic and environmental influences operate through a variety of routes both direct and indirect; that the causal chains often involve multiple indirect links; that important changes can still take place in adult life; and that the influences on antisocial behavior that continues into adult life may not be the same as those that are concerned with the initiation of antisocial behavior in childhood.

Our own work has not, for the most part, focused on the specific circumstances that led someone to commit a delinquent act in a particular situation at a particular time, but those are a key feature of other chapters in this volume (see Heimer & Matsueda; McCord; Patterson & Yoerger; Tedeschi). It is necessary, however, to summarize here some of the operative mechanisms because many are the end product of the longer-term causal processes that we have studied. Thus, criminal activities are more likely to occur when there are good opportunities for them (see Figure 27 for a summary of some of the elements in opportunities, situational "presses," provoking features, and perceptions of cost-benefits). Although we lack sure knowledge on the causes of the major rise in crime over the last half-century, it is likely that the greater range of goods to steal brought about by increasing affluence may have played a role (Rutter & Smith, 1995). The much greater availability and acceptability of hand-

OPPORTUNITIES

Accessible Goods to Steal

Confrontational Situation

Unsupervised Time
(while playing truant, unemployed)

Available Means
(e.g., weapons)

SITUATIONAL 'PRESSES'

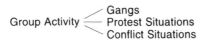

Group Activity
— Gangs
— Protest Situations
— Conflict Situations

Antisocial Models ——— Activities of
Other People

Previous Antisocial
Acts (broken windows,
graffiti, etc.)

■ 185

PROVOKING FEATURES

Anger

Frustration

Lack of Alternative Rewards

Need for
— Material Resources
— Power
— Status

Resentment

PERCEPTION OF COST-BENEFITS

Material Rewards

Respect/Fear/Admiration by Others

Justice Justification

Achievement of Power Control

Figure 27. Opportunities, situational "presses," provoking features, perception of cost-benefits.

guns in the United States is almost certainly a major factor underlying its massively higher homicide rate compared with all European countries. It is not, of course, that having a gun makes people want to kill; rather, when someone feels under threat or wishes to be aggressive, death is more likely to result if the individual has a means of causing death ready to hand. Note, too, that the availability and acceptability of guns may constitute a prime explanation for the between-country differences in homicide rate without their playing much of a role in individual differences within a country (because variations in availability and acceptability within a country are so much smaller).

Doubtless, truancy and unemployment predispose to crime through various different routes, but one of the mechanisms is that both provide unsupervised time during which it is easier to engage in delinquent acts (Osgood et al., 1996).

Another sort of opportunity is provided by confrontational situations, either individual or group. Antisocial individuals tend to quarrel with other people, to challenge aggressively, and to provoke

Motivation and Delinquency. Vol. 44 of the Nebraska Symposium on Motivation, ed. D. W. Osgood, 1997, pp. 44–118

arguments (Robins, 1966). Not surprisingly, these provide increased opportunities for an escalation into assault that contravenes the law. The same applies to the tendency for such individuals to "hang out" with others in groups that seek confrontation in order to assert dominance.

These situations also often provide situational "presses" deriving both from group activities that seem to give "permission" to behave in ways that might not be acceptable in individual circumstances and from models of antisocial behavior. Thus, people acting as members of a gang often undertake acts of violence (including rape and killing) that they might find unacceptable when on their own. Protest marches, similarly, all too often seem to provide legitimacy for violence, looting, and other forms of antisocial behavior. The confrontational situations provided by some soccer matches in Europe, regrettably, seem to serve a similar purpose.

Models of antisocial behavior are also important in both interpersonal and situational terms. Thus, the group situations noted above all provide models of *other* people behaving in antisocial ways that seem to provide a "press" for the individual to do the same. But physical circumstances have been shown to have the same effect (Rutter & Giller, 1983). Thus, buildings that already have broken windows or graffiti are more likely to be vandalized than ones kept in good repair. Our schools research showed the same finding (Rutter et al., 1979).

Provoking features have probably been most investigated in relation to interpersonal aggression. Anger, frustration, and resentment all make violence more likely (Geen, 1995; Zillmann, 1979). One feature of our own research is the finding that a high proportion of antisocial individuals exhibit emotional disturbance and hence may be more vulnerable to these emotion-provoking features. But our results, like those of others, also underline the extent to which adults who were antisocial children frequently are in situations in which they lack alternative rewards (because they are unemployed or in low-paying jobs), they lack status (through work or other activities), and they have financial needs (because of a dependent family, a drug habit, or gambling). All create "incentives" for crime and a lack of incentives for prosocial and socially productive activities.

Finally, people's actions will be influenced by their assessment of the cost-benefits of antisocial behavior. The literature includes many debates on the extent to which antisocial behavior is rational and determined by people's analysis of the rewards to be obtained and the costs to be paid. There is no reason to regard antisocial behavior as different from other behavior in this connection. With the rare exceptions of criminal acts deriving directly from mental illness, antisocial acts are conscious, deliberate, and considered. Accordingly, they will be driven by the perception of material rewards, by the "justified" settling of scores stemming from other people's negative behavior, by the achievement of power and control, and by the earning of other people's fear, respect, or admiration. Research findings, however, put an important perspective on this decision making by their demonstration of the tendency to act for the moment rather than for the future (a lack of "planning"), to make decisions impulsively without a proper appraisal of the cost-benefits, to perceive hostile intent by others on the slightest provocation, and to arrive in situations where there is a limited range of alternative actions. The decision may be no less "rational" than those taken by others, but its outcome is likely to have been shaped to a major extent by both operative situations and by the person's decision-making style. What happens at the moment of deciding to commit an antisocial act is important, but our research emphasizes the crucial lifespan precursors that shape that decision.

Those precursors include genetically influenced individual characteristics. The notion that genes play a role in antisocial behavior has been violently rejected by some social scientists on the wholly mistaken assumption that it represents biological determinism leading to a search for "the gene for crime." Nothing could be further from the truth (Rutter, 1996b, 1996c). Genes play a role in motivation, *not* because there could be a genetic propensity for theft or homicide, but rather because motivation stems from the emotions and thought processes of an individual in a particular social context. Individual characteristics, resulting from the additive and interactive combination of genetic and environmental factors, are important because they influence a person's overall susceptibility to particular emotions and cognitions; because they affect the likelihood of reacting in particular ways as a consequence of social skills, behavioral habits, and social standing; and because individual characteristics also serve to shape and select the social contexts in which the individuals operate. The motivation to commit a certain act at a

• 187

Motivation and Delinquency. Vol. 44 of the Nebraska Symposium on Motivation, ed. D. W. Osgood, 1997, pp. 44–118

specific time and place is the end result of both developmental processes within the individual and of societal forces that are created by the individuals in that society and that, in turn, through social group processes, influence the actions of those individuals.

This overview of our multifaceted research program into antisocial behavior provides just a few frames from a film reel that still has a long way to run. The growth in understanding antisocial behavior from the research undertaken over the last three decades is considerable, but it has to be said that the answers to the questions with which we started have also provided us with a better indication of the many questions still to be tackled in the years to come.

NOTES

1. Research for the Isle of Wight–London comparison was supported by funding from the (U.S.) Foundation for Child Development and the (British) Social Science Research Council. The research workers who played a key role in the work included Michael Berger, Antony Cox, David Quinton, Olwen Rowlands, Michael Rutter, Celia Tupling, Bridget Yule, and William Yule.

2. This research on schools was supported by funding from the (British) Department of Education and Science and the Medical Research Council. The research workers who played a key role in the work included Barbara Maughan, Peter Mortimore, Janet Ouston, and Michael Rutter.

3. The study of families of mentally ill patients was supported by funding from the Invalid Children's Aid Association, the Medical Research Council, and the W. T. Grant Foundation. The research workers who played a key role in the work included Christine Liddle, David Quinton, and Michael Rutter.

4. The study of secular trends was supported by funding from the Johann Jacobs Foundation and the Medical Research Council. David Smith and Michael Rutter were the key workers responsible for the aspects of the study reported here.

5. Follow-up research on children with depressive disorders was supported by funding from the John D. and Catherine T. MacArthur Foundation and the Medical Research Council. The research workers who played a key role in the work included Diana Bredenkamp, Christine Groothues, Hazel Fudge, Richard Harrington, and Michael Rutter. Mayer Ghodsian and Andrew Pickles were responsible for the analyses of the National Child Development Study data.

6. This longitudinal research on London children was supported by funding from the Medical Research Council. The research workers who played a key role included Lorna Champion, Gillian Goodall, Ann Hagell, Barbara Maughan, Andrew Pickles, Michael Rutter, and William Yule.

7. This follow-up of children reared in group foster homes was supported by the Foundation for Child Development, Social Science Research Council, the W. T. Grant Foundation, and the Medical Research Council. The research workers who played a key role in the work included Barbara Maughan, Andrew Pickles, David Quinton, and Michael Rutter.

8. This research on hyperkinetic disorder was supported by the Medical Research Council and the John D. and Catherine T. MacArthur Foundation. The research workers who played a key role in the work included Oliver Chadwick, Susan Giles, Ellen Heptinstall, Michael Rutter, Seija Sandberg, Russell Schachar, Edmund Sonuga-Barke, Geoffrey Thorley, Eric Taylor, and Jody Warner-Rogers.

9. This follow-up research on twins with conduct disorder was funded by the Wellcome Trust and the Medical Research Council. The research workers who played a key role in the work included James Elander, Janet Holmshaw, Robin Murray, Andrew Pickles, Michael Rutter, and Emily Simonoff.

10. The Virginia Twin Study of Adolescent Behavioral Development was funded by NIMH grants, MH 45268 and MH, by the Medical Research Council, and by Junior Faculty Research Awards to Joanne Meyer and Judy Silberg, for the John D. and Catherine T. MacArthur Foundation. The research workers who played a key role in the work included Lindon Eaves, John Hewitt, Rolf Loeber, Hermine Maes, Joanne Meyer, Andrew Pickles, Michael Rutter, Lucinda Shillady, Judy Silberg, and Emily Simonoff.

■189

REFERENCES

Anderson, K. E., Lytton, H., & Romney, D. M. (1986). Mothers' interactions with normal and conduct-disordered boys: Who affects whom? *Developmental Psychology, 22*, 604–609.

Angold, A., Prendergast, M., Cox, A., Harrington, R., Simonoff, E., & Rutter, M. (1995). The Child and Adolescent Psychiatric Assessment (CAPA). *Psychological Medicine, 25*, 739–753.

Bell, R. Q. (1968). A reinterpretation of the direction of effects in studies of socialization. *Psychological Review, 75*, 81–95.

Berger, M., Yule, W., & Rutter, M. (1975). Attainment and adjustment in two geographical areas: 2. The prevalence of specific reading retardation. *British Journal of Psychiatry, 126*, 510–519.

Bock, G. R., & Goode, J. A. (Eds.). (1996). *Genetics of criminal and antisocial behaviour.* Ciba Foundation Symposium No. 194. Chichester, England, & New York: Wiley.

Bohman, M. (1996). Predisposition to criminality: Swedish adoption studies in retrospect. In G. R. Bock & J. A. Goode (Eds.), *Genetics of criminal and antisocial behaviour. Ciba Foundation Symposium 194* (pp. 99–114). Chichester, England, & New York: Wiley.

Brown, G. W., & Harris, T. O. (1978). *Social origins of depression: A study of psychiatric disorder in women.* London: Tavistock.

190 ∎

Cadoret, R. J., Cain, C. A., & Crowe, R. R. (1983). Evidence for gene-environment interaction in the development of adolescent antisocial behavior. *Behavior Genetics, 13*, 301–310.

Cadoret, R. J., Yates, W. R., Troughton, E., Woodworth, G., & Stewart, M. A. (1995). Genetic-environmental interaction in the genesis of aggressivity and conduct disorders. *Archives of General Psychiatry, 52*, 916–924.

Caron, C., & Rutter, M. (1991). Comorbidity in child psychopathology: Concepts, issues and research strategies. *Journal of Child Psychology and Psychiatry, 32*, 1063–1080.

Caspi, A., Elder, G. H., Jr., & Bem, D. J. (1987). Moving against the world: Life course patterns of explosive children. *Developmental Psychology, 23*, 308–313.

———. (1988). Moving away from the world: Life course patterns of shy children. *Developmental Psychology, 24*, 824–831.

Caspi, A., & Moffitt, T. E. (1993). When do individual differences matter? A paradoxical theory of personality coherence. *Psychological Inquiry, 4*, 247–271.

Champion, L. A., Goodall, G. M., & Rutter, M. (1995). Behavioural problems in childhood and stressors in early adult life: A 20-year follow-up of London school children. *Psychological Medicine, 25*, 231–246.

Clarke, R. V. (1985). Jack Tizard memorial lecture: Delinquency, environment and intervention. *Journal of Child Psychology and Psychiatry, 26*, 505–523.

Clarke, R. V. (Ed.). (1992). *Situational crime prevention: Successful case studies*. New York: Harrow & Heston.

Clausen, J. A. (1993). *American lives: Looking back at the children of the Great Depression*. New York: Free Press.

Cloninger, C. R., Adolfsson, R., & Svrakic, N. M. (1996). Mapping genes for human personality. *Nature Genetics, 12*, 3–4.

Cornish, D. B., & Clarke, R. V. (Eds.). (1986). *The reasoning criminal*. New York: Springer-Verlag.

DiLalla, L. F., & Gottesman, I. I. (1989). Heterogeneity of causes for delinquency and criminality: Lifespan perspectives. *Development and Psychopathology, 1*, 339–349.

Dodge, K. A. (1986). A social information processing model of social competence in children. In M. Perlmutter (Ed.), *Eighteenth Annual Minnesota Symposium of Child Psychology* (pp. 77–125). Hillsdale NJ: Lawrence Erlbaum.

Dodge, K. A., Pettit, G. S., Bates, J. E., & Valente, E. (1995). Social information-processing patterns partially mediate the effects of early physical abuse on later conduct problems. *Journal of Abnormal Psychology, 104*, 632–643.

Dodge, K. A., Pettit, G. S., McClaskey, C. L., & Brown, M. (1986). Social competence in children. *Monographs of the Society for Research in Child Development, 51*(2, Serial No. 213).

Eaves, L. J., Last, K. A., Young, P. A., & Martin, N. G. (1978). Model-fitting approaches to the analysis of human behavior. *Heredity, 41*, 249–320.

Eaves, L. J., Silberg, J., Hewitt, J. K., Meyer, J., Rutter, M., Simonoff, E., Neale, M., & Pickles, A. (1993). Genes, personality, and psychopathology: A latent class analysis of liability to symptoms of attention-deficit hyperactivity disorder in twins. In R. Plomin & G. E. McClearn (Eds.), *Nature, nurture, and psychology* (pp. 285–303). Washington DC: American Psychological Association.

Eaves, L. J., Silberg, J. L., Meyer, J. M., Maes, H. H., Simonoff, E., Pickles, A., Rutter, M., Neale, M. C., Reynolds, C. A., Erikson, M. T., Heath, A. C., Loeber, R., Truett, K. R., & Hewitt, J. K. (in press). Genetics and developmental psychopathology: 2. The main effects of genes and environment on behavioral problems in the Virginia Twin Study of Adolescent Behavioral Development. *Journal of Child Psychology and Psychiatry.*

Engfer, A., Walper, S., & Rutter, M. (1994). Individual characteristics as a force in development. In M. Rutter & D. F. Hay (Eds.), *Development through life: A handbook for clinicians* (pp. 79–111). Oxford: Blackwell Scientific.

Farrington, D. P. (1986). Age and crime. In M. Tonry & N. Morris (Eds.), *Crime and justice.* Chicago: University of Chicago Press.

———. (1992). Trends in English juvenile delinquency and their explanation. *International Journal of Comparative and Applied Criminal Justice, 16,* 151–163.

———. (1995a). The challenge of teenage antisocial behavior. In M. Rutter (Ed.), *Psychosocial disturbances in young people: Challenges for prevention* (pp. 83–130). New York: Cambridge University Press.

———. (1995b). The development of offending and antisocial behaviour from childhood: Key findings from the Cambridge Study in Delinquent Development. The Twelfth Jack Tizard Memorial Lecture. *Journal of Child Psychology and Psychiatry, 36,* 929–964.

Felson, R. B., & Tedeschi, J. T. (Ed.). (1993a). *Aggression and violence: Social interactionist perspectives.* Washington DC: American Psychological Association.

———. (1993b). A social interactionist approach to violence: Cross-cultural applications. *Violence and Victims, 8,* 295–310.

Fergusson, D. M., Horwood, L. J., & Lloyd, M. T. (1991). Confirmatory factor models of attention deficit and conduct disorder. *Journal of Child Psychology and Psychiatry, 32,* 257–274.

Fergusson, D. M., Horwood, L. J., & Lynskey, M. T. (1993). The effects of conduct disorder and attention deficit in middle childhood on offending and scholastic ability at age 13. *Journal of Child Psychology and Psychiatry, 34,* 899–916.

Fergusson, D. M., Lynskey, M. T., & Horwood, L. J. (1996). Alcohol misuse and juvenile offending in adolescence. *Addiction, 91,* 483–494.

Geen, R. G. (1995). Human aggression. In A. Tessler (Ed.), *Advanced social psychology* (pp. 383–417). New York: McGraw-Hill.

Glueck, S., & Glueck, E. (1950). *Unraveling juvenile delinquency.* New York: Commonwealth Fund.

Goodman, R. (1995). The relationship between normal variation in IQ and common childhood psychopathology: A clinical study. *European Child and Adolescent Psychiatry, 4*, 187–196.

Goodman, R., Simonoff, E., & Stevenson, J. (1995). The impact of child IQ, parent IQ and sibling IQ on child behavioural deviance scores. *Journal of Child Psychology and Psychiatry, 36*, 409–425.

Gottfredson, M. R., & Hirschi, T. (1990). *A general theory of crime.* Stanford: Stanford University Press.

Graham, P., & Rutter, M. (1973). Psychiatric disorder in the young adolescent: A follow-up study. *Proceedings of the Royal Society of Medicine, 66*, 1226–1229 (Section of Psychiatry, pp. 58–61).

Gray, G., Smith, A., & Rutter, M. (1980). School attendance and the first year of employment. In L. Hersov & I. Berg (Eds.), *Out of school: Modern perspectives in truancy and school refusal* (pp. 343–370). Chichester, England: Wiley.

Greenberg, M. T., Speltz, M. L., & DeKlyen, M. (1993). The role of attachment in the early development of disruptive behavior problems. *Development and Psychopathology, 5*, 191–213.

Hare, R. D. (1986). Twenty years of experience with the Cleckley psychopath. In W. H. Reid, D. Dorr, J. Walker, & J. W. Bonner (Eds.), *Unmasking the psychopath: Antisocial personality and related syndromes.* New York: Norton.

Harrington, R., Bredenkamp, D., Groothues, C., Rutter, M., Fudge, H., & Pickles, A. (1994). Adult outcomes of childhood and adolescent depression: 3. Links with suicidal behaviours. *Journal of Child Psychology and Psychiatry, 35*, 1309–1319.

Harrington, R., Fudge, H., Rutter, M., Pickles, A., & Hill, J. (1991). Adult outcomes of childhood and adolescent depression: 2. Links with antisocial disorder. *Journal of the American Academy of Child and Adolescent Psychiatry, 30*, 434–439.

Harrington, R., Rutter, M., & Fombonne, E. (1996). Developmental pathways in depression: Multiple meanings, antecedents and endpoints. *Development and Psychopathology, 8*, 601–616.

Harris, T., Brown, G. W., & Bifulco, A. (1990). Loss of parent in childhood and adult psychiatric disorder: A tentative overall model. *Development and Psychopathology, 2*, 311–327.

Heimer, K., & Matsueda, R. L. (1994). Role-taking, role-commitment, and delinquency: A theory of differential social control. *American Sociological Review, 59*, 365–390.

Hewitt, J. K., Silberg, J. L., Rutter, M., Simonoff, E., Meyer, J. M., Maes, H., Pickles, A., Neale, M. C., Loeber, R., Erickson, M., Kendler, K. S., Heath, A. C., Truett, K. R., Reynolds, C., & Eaves, L. J. (in press). Genetics and developmental psychopathology: 1. Phenotypic assessment in the Virginia Twin Study of Adolescent Behavioral Development. *Journal of Child Psychology and Psychiatry.*

192 ▪

Hinshaw, S. P. (1992). Externalizing behavior problems and academic underachievement in childhood and adolescence: Causal relationships and underlying mechanisms. *Psychological Bulletin, 111,* 127–155.

Home Office. (1994). *Criminal statistics England and Wales.* London: Author.

Horney, J., Osgood, D. W., & Marshall, I. H. (1995). Criminal careers in the short-term: Intra-individual variability in crime and its relation to local life circumstances. *American Sociological Review, 60,* 665–673.

Jessor, R., Donovan, J. E., & Costa, F. M. (1991). *Beyond adolescence: Problem behavior and young adult development.* Cambridge: Cambridge University Press.

Kagan, J. (1981). *The second year: The emergence of self-awareness.* Cambridge: Harvard University Press.

Kendler, K. S., Neale, M. C., Kessler, R. C., Heath, A. C., & Eaves, L. J. (1993). A longitudinal twin study of 1-year prevalence of major depression in women. *Archives of General Psychiatry, 50,* 843–852.

Lahey, B. B., McBurnett, K., Loeber, R., & Hart, E. L. (1995). Psychobiology of conduct disorders. In G. P. Scholevar (Ed.), *Conduct disorders in children and adolescents: Assessments and intervention* (pp. 27–44). Washington DC: American Psychiatric Press.

Loeber, R., & Hay, D. F. (1994). Developmental approaches to aggression and conduct problems. In M. Rutter & D. F. Hay (Eds.), *Development through life: A handbook for clinicians* (pp. 488–516). Oxford: Blackwell Scientific.

Lytton, H. (1990). Child and parent effects in boys' conduct disorder: A reinterpretation. *Developmental Psychology, 26,* 683–697.

Maughan, B. (1994). School influences. In M. Rutter & D. F. Hay (Eds.), *Development through life: A handbook for clinicians* (pp. 134–158). Oxford, England: Blackwell Scientific.

Maughan, B., Dunn, G., & Rutter, M. (1985). Black pupils' progress in secondary school: 1. Reading attainment between 10 and 14. *British Journal of Developmental Psychology, 3,* 113–121.

Maughan, B., & Hagell, A. (1996). Poor readers in adulthood: Psychosocial functioning. *Development and Psychopathology, 8,* 457–476.

Maughan, B., Hagell, A., Rutter, M., & Yule, W. (1994). Poor readers in secondary schools. *Reading and Writing: An Interdisciplinary Journal, 6,* 125–150.

Maughan, B., Pickles, A., Hagell, A., Rutter, M., & Yule, W. (1996). Reading problems and antisocial behaviour: Developmental trends in comorbidity. *Journal of Child Psychology and Psychiatry, 37,* 405–418.

Maughan, B., Pickles, A., & Quinton, D. (1995). Parental hostility, childhood behavior and adult social functioning. In J. McCord (Ed.), *Coercion and punishment in long term perspectives* (pp. 34–58). New York: Cambridge University Press.

Maughan, B., Pickles, A., Rutter, M., & Ouston, J. (1991). Can schools change? 1. Outcomes at six London secondary schools. *School Effectiveness and School Improvement, 1,* 188–210.

■ 193

Maughan, B., Rutter, M., & Yule, W. (1996). *Reading problems and emotional well-being: The Isle of Wight revisited.* Manuscript submitted for publication.

Meyer, J. M., Rutter, M., Simonoff, E., Shillady, C. L., Silberg, J. L., Pickles, A., Hewitt, J. K., Maes, H. H., & Eaves, L. J. (1996). *Familial aggregation for conduct disorder symptomatology: The role of genes, marital discord and family adaptability.* Manuscript in preparation.

Moffitt, T. E. (1993a). The neuropsychology of conduct disorder. *Development and Psychopathology, 5*, 135–152.

———. (1993b). Adolescence-limited and life-course-persistent antisocial behavior: A developmental taxonomy. *Psychological Review, 100*, 674–701.

Moffitt, T. E., Caspi, A., Dickson, N., Silva, P., & Stanton, W. (1996). Childhood-onset versus adolescent-onset antisocial conduct problems in males: Natural history from ages 3 to 18 years. *Development and Psychopathology, 8*, 399–424.

Mortimore, P. (1995). The positive effects of schooling. In M. Rutter (Ed.), *Psychosocial disturbance in young people: Challenges for prevention* (pp. 333–363). New York: Cambridge University Press.

Office of Population Censuses & Surveys. (1994). *Marriage and Divorce Statistics.* London: Author.

Olsson, D. H., Sprenkle, D. H., & Russel, C. S. (1979). Circumplex model of marital and family systems: 1. Cohesion and adaptability dimensions, family types, and clinical applications. *Family Processes, 18*, 3–28.

Osgood, D. W., Wilson, J. K., O'Malley, P. M., Bachman, J. G., & Johnston, L. D. (1996). Routine activities and individual deviant behavior. *American Sociological Review, 61*, 635–655.

Ouston, J., Maughan, B., & Rutter, M. (1991). Can schools change? 2. Practice at six London secondary schools. *School Effectiveness and School Improvement, 2*, 3–13.

Parker, J. G., & Asher, S. R. (1987). Peer relations and later personal adjustment: Are low-accepted children at risk? *Psychological Bulletin, 102*, 357–389.

Patterson, G. R. (1982). *Coercive family process.* Eugene OR: Castalia.

———. (1996). Some characteristics of a developmental theory for early onset delinquency. In M. F. Lenzenweger & J. J. Haugaard (Eds.), *Frontiers of developmental psychopathology* (pp. 81–124). New York: Oxford University Press.

Patterson, G. R., Reid, J. B., & Dishion, T. J. (1992). *Antisocial boys: A social interactional approach.* Eugene OR: Castalia.

Pickles, A., & Clayton, D. (1996, June). *Logistic regression with mismeasured risk exposures: A latent variable approach.* Paper presented at the meeting of the Danish Society for Theoretical Statistics, Copenhagen, Denmark.

Pickles, A., & Rutter, M. (1991). Statistical and conceptual models of "turning points" in developmental processes. In D. Magnusson, L. R. Bergman, G. Rudinger, & B. Törestad (Eds.), *Problems and methods in longitudinal research: Stability and change* (pp. 133–165). Cambridge: Cambridge University Press.

194

Plomin, R., & Daniels, D. (1987). Why are children in the same family so different from one another? *Behavioral and Brain Sciences, 10,* 1–15.

Quinton, D., Pickles, A., Maughan, B., & Rutter, M. (1993). Partners, peers, and pathways: Assortative pairing and continuities in conduct disorder. *Development and Psychopathology, 5,* 763–783.

Quinton, D., & Rutter, M. (1988). *Parenting breakdown: The making and breaking of inter-generational links.* Aldershot, England: Avebury.

Raine, A. (in press). Antisocial behavior and psychophysiology: A biosocial perspective and a prefrontal dysfunction hypothesis. In D. Stoff, J. Breiling, & J. D. Maser (Eds.), *Handbook of antisocial behavior.* New York: Wiley.

Raine, A., Venables, P. H., & Williams, M. (1996). Better autonomic conditioning and faster electrodermal half-recovery time at age 15 years as possible protective factors against crime at age 29 years. *Developmental Psychology, 32,* 624–630.

Reiss, D., Hetherington, M., Plomin, R., Howe, G. W., Simmens, S. J., Henderson, S. H., O'Connor, T. J., Bussell, D. A., Anderson, E. R., & Law, T. (1995). Genetic questions for environmental studies: Differential parenting and psychopathology in adolescence. *Archives of General Psychiatry, 52,* 925–936.

Robins, L. N. (1966). *Deviant children grown up.* Baltimore: Williams & Wilkins.

Robins, L. N., Tipp, J., & Przybeck, T. (1991). Antisocial personality. In L. Robins & D. A. Regier (Eds.), *Psychiatric disorders in America: The epidemiologic catchment area study* (pp. 258–290). New York: Free Press.

Rutter, M. (1972). *Maternal deprivation reassessed.* Harmondsworth, England: Penguin Books.

———. (1973). Why are London children so disturbed? *Proceedings of the Royal Society of Medicine, 66,* 1221–1226.

———. (1978). Family, area and school influences in the genesis of conduct disorders. In L. Hersov, M. Berger, & D. Shaffer (Eds.), *Aggression and antisocial behaviour in childhood and adolescence* (pp. 95–113). Oxford: Pergamon.

———. (1980). *Changing youth in a changing society: Patterns of adolescent development and disorder.* Cambridge: Harvard University Press. (Original work published 1979)

———. (1989). Psychiatric disorder in parents as a risk factor for children. In D. Shaffer, I. Philips, & N. B. Enzer (Eds.), *Prevention of mental disorders, alcohol and other drug use in children and adolescents* (pp. 157–189). Rockville MD: Office for Substance Abuse Prevention, U.S. Department of Health and Human Services.

———. (1991). Childhood experiences and adult psychosocial functioning. In G. R. Bock & J. A. Whelan (Eds.), *The childhood environment and adult disease* (pp. 189–200). Chichester, England: Wiley.

———. (1994). Beyond longitudinal data: Causes, consequences, changes and continuity. *Journal of Consulting and Clinical Psychology, 62,* 928–940.

———. (1996a). Commentary: Testing causal hypotheses about mechanisms in comorbidity. *Addiction, 91,* 495–498.

■ 195

196 ■

————. (1996b). Concluding remarks. In G. R. Bock & J. A. Goode (Eds.), *Genetics of criminal and antisocial behaviour* (pp. 265–271). Chichester, England, & New York: Wiley.

————. (1996c). Introduction: Concepts of antisocial behaviour, of cause, and of genetic influences. In G. R. Bock & J. A. Goode (Eds.), *Genetics of criminal and antisocial behaviour* (pp. 1–15). Chichester, England, & New York: Wiley.

————. (1996d). Transitions and turning points in developmental psychopathology: As applied to the age span between childhood and mid-adulthood. *International Journal of Behavioral Development, 19,* 603–626.

————. (in press-a). Antisocial behavior: Developmental psychopathology perspectives. In D. Stoff, J. Breiling, & J. D. Maser (Eds.), *Handbook of antisocial behavior.* New York: Wiley.

————. (in press-b). Individual differences and levels of antisocial behavior. In A. Raine, D. Farrington, P. Brennan, & S. A. Mednick (Eds.), *Biosocial bases of violence.* New York: Plenum Press.

Rutter, M., Cox, A., Tupling, C., Berger, M., & Yule, W. (1975). Attainment and adjustment in two geographical areas: 1. The prevalence of psychiatric disorder. *British Journal of Psychiatry, 126,* 493–509.

Rutter, M., Dunn, J., Plomin, R., Simonoff, E., Pickles, A., Maughan, B., Ormel, J. H., Meyer, J., & Eaves, L. (in press). Integrating nature and nurture: Implications of person-environment correlations and interactions for developmental psychopathology. *Development and Psychopathology.*

Rutter, M., & Giller, H. (1983). *Juvenile delinquency: Trends and perspectives.* Harmondsworth, England: Penguin Books.

Rutter, M., Harrington, R., Quinton, D., & Pickles, A. (1994). Adult outcome of conduct disorder in childhood: Implications for concepts and definitions of patterns of psychopathology. In R. D. Ketterlinus & M. Lamb (Eds.), *Adolescent problem behaviors: Issues and research* (pp. 57–80). Hillsdale NJ: Lawrence Erlbaum.

Rutter, M., & Madge, N. (1976). *Cycles of disadvantage: A review of research.* London: Heinemann Educational Books.

Rutter, M., Maughan, B., Mortimore, P., Ouston, J., & Smith, A. (1979). *Fifteen thousand hours: Secondary schools and their effects on children.* London: Open Books.

Rutter, M., & Quinton, D. (1977). Psychiatric disorder—Ecological factors and concepts of causation. In H. McGurk (Ed.), *Ecological factors in human development* (pp. 173–187). Amsterdam: North-Holland.

————. (1984). Parental psychiatric disorder: Effects on children. *Psychological Medicine, 14,* 853–880.

Rutter, M., & Rutter, M. (1993). *Developing minds: Challenge and continuity across the lifespan.* Harmondworth, England: Penguin; New York: Basic Books.

Rutter, M., Silberg, J., & Simonoff, E. (1993). Whither behavior genetics? A developmental psychopathology perspective. In R. Plomin & G. E. Mc-

Clearn (Eds.), *Nature, nurture, and psychology* (pp. 433–456). Washington DC: American Psychological Association.

Rutter, M., & Smith, D. J. (Ed.). (1995). *Psychosocial disorders in young people: Time trends and their causes.* Chichester, England: Wiley.

Rutter, M., Tizard, J., & Whitmore, K. (Eds.). (1970). *Education, health and behaviour.* London: Longmans.

Rutter, M., Yule, B., Quinton, D., Rowlands, O., Yule, W., & Berger, M. (1975). Attainment and adjustment in two geographical areas: 3. Some factors accounting for area differences. *British Journal of Psychiatry, 126,* 520–533.

Sampson, R. J., & Laub, J. H. (1993). *Crime in the making: Pathways and turning points through life.* Cambridge: Harvard University Press.

Schachar, R. J. (1991). Childhood hyperactivity. *Journal of Child Psychology and Psychiatry, 32,* 155–191.

Schachar, R. J., Rutter, M., & Smith, A. (1981). The characteristics of situationally and pervasively hyperactive children: Implications for syndrome definition. *Journal of Child Psychology and Psychiatry, 22,* 375–392.

Schachar, R. J., Tannock, R., & Logan, G. (1993). Inhibitory control, impulsiveness and attention deficit hyperactivity disorder. *Clinical Psychology Review, 13,* 721–739.

Schachar, R. J., Taylor, E., Wieselberg, M., Thorley, G., & Rutter, M. (1987). Changes in family function and relationships in children who respond to methylphenidate. *Journal of the American Academy of Child and Adolescent Psychiatry, 26,* 728–732.

Shepherd, M., Oppenheim, B., & Mitchell, S. (1971). *Childhood behaviour and mental health.* London: University of London Press.

Shillady, L. L., Silberg, J. L., Simonoff, E., Pickles, A., Maes, H. M., Rutter, M. L., Hewitt, J. K., Eaves, L. J., & Meyer, J. M. (1996). *Parental psychopathology as a risk factor for childhood disorder: a latent class analysis of 1,408 families.* Manuscript in preparation.

Silberg, J. L., Meyer, J., Pickles, A., Simonoff, E., Eaves, L., Hewitt, J., Maes, H., & Rutter, M. (1996). Heterogeneity among juvenile antisocial behaviors: Findings from the Virginia Twin Study of Adolescent Behavioural Development. In G. R. Bock & J. A. Goode (Eds.), *Genetics of criminal and antisocial behaviour* (pp. 76–86). Chichester, England, & New York: Wiley.

Silberg, J. L., Rutter, M. L., Meyer, J., Maes, H., Simonoff, E., Pickles, A., Hewitt, J., & Eaves, L. (1996). Genetic and environmental influences on the covariation between hyperactivity and conduct disturbance in juvenile twins. *Journal of Child Psychology and Psychiatry, 37,* 803–816.

Simonoff, E. (1996). Personal communication.

Simonoff, E., Pickles, A., Hewitt, J., Silberg, J., Rutter, M., Loeber, R., Meyer, J., Neale, M., & Eaves, L. (1995). Multiple raters of disruptive child behavior: Using a genetic strategy to examine shared views and bias. *Behavior Genetics, 25,* 311–326.

Simonoff, E., Pickles, A., Meyer, J. M., Silberg, J. L., Maes, H. H., Loeber,

■197

R., Rutter, M., Hewitt, J. K., & Eaves, L. J. (in press). The Virginia Twin Study of Adolescent Behavioral Development: Influences of age, gender and impairment on rates of disorder. *Archives of General Psychiatry*.

Smith, D. J. (1995). Youth crime and conduct disorders: Trends, patterns and causal explanations. In M. Rutter & D. J. Smith (Eds.), *Psychosocial disturbances in young people: Time trends and their causes* (pp. 389–489). Chichester, England: Wiley.

Sonuga-Barke, E. J. S., Taylor, E., Sembi, S., & Smith, J. (1992). Hyperactivity and delay aversion: 1. The effect of delay on choice. *Journal of Child Psychology and Psychiatry, 33*, 387–398.

Spanier, G. B. (1976). Measuring dyadic adjustment: New scales for assessing the quality of marriage and other dyads. *Journal of Marriage and Family, 38*, 15–28.

Sumner, M., & Parker, H. (1995). *Low in alcohol*. Manchester, England: Department of Social Policy and Social Work, University of Manchester.

Taylor, E. (Ed.). (1986). *The overactive child: Clinics in developmental medicine no. 97*. London: MacKeith Press; Oxford, England: Blackwell Scientific.

Taylor, E., Chadwick, O., Heptinstall, E., & Danckaerts, M. (1996). Hyperactivity and conduct problems as risk factors for adolescent development. *Journal of the American Academy of Child and Adolescent Psychiatry, 35*, 1213–1226.

Taylor, E., Sandberg, S., Thorley, G., & Giles, S. (1991). *The epidemiology of childhood hyperactivity*. Oxford: Oxford University Press.

Taylor, E., Schacher, R., Thorley, G., Wieselberg, H. M., Everitt, B., & Rutter, M. (1987). Which boys respond to stimulant medication? A controlled trial of methylphenidate in boys with disruptive behaviour. *Psychological Medicine, 17*, 121–143.

Tedeschi, J. T., & Felson, R. B. (1994). *Aggression and coercive actions: An interactionist perspective*. Washington DC: American Psychological Association.

Tonry, M., & Farrington, D. P. (Eds.). (1995). *Building a safer society: Strategic approaches to crime prevention*. Chicago: University of Chicago Press.

Wartella, E. (1995). Media and problem behaviours in young people. In M. Rutter & D. J. Smith (Eds.), *Psychosocial disorders in young people: Time trends and their causes* (pp. 296–323). Chichester, England: Wiley.

Zillmann, D. (1979). *Hostility and aggression*. Hillsdale NJ: Lawrence Erlbaum.

Zoccolillo, M., Pickles, A., Quinton, D., & Rutter, M. (1992). The outcome of childhood conduct disorder: Implications for defining adult personality disorder and conduct disorder. *Psychological Medicine, 22*, 971–986.

American Journal of Psychiatry, 1982, vol. 139, pp. 21–33

Syndromes Attributed to "Minimal Brain Dysfunction" in Childhood

BY MICHAEL RUTTER, M.D.

The author considers two main concepts of minimal brain dysfunction: 1) a continuum notion, in which minimal brain dysfunction is viewed as a lesser variant of gross traumatic brain damage, and 2) a syndrome notion, in which minimal brain dysfunction constitutes a genetically determined disorder rather than a response to any form of injury. The evidence on the former indicates that subclinical damage to the brain may occur and may involve psychological sequelae—but the damage probably has to be rather severe, and the result is not a homogeneous syndrome. The second alternative remains a possibility, but the claims far outrun the empirical findings that could justify them.

In the first Salmon lecture (1) (published in the December 1981 issue of the *Journal*) I discussed psychological sequelae in terms of the effects of *known* brain damage in childhood—known, that is, either because there was a clear history of brain injury or because there were unequivocal abnormalities on a clinical neurological examination. That was a necessary strategy if soundly based conclusions were to be drawn on the psychiatric consequences of brain damage. However, most of the theorizing about "minimal brain dysfunction" is based on the consideration of disorders in children who *lack* both a history of damage and abnormal neurological signs. This paper focuses on that much broader group.

THE CONCEPT OF MINIMAL BRAIN DYSFUNCTION

There are several accounts of the history of the concept of "minimal brain dysfunction" (2–5). Its

Second Salmon lecture, presented at the New York Academy of Medicine, New York, Dec. 6, 1979. Received March 13, 1980; revised July 18, 1980; accepted Oct. 21, 1980.

From the Institute of Psychiatry, London. Address correspondence to Dr. Rutter, Department of Child and Adolescent Psychiatry, Institute of Psychiatry, de Crespigny Park, Denmark Hill, London SE5 8AF, England.

This paper was prepared while the author was a Fellow at the Center for Advanced Study in the Behavioral Sciences; the author thanks the Grant Foundation, the Foundation for Child Development, the Spencer Foundation, and the National Science Foundation (BNS 78-24671) for financial support.

origins are probably to be found in the reports during the 1920s that hyperactivity, antisocial behavior, and emotional instability commonly developed following encephalitis in childhood. Rather similar symptoms were said to occur after head injuries, and it came to be believed that, as Bond and Partridge (6) put it in 1926, "the intensively hyperkinetic form of reaction . . . seems the most conclusively organic." A few years later, Kahn and Cohen (7), in a seminal paper, coined the term "organic drivenness" to describe this type of hyperkinesis. Shortly afterwards, Bradley (8) found that overactivity often responded to stimulant medication.

The view that the presence of hyperkinesis might itself be used as an indication of damage to the brain drew considerable strength from Strauss's very influential studies of what he regarded as "brain-injured" children (9). In essence, he and his colleagues found that various characteristics, including hyperactivity, disinhibition, and distractibility, differentiated brain-injured mentally retarded children from those who were not brain-injured. On this basis they argued that all brain lesions were followed by a similar kind of behavioral disturbance and, moreover, that this type of behavior was always due to brain damage. Not only is that logic quite seriously faulty but also the signs and symptoms of brain injury on which it was based were of dubious validity. In spite of these grave deficiencies, the "Strauss syndrome" rapidly came to be accepted as one involving organic brain dysfunction.

The next landmark in the story of minimal brain dysfunction was provided by Pasamanick and Knobloch's studies in the 1950s and early 1960s of the association between pregnancy complications and a range of outcomes extending from cerebral palsy and mental retardation to hyperactivity and reading disorders (10). They postulated a "continuum of reproductive casualty" in which the effects of damage to the brain during the prenatal period and the birth process were thought to vary according to the extent of the damage. When the damage was severe, clear-cut neurological disorders resulted, but when it was mild there was a predisposition to behavioral difficulties, which was unaccompanied by any overt signs of neurological abnormality. Thus Pasamanick and Knobloch hypothesized the existence of minimal brain injury, which was similar in kind, but not in degree, to that which gave rise to cerebral palsy and mental retardation.

▪199

American Journal of Psychiatry, 1982, vol. 139, pp. 21–33

Finally, during the last two decades the term "minimal brain dysfunction" has come to be applied increasingly to a broad group of behavioral and learning disabilities in childhood in which the main features are based on the hyperkinetic syndrome, but with the addition of perceptual, cognitive, and specific learning disabilities (4). The extension of this diagnosis to a wider and wider segment of the child psychiatric population is illustrated by Wender's estimate that it applied to about half of all cases (11) and by Gross and Wilson's use of the term for a majority of their patients (12). As Gross and Wilson themselves commented, "It is surely remarkable that three-quarters of over a thousand consecutive child patients were found to have this disorder!" (pp. 142–143).

It would be wrong, however, to suppose that we are now dealing with a single concept of minimal brain dysfunction, for we are not. Many finer distinctions could be made, but perhaps the most basic is that between the view of minimal brain dysfunction as a lesser variant of gross traumatic or infective brain damage and the view of the disorder as something quite different in which the organic origin probably lies in a genetic abnormality rather than in any form of injury to the brain (5).

The former view sees brain damage in quantitative terms as a unitary continuous variable that produces a characteristic set of deficits, the nature of which depends on the *amount* of brain damage rather than on its site or etiology. The arguments for this concept of minimal brain dysfunction were expressed by Gross and Wilson (12) as follows: *"The most compelling evidence for the existence of MBD as an entity is (1) the similarity . . . between its symptoms and symptoms of children with proven brain disease; and (2) the remarkable response to certain medications, a response not found in non-MBD children"* (p. 6). The current concerns that subclinical lead intoxication may lead to impaired intelligence and hyperactive behavior (13) are an extension of that concept from pre- and perinatal hazards to postnatal toxins.

The latter view of minimal brain dysfunction as a different type of disorder is epitomized by Wender's concept of it as a condition involving a diminished capacity for positive and negative affect and abnormalities in cortical arousal (11, 14). The clinical phenomena of this hypothesized diagnostic category are said to approximate those of the hyperkinetic syndrome. Thus Wender (14) stated that Laufer and Denhoff's description (15) provided "as good a summary as any." The etiology is thought to lie in genetically determined abnormalities in the metabolism of serotonin, dopamine, and norepinephrine. As do Gross and Wilson, Wender relies on a distinctive response to stimulants as one of the hallmarks of the syndrome (16) but also invokes family history findings in support of a genetic basis.

As Benton (17) noted, either view of minimal brain dysfunction involves the use of "a behavioral concept with neurological implications." This means that the validity of the concept of minimal brain dysfunction must first be tested by determining whether there is evidence for the existence of a meaningfully distinctive behavioral syndrome that differs from other psychiatric conditions. If such a syndrome can be shown to exist, there is then the secondary question of whether or not it has an organic etiology and, if it has, what specific deficits or abnormalities are involved.

These two major issues constitute the main focus of this paper. However, with the former "continuum" concept of minimal brain dysfunction there is an issue that needs to be discussed first, namely, the problem of whether there can be subclinical brain damage that gives rise to behavioral or cognitive sequelae. In essence, this involves five questions: 1) Can there be brain damage without abnormalities on a neurological examination? 2) If so, does such damage give rise to psychological sequelae? 3) What is the threshold of severity of brain injury above which psychological sequelae can be detected? 4) Under what circumstances can such subclinical brain damage occur? and 5) How may organic brain dysfunction be recognized if the clinical neurological examination is normal?

SUBCLINICAL BRAIN DAMAGE

Brain Damage Without Neurological Abnormalities

The answer to the question of whether it is possible for overt and indisputable brain damage to occur and yet for a careful clinical neurological examination to reveal no definite abnormalities is a clear-cut yes (18). Thus Solomons and associates (19) observed that children who have obvious neurological abnormalities in infancy may appear normal when examined some years later. Similarly, Meyer and Byers (20) noted that the neurological sequelae of encephalitis may clear up completely as the affected children grow older. Also, in Shaffer and associates' study of children with confirmed gross damage to the brain substance (21) only a third showed definite neurological signs at follow-up a few years later, and a third showed no signs whatever of abnormality, dubious or definite. All these findings, together with others, indicate that there are some children with definite brain damage who show no abnormalities on clinical neurological examination. That part of the concept of minimal brain dysfunction has research support.

Psychological Sequelae of Subclinical Brain Damage

To answer the question of whether subclinical brain damage gives rise to psychological sequelae, we need to have a sample of children in which there is both a systematic neurological examination with normal findings and also contemporaneous evidence of brain damage at an earlier age. The prospective study of children with severe head injuries conducted by my associates and myself (22–24) provides just such a group. All of the children we studied had experienced a posttraumatic amnesia of at least 1 week, so that it was reasonable to infer some degree of brain injury, and all were examined by an experienced research neurologist at the follow-up 2¼ years after the accident. The test is the rate of new psychiatric disorders (that is, those with an onset *after* the head injury) in children without neurological abnormalities. The rate of disorder in children with severe head injuries was found to be still substantially above that in the control subjects even in the subgroup with a normal neurological examination (although the rate of psychiatric disorder was highest in those with abnormalities on a clinical examination). Evidently, brain injury (as indicated by posttraumatic amnesia lasting longer than 1 week) *can* lead to psychiatric abnormalities even when there are no discernible neurological sequelae.

The same question may be tackled another way by using our measures of intellectual impairment in the same group. As discussed in the first Salmon lecture (1), the presence of cognitive recovery was used as an index of an initial intellectual impairment, and a score at least one standard deviation below the score of the control group at the final follow-up served to identify persistent (as distinct from transient) impairment. The findings showed that the psychiatric risk was greatest in those children with a persisting cognitive impairment (a subgroup of those with the most severe injuries), but the rate was nevertheless still raised well above the rate for the control group even in children with *no* measurable intellectual impairment.

Yet a third approach is to use the presence of epileptic seizures as an indication of some kind of organic brain dysfunction. In the Isle of Wight general population epidemiological studies (2) my associates and I assessed the rate of psychiatric disorder in epileptic children of normal intelligence and without abnormalities on the systematic neurological examination. The rate of disorder found—whether based on a detailed psychiatric appraisal, on a teacher's questionnaire, or on a parental questionnaire—was several times that found in the randomly selected control group. A variety of methodological checks showed that this was likely to be a valid difference.

We may conclude that there *is* evidence for the existence of psychiatric disorders due to brain injuries that are subclinical to the extent that the children's general intelligence is normal and that there are no abnormalities on a systematic neurological examination. Of course, it has been possible to test the hypothesis only by reliance on groups in which the presence of organic brain dysfunction is known because of a history of head injury or epileptic seizures. We cannot necessarily generalize the finding to groups of children for whom the history gives no evidence of brain injury. Even so, the very existence of such examples of subclinical psychological deficits provides limited support for the notion of minimal brain dysfunction.

Threshold for Psychological Sequelae

There are two ways in which we can obtain a better estimate of how widely the continuum notion of minimal brain dysfunction can be extended. The first is by determining the *threshold* of severity of brain injury above which psychological sequelae can be detected, and the second is by examining the sequelae of possible *causes* of subclinical brain injury. If the threshold is low, wide generalization would be reasonable, whereas if it proves to be high only a very limited generalization would be warranted. Once again, our prospective study of children with head injuries (22–24) provides a means of doing this.

We had two indicators of which psychiatric disorders could be attributed to brain injury—the emergence of new disorders in children who were psychiatrically normal before the accident and a dose-response relationship between the severity of injury and the risk of disorder. With both research strategies there was no indication of any increased psychiatric risk with head injuries that led to posttraumatic amnesia lasting less than a week. The same issue was studied with respect to cognitive impairment—with broadly similar findings. In short, the evidence suggested that there was a rather high threshold.

For any persistent increase in cognitive or behavioral difficulties to be demonstrable, the head injury must have been sufficiently severe to cause posttraumatic amnesia lasting at least 7 days. These findings provide *no* support for the notion that a very mild brain injury causes psychiatric or intellectual problems. In an earlier review of relevant research findings Benton (17) concluded, "This mass of evidence points to the fact that cerebral lesions in children must be either quite extensive or have specific disorganizing properties in order to produce important behavioral abnormalities." Our results are in keeping with that summary: brain damage does greatly increase the psychiatric risk, but for this to happen it seems that the damage must be of some severity. The adjective "minimal" in minimal brain dysfunction seems misleading.

Causes of Subclinical Brain Injury

The fourth question concerns the possible causes of subclinical brain injury. If the concept of minimal brain dysfunction is to be extended at all (and the threshold data suggest that it should not be extended too far), we need to consider what etiologies we should have in mind—apart from the easily recognizable factors such as head injury or encephalitis. There are several, but just two—perinatal hazards and lead intoxication—will be taken as illustrative of the general pattern of findings.

American Journal of Psychiatry, 1982, vol. 139, pp. 21–33

Pregnancy complications and low birth weight constitute an obvious potential source of brain injury, which might affect large numbers of children. It is known that, when severe, they can and do lead to cerebral palsy and mental retardation, and it seems reasonable to suppose, as suggested by Pasamanick and Knobloch (10), that in lesser degree they might lead to less devastating but still important psychological sequelae. The evidence on whether this in fact happens has been well reviewed by several writers. Because these authors have approached the topic from varying viewpoints (25, 26), only their main conclusions will be summarized here.

One of the major difficulties in any assessment of the long-term sequelae of perinatal brain injury is the uncertainty as to whether such injury has actually occurred. This is a double problem in that pregnancy complications and low birth weight tend to be much more frequent in socially disadvantaged groups, so that such sequelae as do occur may be a consequence of the social adversities rather than the physical injury. Indeed, the large-scale studies, such as the British National Child Development Study (27) or the American Perinatal Collaborative Study (28), show that the intellectual and behavioral consequences are quite minor in the general population of children who do not have overt cerebral palsy or mental retardation, once statistical controls for social variables have been introduced. Also, however, there may be false negative findings simply because the few children with real brain injuries resulting from perinatal factors may have been diluted by the larger number who experienced perinatal hazards but who escaped cerebral damage. In order to deal with this problem, several investigations have concentrated on infants with anoxia or with neurological abnormalities in the neonatal period (29). Once again, the long-term sequelae have usually turned out to be quite minor: the case-control differences are very small after the preschool years. A further point, however, is that the outcome for children at perinatal risk has usually been found to be worse for those reared with social disadvantages (26, 30). It seems that the biological hazards are most likely to lead to later sequelae when they are combined with psychosocial adversity. Altogether, the findings suggest that perinatal traumata *can* occasionally lead to psychological sequelae even when there is no overt neurological disorder, but, equally, the results indicate that this is *not* the usual outcome.

During the last decade increasing attention has come to be paid to the possible neurotoxic effects of lead at levels hitherto regarded as safe or acceptable (13). The general argument is that it has been known since the beginning of this century that lead poisoning can cause encephalopathy and, moreover, that the survivors often show serious mental impairment. It is suggested that lesser increases in the overall body burden of lead may similarly lead to psychological sequelae through a neurotoxic effect, even if there are no signs of encephalopathy or clinical evidence of neurological damage. As with low birth weight, there is the problem of overlap with psychosocial adversity. Children are often exposed to lead because of pica, and pica is more frequent in less intelligent and behaviorally disturbed children. Other children have raised lead levels because of lead hazards in the areas in which they live—but where people live is strongly associated with their psychosocial characteristics and circumstances. Not surprisingly, therefore, it has proved quite difficult to sort out causes and consequences, and the research findings are not by any means decisive. Because the evidence has been reviewed in detail elsewhere (13), I will simply restate the main conclusions here. Although the findings are somewhat contradictory, the evidence suggests that persistently raised blood lead levels in the range above 40 μg/100 ml may cause slight cognitive impairment (a reduction of 1 to 5 points on average) and, less certainly, may increase the risk of behavioral difficulties in children without neurological signs or symptoms. There are indications that there may also be psychological risks with lead levels below 40 μg/100 ml, but the evidence on this point is inconclusive so far.

In short, the findings on the sequelae of these two possible causes of subclinical brain injury are in keeping with the head injury data in suggesting that indeed there may be psychological sequelae in children without neurological signs. But they also indicate that in general such sequelae are probably neither common nor severe unless the brain injury is also severe or the injury coexists with psychosocial hazards. However, the evidence is not particularly satisfactory, and any conclusions are necessarily rather tentative.

Indications of Organic Brain Dysfunction

The fifth and last question on the continuum concept of minimal brain dysfunction concerns the issue of how organic brain dysfunction may be recognized if the clinical neurological examination is normal. The proponents of the concept have usually suggested that the form of the child's behavior is itself diagnostic—on the grounds of the supposed close similarity with the behavioral symptoms of children with proven brain disease. This claim can be firmly dismissed on two grounds. In the first place, the symptoms of children with known brain damage are far from homogeneous and, with the exception of social disinhibition, do not constitute any recognizable psychiatric or cognitive syndrome (1). In the second place, studies of children with possible subclinical brain damage (in terms of head injury, perinatal hazards, lead intoxication, or any other postulated etiology) equally do not indicate any consistent behavioral or cognitive outcome. The behavioral diagnosis of brain damage is invalid.

Alternatively, so-called "soft" neurological signs have been used as evidence of organic brain dysfunc-

202 ■

tion. Most of these concern immaturities in developmental functions such as language, motor coordination, or perception (2). They are regarded as "soft" signs not because they are unreliable (to the contrary, if appropriately assessed, many can be measured with considerable precision) but, rather, because their interpretation and meaning remain somewhat uncertain. On the one hand, children with known brain dysfunction (as, for example, children with epilepsy) frequently exhibit no "soft" signs, so that the assessment produces many false negatives. On the other hand, a substantial minority of the general population *do* have "soft" signs of neurodevelopmental dysfunction—in spite of a complete lack of history of anything that is likely to have led to brain injury. Accordingly, there are also many false positives. Also, neurologists tend to differ in their threshold for the recognition of "soft" signs (31) and the signs show rather low temporal stability (32). It is true that several studies have shown "soft" signs to be more frequent in groups of children with behavior or learning problems than in the general population, but it is not at all clear just what these associations mean. Moreover, as Nichols and Chen's detailed analysis of the Collaborative Perinatal Project data (31) shows, there are only weak associations between neurological "soft" signs, hyperactivity, and learning disorders and even weaker associations between these variables and perinatal complications.

Precisely the same problems apply to the use of EEG abnormalities to diagnose brain dysfunction (5). Many of the abnormalities not only occur in a lot of apparently normal children but also show rather weak associations with neurological signs of structural brain disease. As Werry (5) put it, "Although children with psychiatric disorders often have abnormal EEGs, . . . most . . . fall in a no-man's land between normality and undeniable pathology." Thus Ritvo and associates (33) found EEG abnormalities in 35% of children with psychiatric disorders thought to be definitely or probably organic but in 19% of those with conditions considered nonorganic. In neither group did the EEG abnormality correlate with the type of psychiatric disorder—a negative finding in keeping with nearly all other studies (34).

In the last few years there have been important developments in quantitative computer analysis of the EEG and of sensory-evoked potentials, giving rise to what Roy John and his colleagues (35) have termed "neurometrics." Promising findings have been reported in terms of the ability of these techniques to differentiate children with learning disabilities. It may be that in the future they will come to provide the most satisfactory measures of brain functioning. However, so far it remains a research tool whose potential has still to be adequately evaluated.

Finally, there are the psychometric measures of brain dysfunction. Reitan and Boll (36) have shown that their battery of tests successfully differentiated normal children from those with overt brain damage. They also showed that the results for children with minimal brain dysfunction (with either learning deficits or behavioral abnormalities) were intermediate. However, there are two major drawbacks to this approach. First, it is possible to pick out all the children with minimal brain dysfunction only at the cost of also picking out over a third of normal children, with the consequence of considerable misclassification. Second, the deficits on the highly specific tests of the Reitan battery tend to parallel the overall IQ findings (37). As Chadwick and I also found out in our head injury study (38), there is no specific pattern of cognitive deficits that is diagnostic of brain injury. Thus Knights and Tymchuck (39) found that children's performances on the Reitan battery of tests were significantly correlated with IQ and that the tests appeared to be sensitive to impairment, regardless of whether the impairment was due to a brain lesion or some other factor.

In short, we must conclude that we still lack adequate tools with which to diagnose organic brain dysfunction when the clinical neurological examination is normal and when the history reveals no cause for brain injury. The various approaches mentioned, of course, have other uses, which justify their existence, and they can also provide useful pointers to the possibility of brain injury. Still, at best, they provide only circumstantial evidence, which is inadequate for individual diagnosis.

The one test not mentioned so far is that of drug response. Because this is also invoked in support of the other, *non*continuum concept of minimal brain dysfunction, detailed discussion will be postponed until later in the paper. However, it may be stated here that it does not provide the crucial link in the argument that is required.

Conclusions on the Continuum Concept

Clearly, the postulate that there can be subclinical damage to the brain is valid. Moreover, there is also evidence that such damage may give rise to behavioral and cognitive sequelae. However, although the evidence is not such as to give rise to firm conclusions, it seems that fairly severe brain injuries are required for this to occur and, therefore, that such minimal brain dysfunction syndromes are probably relatively uncommon. We have no good guidelines to their frequency, but it seems extremely unlikely that they account for the majority of child psychiatric referrals, as suggested by some writers. Most important of all, the psychological outcome of subclinical brain damage does *not* constitute a homogeneous syndrome, and so far we lack the means to diagnose such syndromes with any accuracy. In short, the notion of a continuum of brain injury probably has some validity, but it does not lead to a particular psychiatric syndrome. As a result, the diagnosis of minimal brain dysfunction, at best, is just

American Journal of Psychiatry, 1982, vol. 139, pp. 21–33

an uncertain hypothesis, which usually is not open to testing in the individual child, and, at worst, creates a neuromythology, which provides a rather pretentious cloak to cover ignorance.

THE HYPERKINETIC SYNDROME

Wender (11) has put forward a rather different concept of minimal brain dysfunction as a qualitatively distinct syndrome, which is thought to be due to a genetically determined biochemical abnormality rather than to any form of brain damage, major or minor. As indicated here, in order to test this concept we need first to examine the validity of the behavioral syndrome before considering its etiology. The clinical descriptions of the syndrome provided by various writers cover a wide range of symptoms, but the central features usually involve the phenomena of hyperactivity, impulsivity, and attentional deficits; therefore, the notion of a hyperkinetic syndrome will be used as a starting point (11, 40, 41).

Clinical Picture

The clinical picture of the hyperkinetic syndrome looks very striking. Hyperkinetic children are said to show a very short attention span, high distractibility, an inability to cut out extraneous stimuli when attempting to concentrate on a task, and impulsivity such that they attempt to solve problems too quickly without pausing to think and in consequence make many errors—the characteristics of an attentional deficit. When young, but less often when older, the children are thought to be overactive, unable to sit still for long, rushing restlessly about in a disorganized way, apparently unable to modulate or regulate their activity level to fit in with social requirements. Impulsive behavior is also manifest by frequent speaking out of turn in class, interruptions of or intrusions into other children's activities, poor frustration tolerance, and difficulties in waiting for their turn in group situations. One would think that such a dramatic disorder of behavior ought to be very easily recognizable and that there would be very good agreement among observers. But this has not proved to be the case.

In the first place, several studies in the United States (42, 43) have shown relatively low levels of agreement among parents, teachers, and clinicians on which children should be regarded as hyperkinetic. There are also the most amazing differences in the frequency with which the syndrome is diagnosed on either side of the Atlantic. In North America, the hyperkinetic syndrome (or minimal brain dysfunction) is diagnosed in up to half, or even more than half, of all children referred to psychiatric clinics (11, 12, 44). In Britain, on the other hand, the diagnosis is made in only about 1% of child patients of normal intelligence

(45). What is the meaning of this *50-fold* difference in diagnostic usage? Direct international comparisons are much needed to elucidate the matter, but it seems highly likely that clinicians in the two countries are using different concepts of the hyperkinetic syndrome. Certainly, when the same questionnaire to measure hyperactivity is used, not only are the factor structures obtained broadly similar but also the distributions of scores are generally comparable (46). In other words, it appears that children in the United Kingdom and in the United States are equally likely to show overactive behaviors—the difference lies in the frequency with which these are regarded as constituting the hyperkinetic syndrome.

A second problem is posed by the repeated finding that different measures of hyperactivity intercorrelate quite weakly (47–50). Moreover, when factor analytic techniques are applied to the results of several different measures of hyperkinesis, no overall hyperactivity factor is obtained (51). There seems to be some kind of coherence to the concept of a grouping of overactivity, inattention, and impulsiveness when these are all measured by the *same* rating instrument but not when they are measured by different instruments. Moreover, there is only rather modest agreement between different questionnaires that purport to measure hyperactivity (46, 52).

A third problem is that it has proved very difficult to obtain any questionnaire measure of overactivity that does not also correlate highly with measures of general conduct disturbance (46, 52). In other words, in practice, children who are hyperactive are also usually socially disruptive, aggressive, or antisocial. Ratings of motor activity overlap greatly with assessments of socially unacceptable behavior. This has given rise to questions as to whether judgments of hyperactivity are saying anything more than that the child is behaving in ways that the rater finds disturbing or disruptive (53).

The whole notion of a hyperkinetic syndrome begins to look rather illusory, and it has been easy for critics to dismiss the concept as just a myth, an artifact of medical labeling, or a way for professionals to conceal their lack of knowledge (53). But is the situation really as muddled as it seems and are the hypotheses really as insubstantial as they appear? I think not, but to answer these questions we need to turn our critical attention to the issues involved in measurement.

Measurement

As is evident in Sandoval's review of the topic (54), a wide range of measures of hyperactivity are available. These include a variety of mechanical devices such as actometers that can be attached to limbs, ballistographic cushions, ultrasonic or photoelectric systems, and telemetric transmitters.

In addition, there are observational techniques, various psychometric tests, and several questionnaires for completion by teachers, parents, or professionals.

204

The measures vary in the extent to which they have been adequately evaluated, but a number have been shown to be both reliable and valid in the sense that they measure what they purport to measure. Hence, the finding that they intercorrelate only weakly is not a reflection of their inadequacy as measures. Rather, the findings are explicable in terms of two other features.

First, it is apparent that neither hyperactivity nor inattention constitutes a unitary variable (54, 55). The child who is fidgety and squirmy is not necessarily the same child who runs up and down stairs all day long. Similarly, the child who is distracted by extraneous stimuli need not necessarily be impersistent, impulsive, or prone to cognitive error. Moreover, these various different facets of hyperactivity do not necessarily all show the same response to stimulant medication (56). It is necessary to add that it is also not self-evident which is the "best" or most appropriate measure. Sometimes there is an assumption that if teacher ratings do not agree with the more accurately quantitative mechanical devices, then the teacher ratings must be wrong. But it is equally plausible that the teachers are truly picking out the most relevant behaviors and that it is the labels they apply that are misleading. Perhaps the important thing is not the sheer amount of limb movement but the inappropriate or inadequate *modulation* of activity level (57), or perhaps the key feature concerns some aspect of attention rather than activity. The issue needs to be tackled in several different ways, but one essential preliminary is to determine precisely which aspects of behavior are being identified by teachers, parents, or professionals as "hyperactive." So far this has been attempted rather infrequently, although the studies by Rapoport and associates (58), by Abikoff and associates (59), by Copeland and Weissbrod (60), and by Whalen and associates (57) provide an important start.

The second issue that is relevant to the rather low agreement between measures is the extent to which hyperactivity is situation-specific. Thus Whalen and associates (57, 61) showed that hyperactive boys were most inattentive and disrupting during classroom conditions of high ambient noise or when they were expected to tackle difficult tasks at a pace dictated by the teacher. Stevens and associates (49) also showed that clinical staff ratings correlated best with acto-meter activity in classroom situations, whereas mothers' ratings did so best in the more informal settings of the gymnasium and the workshop. This finding suggests that different *facets* or *types* of hyperactivity may be evident in different settings; this may be one reason why parent and teacher ratings usually agree so poorly, as they do (46, 62). The converse of situation specificity is evident in Jacob and associates' finding that hyperactive children were most different from control children in a formal classroom setting and not very different from control children in an informal situation (63). The explanation of why this is the converse of specificity is that the reason for the difference between situations lay in the control subjects and not the hyperactive group. The hyperactive children were equally hyperactive in both situations, whereas the control children showed much more activity in the informal setting.

Situational Versus Pervasive Overactivity

The findings with respect to situational effects on hyperactivity are still rather fragmentary, and no succinct conclusions of a general kind are yet possible. Obviously, further research on this issue would be most worthwhile. However, the most important question is *not* whether hyperactivity is most likely to be manifest under these circumstances rather than those. Rather, we ought to ask, Are there differences between hyperactivity that is only shown in some situations and hyperactivity that is relatively pervasive across all situations? The possible relevance of this distinction was first brought out by Campbell and associates' follow-up of hyperactive preschoolers into elementary school (64). Situationally hyperactive children had fewer difficulties at the time of the follow-up at age 6½ years than those with pervasive hyperactivity; in particular, the situational group showed less inattentive off-task behavior.

The importance of this distinction has recently been further investigated by Schachar and associates (62), who used data from the Isle of Wight longitudinal study of all the 10-year-olds living on the island. This group of children were followed to age 15 years, and comparable psychoeducational and behavioral assessments were made at both ages. The hyperactivity factor scores on the Rutter parent and teacher scales were used to assess hyperactivity.

The hyperactivity scores were then used to divide the total group of children into three nonoverlapping groups. First, there were those few children with high scores on *both* the parent and teacher scales; this group with "pervasive" hyperactivity constituted about 22% of all the 10-year-olds. Second, 14% of the children had high scores on one questionnaire but not the other—the situational hyperactivity group. The third group, which made up the bulk of the children studied, was not hyperactive on either measure. The question, then, is how these three groups differ, after we have taken into account other relevant variables.

The first very striking finding was that whereas pervasive hyperactivity was strongly associated with the presence of cognitive deficits, situational overactivity was not. This was so regardless of whether the assessment concerned tests of general intelligence or of scholastic attainment. The result suggests that pervasive and situational hyperactivity may reflect rather different types of behavioral disturbance.

The second finding was that pervasive overactivity was strongly associated with the persistence of psychiatric disorder, however this was measured. The asso-

■ 205

American Journal of Psychiatry, 1982, vol. 139, pp. 21–33

ciation with situational overactivity was similar but less marked. These two findings, taken in combination, suggest that pervasive, but not situational, hyperactivity might constitute a meaningfully distinct behavioral syndrome that is distinctive in terms of both its association with cognitive impairment and its chronicity and persistence into adolescence.

However, a further methodological check was needed before we could conclude that the associations were specific to pervasive hyperactivity. It was necessary to determine whether a comparable distinction between pervasive and situational disorders would be found with any other constellation of behaviors. Because poor peer relationships are known to have both a strong association with general behavioral disturbance and a poor prognosis (65), this behavioral pattern seemed an appropriate one to compare with hyperactivity. The same approach as used with hyperactivity was followed to produce an "unsociability" score that could be employed to define situational and pervasive unsociability.

The findings showed that there were no differences between the situationally unsociable and the situationally overactive children in terms of the persistence of behavioral problems between 10 and 15 years. On the other hand, the pervasively hyperactive group stood out in terms of their worse prognosis. This strong persistence into adolescence was *not* found with pervasive unsociability.

The cognitive findings showed the same group differentiation. The pervasive hyperactivity group had a mean nonverbal IQ of about 80, whereas all the other groups had scores that were average for the general population. We may conclude that the characteristics associated with *situational* hyperactivity were probably nonspecific and hence of no particular diagnostic significance. On the other hand, the very small group of children with *pervasive* hyperactivity did seem distinctively different.

Of course, the findings derive from just one study and in any case refer only to questionnaire measures of hyperactivity. However, if taken in conjunction with the earlier findings on situation specificity from other investigations, they begin to make a case for a better differentiation *within* the large heterogeneous group of children with inattentive, overactive, socially disruptive behavior. Rather than deal with them all as if they all had the same syndrome, perhaps we should focus on the very much smaller subgroup who show these features in a wider range of circumstances.

Hyperactivity and Conduct Disorder

The suggestion that the broad heterogeneous group of overactive children should be subdivided raises the broader question of how we may determine whether hyperactivity (pervasive, situational, or any other variety) does or does not constitute a valid, meaningfully distinct clinical condition.

Most of the research into hyperactivity has been concerned with some type of comparison between hyperactive children and normal children. The results of these comparisons are informative and useful, but it is important to appreciate that they are of no relevance whatever to the question of syndrome definition. The issue is *not* whether hyperkinesis differs from normality (which obviously it does) but, rather, whether it differs from *other* psychiatric conditions. For a diagnostic category to have scientific meaning it must be shown to be distinctive in terms of etiology, course, response to treatment, or some variable *other than the symptoms that define it* (66). Thus it is of no help to assert that what differentiates the hyperkinetic syndrome is the presence of hyperactivity. The key issue is whether the constellation of hyperkinetic behaviors constitutes a syndrome that differs from conduct disorders, depression, schizophrenia, sociopathy, and the like.

In this connection, the most obvious potential overlap is that between hyperactivity and other forms of conduct disturbance. Factor-analytic studies show that hyperactivity, aggressivity, and conduct disturbance tend to occur together (53). Moreover, the hyperkinetic syndrome is not only strongly associated with the development of antisocial behavior in childhood, adolescence, and adult life; it is also associated with a family history of antisocial personality and alcoholism (67). The question then is whether the hyperactive syndrome differs in any way from other varieties of conduct disorder or antisocial disturbance.

Sandberg and associates (50) tackled this problem in a study of 5- to 11-year-old boys referred to the Maudsley Hospital. The research design involved the comparison of two groups of disorders: first, those in which the symptoms of overactivity or inattention occurred in marked degree and, second, all other psychiatric conditions (excluding psychosis). In short, the purpose was to determine whether any clinical significance could be attached to the presence of these hyperkinetic symptoms. Hyperactivity was assessed both through the Conners' parent and teacher questionnaires and by means of systematic observations of the child during psychological testing. The dependent variables were chosen on the basis of the features generally supposed to be associated with the hyperkinetic syndrome—namely, congenital stigmata, neurodevelopmental abnormalities, impulsivity (assessed on the Matching Familiar Figures test), a history of perinatal complications, and tests of general intelligence and scholastic achievement.

Four main findings derive from the data analysis. First, as others have found, there were only quite low correlations between different measures of overactivity. Second, not only did a high proportion of children with psychiatric problems show overactivity and inattention, but also there was a very substantial overlap between hyperactivity and general disturbances of conduct. Third, the presence of hyperactivity, as defined by a very high score on any single instrument, was of no clinical significance. The disorders with hyperactivity looked much the same as those without hyperactivity.

However, this conclusion refers to hyperkinesis assessed on just one measure. The fourth finding suggests that the implications may be different if pervasive overactivity is considered instead. To examine that possibility, hyperactivity was redefined in terms of abnormality on all measures—the teachers' scale, the parents' scale, and the observational measures. This left only 7 children, which emphasizes the rarity of pervasive hyperkinesis. These children were then compared with 7 normally active control children individually matched for age and IQ. The pervasively hyperactive children differed significantly in having been overactive from the preschool years, in showing more errors on the Matching Familiar Figures Test, and in being more likely to have neurodevelopmental abnormalities. Accordingly, there is the implication that this rarer group of children with pervasive hyperactivity might constitute a valid diagnostic entity. The numbers are far too small for this to be anything more than a very tentative and provisional suggestion, but the possibility warrants further exploration. On the other hand, the study provided *no* evidence to support the more usual wider concept of the hyperkinetic syndrome.

Firestone and Martin (68) have also recognized the crucial importance of determining whether the reported deficits attributed to hyperactivity are indeed specific to the syndrome or apply to most forms of emotional and behavioral disturbance. They tackled the question by comparing hyperactive children, children with conduct disorders, asthmatic children, and control subjects. In brief, the hyperactive group stood out as quite different from the control group but appeared rather similar to the other disturbed groups. Again, hyperactivity did not appear to pick out any valid diagnostic grouping. However, pervasive hyperactivity was not specifically studied in this investigation. Stewart and associates (69) have also investigated the same problem—again finding substantial overlap between hyperactive and unsocialized aggressive children.

Family History Findings

This issue arises particularly strongly with respect to the family history findings used by Wender (11) and others to argue that the syndrome has a genetic basis and that it is a distinct clinical entity. It should be appreciated that these two claims are not the same. The two questions of 1) whether there are hereditary influences and 2) if there are, whether what is inherited differentiates the hyperkinetic syndrome from other psychiatric conditions need to be considered separately.

Cantwell (70) has recently provided a succinct summary of the family history data relevant to the first question. However, the two key studies are his own (71) and that of Morrison and Stewart (72), both of which showed an increase not only in hyperactivity but also in alcoholism, sociopathy, and hysteria in the biological but not the adoptive parents of children with the hyperkinetic syndrome. The finding certainly suggests a genetic transmission, but the results are inconclusive in the absence of data on the biological parents of adopted hyperkinetic children and on the adoptive parents of nonhyperkinetic children. The point is that the biological-adoptive parent differences could just mean that adoptive parents tend to be more mentally healthy because those with psychiatric problems have been refused adoption. This explanation is quite independent of hyperactivity.

However, let us suppose that genetic factors could be confirmed (and it is quite likely that they would be); there is still the question of what is being inherited. As Stewart and associates (69) have rightly recognized, the key question is whether the family history associated with the hyperkinetic syndrome is different from that associated with nonoveractive conduct disorders. This comparison is especially important because the family history data reported for delinquent and antisocial boys in other investigations sounds remarkably similar to that linked with hyperkinesis (67, 73, 74). Could it be that the family history findings are a function of antisocial disorder and have nothing to do with hyperkinesis at all? That is just what Stewart and his colleagues (69) found. The presence of antisocial disorders or alcoholism in the parents was *not* associated with hyperkinesis in the children but *was* associated with aggressive conduct disorders irrespective of the presence or absence of overactivity.

The finding needs to be replicated, but the evidence available to date provides no support for the notion of the hyperkinetic syndrome as a meaningfully distinct genetic entity.

Biochemical and Physiological Findings

Of course, it could be that the wrong hereditary features are being studied. After all, Wender's basic hypothesis has been that biochemical and/or physiological abnormalities underlie the clinical phenomena (11). Again, the same two issues arise that do with the family history—namely, first, which biochemical and physiological features are associated with hyperkinesis and, second, are these different from those associated with other psychiatric disorders in childhood? The hypotheses on physiological features have suggested underarousal, overarousal, and also poorly modulated arousal (75–77). In fact, different studies have found all three, although many have found no consistent differences from normal (78, 79). No unambiguous conclusions are possible on arousal, but, since the comparisons have generally been with normal

■207

American Journal of Psychiatry, 1982, vol. 139, pp. 21–33

children rather than those with other psychiatric conditions, the findings are in any case of no help in syndrome definition.

The same problems face us with respect to biochemical findings. The hypotheses are varied, the empirical findings contradictory and inconclusive, and such differences as have been found serve to differentiate hyperkinetic from normal children and not from those with other psychiatric disorders. The key studies are well received by Shaywitz and her colleagues (80), who took the view that brain monoaminergic mechanisms may ultimately prove to be important in the genesis of minimal brain dysfunction, although clearly this has not yet been shown. However, whether or not this turns out to be the case, once more the question will be whether the findings are specific to the hyperkinetic syndrome. Thus, for example, Shekim and his associates (81, 82) have reported decreased urinary MHPG in samples of hyperkinetic children, but Young and his coworkers (83) have found the same with autistic children. Of course, there are immense problems in knowing how best to study the biochemistry of the brain in that there is an uncertain relationship between blood and urine metabolites and CNS activity (84). Clearly, it would be premature to conclude that biochemical abnormalities do not constitute the basis of the hyperkinetic syndrome. Equally obviously, there is no good evidence as yet that they do, and, more importantly, there is no indication of any biochemical feature that is specific to the hyperkinetic syndrome.

Much the same has also to be said with respect to other so-called ''organic'' features. Dubey (85), in his review of the topic, usefully brought out many of the research issues and emphasized, as I have done, that the crucial question is whether any abnormality (be it EEG abnormalities, soft neurological signs, perinatal complications, or congenital stigmata) is *specifically* associated with hyperkinesis in a way not found with other psychiatric conditions. Such comparisons have been few and often not very adequate, but to date no feature has been isolated that is in any way specific to the hyperkinetic syndrome.

Response to Stimulants

Finally, we need to consider the question in response to stimulant medication. As noted here, both main varieties of the concept of minimal brain dysfunction have relied on a distinctive and qualitatively different response to stimulants as one of the main buttresses in the arguments for the existence of some kind of syndrome of minimal brain dysfunction. Undoubtedly, if hyperkinetic children could be shown to differ from other children in their response to stimulants, this would indeed be a most useful validating feature (86). However, in spite of continuing claims regarding a specific drug response (11, 16), there is no good evidence that it exists. Of course, numerous drug

studies attest to the short-term benefits of stimulant medication in hyperkinetic children (87), but that is not what matters. The question is whether the response is *different* from that in other psychiatric conditions. The problem has not yet been adequately studied, but so far the findings run counter to this suggestion. With the possible exception of anxiety reactions, most disorders seem to respond well to stimulants (88, 89). The response is not really paradoxical (90), and recent studies have shown that both normal children (91–93) and enuretic children (94) respond in much the same way as do hyperkinetic children. Furthermore, drug response does not appear to relate to differences in autonomic arousal—one hypothesized specific mechanism (95)—and, in spite of very different pharmacologic actions, it appears that amitriptyline and methylphenidate may have rather comparable effects on hyperactivity (96, 97, 98). It is still worth pursuing the idea that a distinctive response to stimulants may relate to clinical features, but the evidence so far does not support the suggestion that this is a characteristic of the hyperkinetic syndrome.

Minimal Brain Dysfunction as a Qualitatively Distinct Syndrome

It is all too obvious that none of the features considered serve to validate a syndrome concept of minimal brain dysfunction. However, before dismissing the whole idea, it is important to recognize that nearly all of the studies have been concerned with rather broad, often ill-defined, and almost certainly heterogeneous groups of fidgety, restless, disruptive, and inattentive children. It may be that real differences have been concealed by the unhelpfully global nature of the categories studied. As is evident from the studies of pervasive and situational hyperactivity, there is no good support for the very broad concept of a hyperkinetic syndrome, but there are pointers that there may be a rarer but valid syndrome of hyperkinesis if this is defined in narrower terms demanding the existence of abnormalities that persist across a range of situations or circumstances. Whether such a syndrome, if it exists, is due to genetically based biochemical abnormalities is quite another matter, but it remains a possibility worth investigating.

CONCLUSIONS

Before concluding, I should note that my discussion has been limited to the hyperkinetic syndrome, although many clinicians now regard attentional deficits as the central feature of the disorder. Although the suggestion is plausible, so far it lacks empirical support; moreover, just as with hyperactivity, attentional problems are common in many different types of psychiatric disorder (55), and there is the same problem of lack of agreement between measures (55).

Similarly, many consider learning disorders to constitute part of the concept of minimal brain dysfunction. However, they show only weak associations with perinatal complications, with neurological impairment, and with hyperkinesis (31). Also, there is reason to suppose that they include several meaningful subcategories (99, 100). Hence, if I had considered either attentional deficits or learning deficits in this review, my conclusions would have been similar—namely, that it is both unhelpful and invalid to group them all together under the umbrella of minimal brain dysfunction.

Where, then, does all this leave the concept, or rather the several concepts, of minimal brain disorder? So far as the continuum concept is concerned, we may conclude that there is no doubt that subclinical damage to the brain does occur and that it may involve psychological sequelae. On the other hand, it is probable (but not certain) that rather severe damage is needed to give rise to persistent behavioral and cognitive sequelae. Moreover, such damage does not result in any kind of homogeneous, recognizable clinical syndrome.

So far as the second, noncontinuum, qualitatively distinct type of minimal brain dysfunction concept is concerned, we need to have recourse to the Scottish-style judicial verdict of "not proven." Undoubtedly, claims regarding this type of minimal brain dysfuncton syndrome have far outrun the empirical findings that could justify it. However, until the last few years most of the research has been rather tangential to the issue of syndrome definition, and it is only now that some of the crucial studies are being undertaken. All too often speculations about minimal brain dysfunction have given rise to postures of certainty when only ignorance exists. Nevertheless, these speculations have been surprisingly fruitful in their stimulation of research. Perhaps out of that research may eventually emerge new concepts with a better empirical base.

REFERENCES

1. Rutter M: Psychological sequelae of brain damage in childhood. Am J Psychiatry 138:1533–1544, 1981
2. Rutter M, Graham P, Yule W: A Neuropsychiatric Study in Childhood: Clinics in Developmental Medicine 35/36. London, William Heinemann Medical Books/SIMP, 1970
3. Strother CR: Minimal cerebral dysfunction: a historical overview. Ann NY Acad Sci 205:6–17, 1973
4. Rie HE, Rie ED (eds): Handbook of Minimal Brain Dysfunctions: A Critical View. New York, Wiley-Interscience, 1980
5. Werry JS: Organic factors, in Psychopathological Disorders of Childhood, 2nd ed. Edited by Quay HC, Werry JS. New York, John Wiley & Sons, 1979
6. Bond ED, Partridge GE: Post-encephalitic behavior disorders in boys and their management in a hospital. Am J Psychiatry 83:25–103, 1926
7. Kahn E, Cohen LH: Organic drivenness—a brain stem syndrome and an experience—with case reports. N Engl J Med 210:748–756, 1934
8. Bradley C: The behavior of children receiving benzedrine. Am J Psychiatry 94:577–585, 1937
9. Strauss AA, Lehtinen V: Psychopathology and Education of the Brain-Injured Child, vol I. New York, Grune & Stratton, 1947
10. Pasamanick B, Knobloch H: Retrospective studies on the epidemiology of reproductive casualty: old and new. Merrill-Palmer Quarterly of Behavioral Development 12:7–26, 1966
11. Wender P: Minimal Brain Dysfunction in Children. New York, John Wiley & Sons, 1971
12. Gross MD, Wilson WC: Minimal Brain Dysfunction: A Clinical Study of Incidence, Diagnosis and Treatment in Over 1,000 Children. New York, Brunner/Mazel, 1974
13. Rutter M: Raised Lead Levels and Impaired Cognitive/Behavioral Functioning: A Review of the Evidence. Dev Med Child Neurol Suppl 42, 1980
14. Wender PH: Some speculation concerning a possible biochemical basis of minimal brain dysfunction. Ann NY Acad Sci 205:18–28, 1973
15. Laufer MW, Denhoff E: Hyperkinetic behavior syndrome in children. J Pediatr 50:463–474, 1957
16. Wood DR, Reimherr FW, Wender PH: Diagnosis and treatment of MBD in adults. Arch Gen Psychiatry 33:1453–1460, 1976
17. Benton AL: Minimal brain dysfunction from a neuropsychological point of view. Ann NY Acad Sci 205:29–37, 1973
18. Rutter M, Chadwick OPD: Neuro-behavioral associations and syndromes of "minimal brain dysfunction," in Clinical Neuro-Epidemiology. Edited by Rose FC. Tunbridge Wells, England, Pitman, 1980
19. Solomons G, Holden RH, Denhoff E: The changing picture of cerebral dysfunction in early childhood. J Pediatr 63:113–120, 1963
20. Meyer E, Byers RK: Measles encephalitis: a follow-up study of sixteen patients. Am J Dis Child 84:543–579, 1952
21. Shaffer D, Chadwick O, Rutter M: Psychiatric outcome of localized head injury in children, in Outcome of Severe Damage to the Central Nervous System: Ciba Foundation Symposium 34. Edited by Porter R, FitzSimmons DW. Amsterdam, Elsevier-Excerpta Medica-North Holland, 1975
22. Rutter M, Chadwick O, Shaffer D, et al: A prospective study of children with head injuries, I: design and methods. Psychol Med 10:633–645, 1980
23. Chadwick O, Rutter M, Brown G, et al: A prospective study of children with head injuries, II: cognitive sequelae. Psychol Med 11:49–61, 1981
24. Brown G, Chadwick O, Shaffer D, et al: A prospective study of children with head injuries in adulthood, III: psychiatric sequelae. Psychol Med 11:63–78, 1981
25. Birch HG, Gussow JD: Disadvantaged Children: Health, Nutrition, and School Failure. New York, Grune & Stratton, 1970
26. Sameroff A, Chandler M: Reproductive risk and the continuum of caretaking casualty, in Review of Child Development Research, vol 4. Edited by Horowitz F, Hetherington M, Scarr-Salapatek S, et al. Chicago, University of Chicago Press, 1975
27. Davie R, Butler NR: From Birth to Seven: The Second Report of the National Child Development Survey. Atlantic Highlands, NJ. Humanities Press, 1972
28. Broman SH, Nichols PL, Kennedy WA: Preschool IQ: Prenatal and Early Development Correlates. Hillsdale, NJ, Lawrence Erlbaum Associates, 1975
29. Corah N, Anthony E, Painter P, et al: Effects of Perinatal Anoxia After Seven Years. Psychological Monograph 79 (596), 1965
30. Werner EE, Bierman JM, French FE: The children of Kauai. Honolulu, University Press of Hawaii, 1971
31. Nichols PL, Chen T-C: Minimal Brain Dysfunction: A Prospective Study. Hillsdale, NJ, Lawrence Erlbaum Associates, 1980
32. McMahon SA, Greenberg LM: Serial neurologic examination of hyperactive children. Pediatrics 59:584–587, 1977
33. Ritvo ER, Ornitz EM, Walker RD, et al: Correlation of psychiatric diagnoses and EEG findings: a double-blind study of 184 hospitalized children. Am J Psychiatry 126:988–996, 1970
34. Harris R: The EEG, in Child Psychiatry: Modern Approaches.

American Journal of Psychiatry, 1982, vol. 139, pp. 21–33

Edited by Rutter M, Hersov L. London, Blackwell Scientific, 1977

35. John ER, Karmel BZ, Corning WC, et al: Neurometrics. Science 196:1393–1410, 1977
36. Reitan RM, Boll TJ: Neuropsychological correlates of minimal brain dysfunction. Ann NY Acad Sci 205:65–88, 1973
37. Reitan RM, Davison LA: Clinical Neurophysiology: Current Status and Applications. New York, John Wiley & Sons, 1974
38. Chadwick O, Rutter M, Shaffer D, et al: A prospective study of children with head injuries, IV: specific cognitive deficits. Journal of Clinical Neuropsychology 3:101–120, 1981
39. Knights RM, Tymchuck AJ: An evaluation of the Halstead-Reitan category tests for children. Cortex 4:403–414, 1968
40. Cantwell DP: The hyperkinetic syndrome, in Child Psychiatry: Modern Approaches. Edited by Rutter M, Hersov L. London, Blackwell Scientific, 1977
41. Weiss G, Hechtman L: The hyperactive child syndrome. Science 205:1348–1354, 1979
42. Kenny TJ, Clemmens RL, Hudson BW, et al: Characteristics of children referred because of hyperactivity. J Pediatr 79:618–622, 1971
43. Lambert NM, Sandoval J, Sassone D: Prevalence of hyperactivity in elementary school children as a function of social system definers. Am J Orthopsychiatry 48:446–463, 1978
44. Huessy HR, Gendron RA: Prevalence of the so-called hyperkinetic syndrome in public school children in Vermont. Acta Paedopsychiatr (Basel) 31:243–248, 1970
45. Rutter M, Shaffer D, Shepherd M: A Multi-Axial Classification of Child Psychiatric Disorders: An Evaluation of a Proposal. Geneva, World Health Organization, 1975
46. Sandberg ST, Wieselberg M, Shaffer D: Hyperkinetic and conduct problem children in a primary school population: some epidemiological considerations. J Child Psychol Psychiatry 21:293–311, 1980
47. Shaffer D, McNamara N, Pincus JH: Controlled observations on patterns of activity, attention, and impulsivity in brain-damaged and psychiatrically disturbed boys. Psychol Med 4:4–18, 1974
48. Schulman J, Kaspar J, Throne F: Brain Damage and Behavior: A Clinical-Experimental Study. Springfield, Ill, Charles C Thomas, 1965
49. Stevens TM, Kupst MJ, Suran BG, et al: Activity level: a comparison between actometer scores and observer ratings. J Abnorm Child Psychol 6:163–173, 1978
50. Sandberg ST, Rutter M, Taylor E: Hyperkinetic disorder in psychiatric clinic attenders. Dev Med Child Neurol 20:279–299, 1978
51. Langhorne JE, Loney J, Peternite CE, et al: Childhood hyperkinesis: a return to the source. J Abnorm Psychol 85:201–209, 1976
52. Quay HC: Classification, in Psychopathological Disorders of Childhood, 2nd ed. Edited by Quay HC, Werry JS. New York, John Wiley & Sons, 1979
53. Shrag P, Divoky D: The Myth of the Hyperactive Child. New York, Dell Publishing Co, 1975
54. Sandoval J: The measurement of the hyperactive syndrome in children. Review of Educational Research 47:293–318, 1977
55. Taylor E: Development of attention, in Scientific Foundations of Developmental Psychiatry. Edited by Rutter M. London, William Heinemann Medical Books, 1980
56. Conners CK, Werry JS: Pharmacotherapy, in Psychopathological Disorders of Childhood, 2nd ed. Edited by Quay HC, Werry JS. New York, John Wiley & Sons, 1979
57. Whalen CK, Collins PE, Henker B, et al: Behavior observations of hyperactive children and methylphenidate (Ritalin) effects in systematically structured classroom environments: now you see them, now you don't. Journal Pediatric Psychology 3:177–187, 1978
58. Rapoport J, Abramson A, Alexander D, et al: Playroom observation of hyperactive children on medication. J Am Acad Child Psychiatry 10:524–534, 1971
59. Abikoff H, Gittelman-Klein R, Klein DF: Validation of a classroom observation code for hyperactive children. J Consult Clin Psychol 45:772–783, 1977
60. Copeland AP, Weissbrod CS: Behavioral correlates of the hyperactivity factor of the Conners teacher questionnaire. J Abnorm Child Psychol 6:339–343, 1978
61. Whalen CK, Kenker B, Collins BE, et al: A social ecology of hyperactive boys: medication effects in structured classroom environments. J Appl Behav Anal 12:65–81, 1979
62. Schachar R, Rutter M, Smith A: The characteristics of situationally and pervasively hyperactive children: implications for syndrome definition. J Child Psychol Psychiatry (in press)
63. Jacob RG, O'Leary KD, Rosenblad C: Formal and informal classroom settings: effects on hyperactivity. J Abnorm Child Psychol 6:47–59, 1978
64. Campbell SB, Endman MW, Bernfeld G: A three-year follow-up of hyperactive preschoolers into elementary school. J Child Psychol Psychiatry 18:239–249, 1977
65. Roff M, Sells SB, Golden MM: Social Adjustment and Personality Development in Children. Minneapolis, University of Minnesota Press, 1972
66. Rutter M: Diagnostic validity in child psychiatry, in Advances in Biological Psychiatry, vol 2. Basel, S Karger, 1978
67. Cantwell DP: Hyperactivity and antisocial behavior revisited: a critical review of the literature, in Biopsychosocial Vulnerabilities in Delinquency. Edited by Lewis D. Jamaica, NY, Spectrum Publications, 1980
68. Firestone P, Martin JE: An analysis of the hyperactive syndrome: a comparison of hyperactive, behavior problem, asthmatic, and normal children. J Abnorm Child Psychol 7:261–273, 1979
69. Stewart MA, de Blois CS, Cummings C: Psychiatric disorder in the parents of hyperactive boys and those with conduct disorder. J Child Psychol Psychiatry 21:283–292, 1980
70. Cantwell DP: Minimal brain dysfunction in adults: evidence from studies of psychiatric illness in the families of hyperactive children, in Psychiatric Aspects of Minimal Brain Dysfunction in Adults. Edited by Bellak L. New York, Grune & Stratton, 1979
71. Cantwell D: Genetic studies of hyperactive children: psychiatric illness in biologic and adopting parents, in Genetic Research in Psychiatry. Edited by Fieve R, Rosenthal D, Brill H. Baltimore, Johns Hopkins University Press, 1974
72. Morrison J, Stewart M: The psychiatric status of the legal families of adopted hyperactive children. Arch Gen Psychiatry 28:888–891, 1973
73. Robins LN: Deviant Children Grown Up. Baltimore, Williams & Wilkins Co, 1966
74. West DJ, Farrington DP: Who Becomes Delinquent? London, William Heinemann Educational Books, 1973
75. Satterfield JH, Dawson ME: Electrodermal correlates of hyperactivity in children. Psychophysiology 8:191–197, 1971
76. Satterfield JH, Atonian G, Brashears GC, et al: Electrodermal studies of minimal brain dysfunction in children, in Clinical Use of Stimulant Drugs in Children: International Congress Series 313. Edited by Conners CK. Amsterdam, Excerpta Medica, 1974
77. Zahn TP, Little BC, Wender PH: Pupillary and heart rate activity in children with minimal brain dysfunction. J Abnorm Child Psychol 6:135–147, 1978
78. Hastings JE, Barkley RA: A review of psychophysiological research with hyperkinetic children. J Abnorm Child Psychol 6:413–447, 1978
79. Rosenthal RH, Allen TW: An examination of attention, arousal, and learning dysfunctions of hyperkinetic children. Psychol Bull 85:689–715, 1978
80. Shaywitz SE, Cohen DJ, Shaywitz BA: The biochemical basis of minimal brain dysfunction. J Pediatr 92:179–187, 1978
81. Shekim WO, Dekirmenjian H, Chapel JL: Urinary catecholamine metabolites in hyperkinetic boys treated with d-amphetamine. Am J Psychiatry 134:1276–1979, 1977
82. Shekim WO, Dekirmenjian H, Chapel JL: Urinary MHPG excretion in minimal brain dysfunction and its modification by d-amphetamine. Am J Psychiatry 136:667–671, 1979
83. Young JG, Cohen DJ, Caparulo BK, et al: Decreased 24-hour urinary MHPG in childhood autism. Am J Psychiatry 136:1055–1057, 1979

210■

84. Boullin DJ: Biochemical indications of central serotonin function, in Serotonin in Mental Abnormalities. Edited by Boullin DJ. Chichester, England, Wiley, 1978

85. Dubey DR: Organic factors in hyperkinesis: a critical evaluation. Am J Orthopsychiatry 46:353–366, 1976

86. Klein D, Gittelman-Klein R: Problems in the diagnosis of minimal brain dysfunction and the hyperkinetic syndrome. International Journal of Mental Health 4:45–60, 1975

87. Barkley RA: A review of stimulant drug research with hyperactive children. J Child Psychol Psychiatry 128:127–165, 1977

88. Barkley RA: Predicting the response of hyperkinetic children to stimulant drugs: a review. J Abnorm Child Psychol 4:327–348, 1976

89. Sroufe LA: Drug treatment of children with behavior problems, in Review of Child Development Research, vol 4. Edited by Horowitz FD. Chicago, University of Chicago Press, 1976

90. Sahakian BJ, Robbins TW: Are the effects of psychomotor stimulant drugs on hyperactive children really paradoxical? Med Hypotheses 3:154–158, 1977

91. Rapoport JL, Buchsbaum MS, Zahn TP, et al: Dextroamphetamine: cognitive and behavioral effects in normal prepubertal boys. Science 199:560–563, 1978

92. Rapoport JL, Buchsbaum MS, Weingartner H, et al: Dextroamphetamine: its cognitive and behavioral effects in normal and hyperactive boys and normal men. Arch Gen Psychiatry 37:933–943, 1980

93. Zahn TP, Rapoport JL, Thompson CL: Autonomic and behavioral effects of dextroamphetamine and placebo in normal and hyperactive prepubertal boys. J Abnorm Child Psychol 8:145–160, 1980

94. Werry JS, Aman MG: Methylphenidate in hyperactive and enuretic children, in The Psychobiology of Childhood: Profile of Current Issues. Edited by Shopsin B, Greenhill L. Jamaica, NY, Spectrum Publications, 1979

95. Barkley RA, Jackson TL: Hyperkinesis, autonomic nervous system activity and stimulant drug effects. J Child Psychol Psychiatry 18:347–357, 1977

96. Winsberg BG, Bialer I, Kupietz D, et al: Effects of imipramine and dextroamphetamine on behavior of neuropsychiatrically impaired children. Am J Psychiatry 128:1425–1431, 1972

97. Rapoport JL, Quinn PO, Bradbard G, et al: Imipramine and methylphenidate treatments of hyperactive boys. Arch Gen Psychiatry 30:789–793, 1974

98. Yepes L, Balka B, Winsberg B, et al: Amitriptyline and methylphenidate treatment of behaviorally disordered children. J Child Psychol Psychiatry 18:39–52, 1977

99. Benton AL, Pearl D: Dyslexia: An Appraisal of Current Knowledge. New York, Oxford University Press, 1978

100. O'Rourke BP: Reading, spelling, arithmetic disabilities: a neuropsychologic perspective, in Progress in Learning Disabilities, vol IV. Edited by Myklebust HR. New York, Grune & Stratton, 1978

American Journal of Psychiatry, 1981, vol. 138, pp. 1533–1544

Psychological Sequelae of Brain Damage in Children

BY MICHAEL RUTTER, M.D.

212 ∎

The author reviews the empirical evidence on the psychological sequelae of brain damage in childhood, concluding that brain injury causes a markedly increased risk in both intellectual impairment and psychiatric disorder. The risk is related to the severity of the brain damage, but there is little indication of locus effects. Psychiatric disorder is probably most likely to occur when there is abnormal neurophysiological activity; to some extent it may be influenced by the nature of the basic medical condition. Psychiatric consequences of brain injury are also substantially affected by the child's pre-injury behavior, psychosocial circumstances, and cognitive level. However, there are few psychological sequelae that are specific to brain damage.

To workers in other fields, the topic of this paper and its companion (1) (to be published in the January 1982 issue of the *Journal*) must seem curiously vague and unhelpfully broad. Surely, it is obvious that brain damage must result in psychological sequelae. After all, the brain is the organ of the mind and injury to that organ must inevitably have behavioral and cognitive consequences, one would suppose. The interest could lie only in the specifics—in the various particular ways in which different types of pathology, in different parts of the brain, lead to specific psychiatric syndromes. But if that were so, what possible

First Salmon lecture, presented at the New York Academy of Medicine, New York, Dec. 6, 1979. Received March 13, 1980; revised July 18, 1980; accepted Oct. 21, 1980.

From the Institute of Psychiatry, London. Address correspondence to Dr. Rutter, Department of Child and Adolescent Psychiatry, Institute of Psychiatry, de Crespigny Park, Denmark Hill, London SE5 8AF, England. Reprints are not available.

This paper was prepared while the author was a Fellow at the Center for Advanced Study in the Behavioral Sciences, Stanford, Calif.; the author thanks the Grant Foundation, the Foundation for Child Development, the Spencer Foundation, and the National Science Foundation (BNS 78-24671) for financial support.

purpose could there be in considering syndromes defined only in terms of the "minimal" nature of the brain dysfunction?

It is all too easy to mock and cast scorn on the terms and concepts. Yet a vast literature has grown up around the notion of behavioral syndromes of "minimal brain dysfunction," and vigorous controversies continue on just what are the psychological sequelae of brain damage in childhood. In part, the difficulties stem from our continuing ignorance of brain-behavior relationships and from the inadequacy of our tools to assess brain functioning. However, in part too, the problems have arisen from a confusion on the *clinical* issues that arise in relation to the possible psychological sequelae of brain damage, minimal or maximal. Unless we are clear on the clinical concepts and questions, we will be in no position to take advantage of the advances in the basic neurosciences that are likely to come in the next few decades. This paper and its companion (1) focus on those clinical issues.

In the first, I consider the problems from the starting point of identified brain pathology, asking, What are the behavioral and cognitive consequences of known brain injury in its various forms? In the second, I grasp the other end of the same stick by using the psychiatric and psychological syndromes sometimes attributed to organic brain dysfunction as the point of origin. The key questions then become, first, What is the evidence that they constitute discrete and meaningfully distinct conditions and, second, What is the evidence that they are due to brain damage, disease, or malfunction? The conceptual issues involved in these two separate but essentially complementary approaches are rather different.

RISKS OF PSYCHIATRIC DISORDER AND INTELLECTUAL IMPAIRMENT

The most basic question is to what extent there are any psychological sequelae of brain damage. Before considering the empirical findings we need to ask *why* this question has taken so long to be answered satisfactorily, for indeed it has. At first sight, it would seem to be a very straightforward matter. After all, it has been well demonstrated that very gross brain lesions can cause severe mental retardation. Indeed, it is known that severe retardation is virtually always due to some identifiable structural brain abnormality (2). Similarly, disintegrative psychoses occurring as a consequence of widespread brain disease are also recognized (3). It would appear that it is just a matter of determining similar associations with some of the less devastating varieties of brain pathology.

The problems arise from at least five different sources, most of which were identified as long ago as 1902 by Still (4) in his classic paper "Some Abnormal Psychical Conditions in Children." First, both psychiatric disorders and intellectual impairment have many causes, including psychosocial stresses as well as constitutional factors. As a result, it is essential to compare rates of disorder in groups of children with brain damage with the rates in the general population, in order to be sure that rates of disorder are above base level. Second, children with brain damage are frequently also physically handicapped, and it could be that the psychological sequelae stem from the physical handicap rather than from the brain lesion. Again, comparative studies are called for in order to check which is the crucial factor.

Third, brain damage often leads to *both* intellectual impairment and psychiatric disorder, and it could be that the emotional and behavioral problems stem from the low IQ rather than brain damage—an important possibility because intelligence may be low for a host of reasons other than brain damage. The implication is that IQ controls are crucial in order to determine whether the high rates of disorder in children with brain damage are just a function of low IQ.

Fourth, attention must be paid to the causes of the brain injury, because they could also constitute the causes of the psychological difficulties. Thus disruptive children of limited intelligence may be more likely to receive head injuries or to develop lead intoxication as a result of pica. The need is for longitudinal studies of change *following* brain injury.

Fifth, children with brain damage are often disadvantaged in many other ways, so that their problems may stem as much from the associated psychosocial deprivation as from the brain pathology. Careful study of and control for psychosocial variables are essential.

Intellectual Impairment

The overall findings on intellectual impairment are reasonably well established. We may conclude that *bilateral* damage of a widespread kind is usually associated with a substantial cognitive retardation—as shown, for example, by the findings from all surveys of cerebral palsy (5). On the other hand, *unilateral*

lesions, even when present from the infancy period, are much less likely to result in intellectual impairment (6). Most children with hemiplegia have an IQ in the normal range. Moreover, brain disorders that are unassociated with gross structural lesions may involve no intellectual impairment at all. Thus the IQ distribution of children with uncomplicated epilepsy is roughly normal (5).

Clearly, then, although severe and especially bilateral brain pathology may lead to mental retardation, there are many organic brain disorders without identifiable cognitive sequelae. It is that observation which has been the source of the controversy over the more subtle intellectual deficits associated with brain injury. The problem has been how to determine whether mild cognitive impairments are in fact due to brain injury rather than to associated genetic or experiential factors. One solution lies in the study of change—as shown by our prospective study of children with head injuries (7–9).

A sample of 28 children with head injuries that resulted in a posttraumatic amnesia lasting at least 1 week were compared with an individually matched control group of children with orthopedic injuries that involved no damage to the head and no loss of consciousness. A third group of 29 children with mild head injuries, involving a posttraumatic amnesia lasting more than an hour but less than a week, were studied in comparable fashion. This group of children with mild head injuries was not individually matched in the same way (as a result of limited resources) and, as it happened, came from a somewhat more disadvantaged background.

It is a general rule, with acute damage to the brain, that the intellectual deficit is greater immediately after the damage and that progressive improvement occurs during the following months. The presence of this pattern of recovery, therefore, provides a strong indication that the initial deficit was a consequence of acute damage. Conversely, the absence of any recovery phase provides strong circumstantial evidence that the initial deficit was *not* due to acute brain damage. It was found that there was a marked cognitive recovery phase in the group with severe head injuries but none in the group with mild injuries. The implication is that the deficit in the former group *was due* to brain injury, whereas that in the latter group was *not*. Although the IQ scores of the children with mild head injuries remained below those of the control children, the lack of recovery implied that the cognitive deficit antedated the injury (and presumably was a function of their more disadvantaged social background).

Another approach to the question of the extent to which brain damage *causes* intellectual impairment is to determine whether there is a consistent relationship between the severity of the brain injury and the extent of the intellectual deficit *within* the group with head injuries—in other words, a "dose-response" relation-

■213

American Journal of Psychiatry, 1981, vol. 138, pp. 1533–1544

ship. For this purpose, three subgroups, all within the group with severe head injuries, were compared. These groups were defined in terms of the presence or absence of two features—cognitive recovery as assessed by change over the first year and persisting impairment as assessed by the deficit at the 2¼-year follow-up. It was found that there was indeed a strong dose-response relationship between the severity of brain injury (as reflected in the duration of posttraumatic amnesia) and the presence of intellectual impairment. Children who experienced a posttraumatic amnesia lasting 3 weeks or more usually had persistent intellectual impairment; those with a posttraumatic amnesia lasting 2–3 weeks were most likely to show just a transient impairment (although in a few children it was persistent); finally, in those with a posttraumatic amnesia lasting less than 2 weeks, intellectual impairment, either transient or persistent, was distinctly unusual.

214■

Various other analyses, including associations with neurological abnormalities, confirmed these findings (8). Moreover, other studies have similarly shown that cognitive sequelae are most marked following injuries resulting in prolonged unconsciousness (10–12). We may conclude that acquired brain injuries may cause substantial intellectual impairment. However, it should be noted that we were able to show this only with rather severe head injuries resulting in a posttraumatic amnesia of at least 1, if not 2, weeks. This point is discussed in more detail in my companion paper as part of a consideration of the threshold above which brain damage results in adverse psychological sequelae (1). However, for the moment, we may observe that these findings suggest a rather high threshold.

Psychiatric Disorder

Comparable questions arise with regard to psychiatric disorder. What is the evidence that brain damage causes an increased risk of emotional and behavioral problems? Several epidemological studies have clearly demonstrated the rather high risk of disorder among children with neuroepileptic conditions. We first examined the matter using data from the Isle of Wight studies of school-age children (5). As assessed on both a teachers' questionnaire and a clinical psychiatric interview, children of normal intelligence with an organic brain condition were twice as likely as children with other physical handicaps (such as asthma, diabetes, or heart disease) to show behavioral deviance or disorder. The difference between the groups suggested that it was specifically brain injury which increased the psychiatric risk. However, this remained an uncertain inference in that the other physical handicaps were less likely to be accompanied by visible crippling. Circumstantial evidence suggested that it was the brain damage rather than the crippling which was crucial, but a doubt necessarily remained.

This doubt was resolved by means of a study we carried out in North London with Eric Seidel (13). Thirty-three normally intelligent school-age children with brain disorders (mostly cerebral palsy) were compared with 42 children with handicapping conditions due to lesions below the brain stem (e.g., polio and muscular dystrophy). In spite of the fact that the groups were comparable in terms of visible crippling, psychiatric disorder was found to be twice as frequent in the group whose handicap was attributable to brain damage. The inference of a causal relationship was strong in that the two groups were matched in other respects. But inferences on cause from cross-sectional associations (however good the statistical controls) are inevitably based on circumstantial evidence with all the uncertainties that this implies (14). Longitudinal data showing *changes* in behavior following brain injury would provide a more convincing and powerful demonstration of a causal effect.

To undertake that analysis we need to return to the prospective study of children with head injuries (7–9) described above. There were three groups of children: those with severe head injuries, those with mild head injuries, and control subjects with orthopedic injuries only. The parents of all three groups of children were interviewed as soon as possible after the injury to obtain an assessment of the child's behavior *before* the accident. Because the interviews were undertaken before it could be known how the child would be affected, the data on pre-injury behavior were likely to be as accurate and unbiased as data of this kind can ever be. Similar information was obtained from school teachers by means of a standardized questionnaire. All three groups were followed up for 2¼ years with further standardized assessments at 4 months, 1 year, and 2¼ years after the accident. It will readily be appreciated that the question of whether brain damage *causes* psychiatric disorder can be tested by determining whether the groups differed in terms of *changes* in behavior following the injury.

The results showed that the rates of disorder were closely similar in the children with severe head injuries and their matched controls *before* the accident but that, by 4 months after the injury, the rate of disorder in the group with severe head injuries had greatly increased to a level well above that in the children who suffered orthopedic injuries. Moreover, the rate of disorder in the group with severe head injuries remained high and well above that in the control group throughout the whole of the 2¼-year follow-up.

The findings for the group of children with mild head injuries were quite different in two crucial respects. First, these children showed an unusually high rate of behavioral disturbance *before* the accident—the rate was well above that in the control group. The implication is that the children with mild head injuries (unlike those with severe injuries) were behaviorally different (and more disturbed) *before* they sustained their head injury. Previous studies have produced closely comparable findings (15). Impulsive, overactive children are more likely to engage in dangerous play activities, which result in head injuries (16, 17). In a sense, it was their behavior that caused the head injury rather than the other way round.

Second, the rate of psychiatric disorder in the group with mild head injuries showed *no* tendency to increase after the injury. The inference is that the psychiatric problems in that group were not caused by the head injury. It appears that whereas severe head injuries increase the risk of psychiatric disorder, mild head injuries do not.

This conclusion may be examined more closely by confining attention to those disorders which arose only *after* the injury, in children who were *without* disorder before the accident. A certain number of problems may be expected to arise simply as a consequence of the passage of time and the stresses this may involve. In particular, some problems may develop as a result of the stresses of the accident and of the hospital admission that followed. However, these could occur in the control subjects to roughly the same extent as in the children with head injuries, because all but a few had had a hospital admission as a result of their accident. The *difference* between the children with head injuries and their controls in rates of *new* psychiatric disorder should represent the disorders *specifically* due to brain injury. The findings are conclusive in indicating the substantial psychiatric risk that follows severe head injury but *not*, it should be noted, mild head injury. The rate of disorders arising de novo after the accident, in children without psychiatric disorder before the injury, was about 10%–20% in both the control subjects and the children with mild head injuries but was three times as high in the group with severe head injuries. An additional methodological check was achieved by using independent psychiatric assessments made on the basis of interview protocols, from which all identifying data had been deleted, made by a rater who was blind to whether the child was a study subject or a control subject. This confirmed the much-increased rate of "new" disorder in the group with severe head injuries (9).

A further way of testing whether this represents a *causal* effect of brain injury is to determine the extent to which the head-injury–psychiatric-disorder association follows a consistent "dose-response" relationship. In other words, if it could be shown that the more severe the brain injury the greater the likelihood of psychiatric disorder, this would considerably strengthen the causal inference. This possibility was tested in three separate ways by using different indices of brain injury—the duration of posttraumatic amnesia, neurological abnormalities found on a systematic clinical examination by a research neurologist at the 2¼-year follow-up, and the presence of intellectual impairment. The analyses showed a statistically significant association between the rate of psychiatric disorder and the duration of posttraumatic amnesia, but weaker and less consistent associations with both of the other indices of brain injury (9). In short, there was some kind of dose-response relationship, but the relationship was of only moderate strength and consistency. These analyses give rise to two conclusions: 1) they confirm that there is indeed a truly *causal* effect by which severe head injury greatly increases the risk of psychiatric disorder, but, also, 2) they suggest that the effect is often *indirect* rather than direct. In this connection, of course, the psychological meaning to the family and to the child of having suffered a head injury (rather than trauma to the limbs) is likely to have played an important role in addition to the effects of brain damage per se. Incidentally, this suggests a difference between psychiatric disorder and intellectual impairment with respect to the etiological role of brain injury. The dose-response relationship with cognitive deficits is strong and consistent, indicating a *direct* causal effect.

■215

MECHANISMS INVOLVED IN THE GENESIS OF PSYCHIATRIC DISORDER

Severity of Brain Damage

With respect to possible neurological features, I have already noted that in the prospective head injury study (7–9) there was only a somewhat inconsistent association with the severity of the injury. Other investigations confirm this finding. For example, in the Isle of Wight epidemological study (5), psychiatric disorder was significantly more common when there was evidence of a bilateral brain disorder than when the condition was strictly one-sided. On the other hand, in Shaffer and colleagues' study of children with localized head injuries (18), no association was found between duration of coma and rate of psychiatric disorder. This negative finding may be in part a consequence of the fact that few of the children had prolonged unconsciousness. On the other hand, in this same group, duration of unconsciousness and treatment for cerebral edema *were* significantly related to cognitive performance (12), so that again it appears that the overall severity of brain injury has a stronger relationship with cognition than with behavior. Other studies, too, have found that duration of coma is associated with the severity of later educational difficulties (11).

Locus of Injury

The possible relevance of the locus of the brain injury was the major objective of Shaffer and associates' study (18) of children with a localized cortical lesion that resulted from a unilateral, compound, depressed fracture of the skull with an associated dural tear; gross damage to the underlying brain substance

American Journal of Psychiatry, 1981, vol. 138, pp. 1533–1544

had been confirmed at the time of the child's operation. Ninety-eight school-age children who had been injured at least 2 years previously were studied. No association was found between the locus of injury and the presence of either psychiatric disorder (18) or intellectual impairment (12). Four caveats are necessary, however, before it can be assumed that the site of brain injury is of no importance. First, because it was a follow-up rather than a prospective study we could not determine which disorders had arisen only after the injury. Without this information it was impossible to provide any identification of psychiatric problems specifically due to brain injury. Accordingly, it may be that nonspecific effects obscured associations with locus. Second, the lesions mainly involved cortical damage, and it could be that subcortical lesions might give rise to more differentiated behavioral sequelae. This possibility is certainly suggested by the finding from other studies that deep intrinsic damage due to vascular lesions and to tumors are more likely than external trauma to give rise to persisting aphasia in both children and adults (19–22). Third, real locus effects may have been obscured by contrecoup injuries or other distant effects (23), although the choice of subjects with a penetrating injury but without second complications makes this unlikely (24). Fourth, whereas the overall risk of disorder may not show much relationship with site of brain damage, the *type* of psychiatric or cognitive disorder may be more strongly associated with locus.

This last possibility has so far received rather little attention, but recently Shaffer and associates (unpublished 1981 data) examined it in connection with the effects of localized head injuries. Most psychiatric symptoms showed no association with locus, but there was a significant tendency for depression to be most common when the lesions were in the right frontal or left parieto-occipital areas. The finding is, perhaps, broadly in keeping with the observation that, in adults, affective disorders are most frequent after right hemisphere lesions, particularly if they involve the frontal lobe (25–27), but the apparent "axis" between the right frontal and left parieto-occipital lobes (25) requires further empirical validation before much weight can be attached to it.

Previous studies using EEG foci to identify the site of lesion have not produced very consistent findings in children (5, 28, 29). Psychiatric problems, and perhaps especially those involving aggressivity, seem to be most frequent among epileptic children with psychomotor seizures. This finding has been used to infer that temporal lobe pathology may be particularly associated with aggression. That could turn out to be so, but it should be appreciated that there is only a rather modest association between type of fit and site of EEG focus. Moreover, the site of focus need not be identical with the locus of brain lesion. Thus far the findings on possible connections between site of brain damage and

the nature of the behavioral sequelae in children can only be regarded an inconclusive.

Rather more attention has been paid to the possible effects of site of lesion on cognition. Several studies have shown a tendency for lesions in the right hemisphere to be particularly associated with impairment on visuospatial tasks and (to a lesser extent) lesions in the left hemisphere to be accompanied by verbal deficits (6, 30–34) and by reading difficulties (35). However, the effects were quite minor in our own study of children with cortical injuries (12), and the general impression is that the effects of site and laterality of lesion are possibly less consistent and less marked in children than in adults.

This apparent age difference may, at least in part, be an artifact resulting from three different factors. First, the lack of locus effect in the head injury study may have been because deeper lesions were necessary (19–22). There is some evidence in both children and adults that recovery from aphasia tends to be better in the case of lesions due to external trauma than with those due to intracerebral pathology (as with vascular lesions or tumors). Moreover, the effect of site of lesion on the pattern of cognitive deficit in adults is also more marked with deep lesions (36). Second, in adults there is some suggestion that the specific effects of locus may be rather greater soon after the brain injury than they are some years later (37), although they can persist for several decades (33, 34). To *some* extent the apparent age difference in the importance of the site of injury may be a consequence of the fact that the sequelae in children have usually been studied many years after the damage (this is necessarily so, of course, in the case of infantile cerebral palsy), whereas in adults most studies have looked at short-term sequelae (38–40). However, this does not seem to account for all the findings, and we may tentatively conclude that the effects of laterality are probably less marked in children than in adults. Finally, the type of pathology may be important, either on its own or in connection with locus.

Type of Pathology

Although the differences in individual studies have not always reached statistical significance, there has been a general tendency for psychiatric disorder to be more frequent when brain lesions have been accompanied by active physiological disturbance (as indicated by the occurrence of epileptic fits or by abnormal EEG discharges) than when it has been simply a matter of a loss of function. For example, in the Isle of Wight study (5) the highest rate of psychiatric disorder was found in children with structural disorders of the brain accompanied by fits. It is also relevant that the rate of disorder in children with uncomplicated epilepsy was several times that in the general population in spite of the fact that the children were of normal intelligence and showed no abnormalities on neurological examination. Similarly, in Shaffer and associates' localized head injury study (18) disorder was most frequent among children with seizures starting late after the head injury. In adults, too, psychiatric disability is more likely to follow head injury when epileptic fits occur (28). In addition, studies of temporal lobectomy in adults show a close relationship between a reduction in the number of fits and a decrease in aggressive behavior (41, 42). In childhood, a similar phenomenon may be evident in the improvements in behavior and cognition that sometimes follow the operation of hemispherectomy (43–45). Further studies are needed to elucidate the matter, but the rather slender evidence available so far points to the probability that the behavioral consequences of *abnormal* brain function may often be greater than those of *loss* of brain function. To some extent, this may also apply to cognitive functioning. Several studies have noted that the intelligence of hemiplegic children tends to be lower when the lesion is also associated with persistent epileptic seizures (6).

The importance of the type of pathology is also shown by the pattern of associations with the syndrome of infantile autism within populations of mentally retarded children (46). Although there is a pronounced general tendency for autism to be much more frequent in children of low IQ than in those of normal intelligence, the nature of the underlying brain disease appears crucial. Thus infantile autism occurs relatively often in association with infantile spasms and hypsarhythmia, with tuberose sclerosis, with congenital rubella, and with phenylketonuria. On the other hand, it is quite rare in children with either Down's syndrome or cerebral palsy. It is not at all obvious just what is the crucial pathological feature that differentiates those medical conditions associated with autism from those *not* so associated, in spite of comparable degrees of mental retardation. But there *is* a difference and it must have some meaning, even if we do not yet know what it is.

There is also a variety of prevailing stereotypes in the nonautistic behaviors supposed to be characteristic of particular mental retardation syndromes. Children with Down's syndrome are thought to be friendly and nonaggressive, and hydrocephalic children to be verbose and superficial. On the whole, the empirical findings suggest that there is only a little substance to these stereotypes (47). However, there are a few exceptions to this generally negative picture, of which the most striking concerns the Lesch-Nyhan syndrome (48). This is a rare disease with the very striking characteristic of a severe and distinctive pattern of self-injurious behavior involving highly traumatic biting of the child's own lips and fingers. The mechanisms remain ill-understood, but it appears that the syndrome represents a rather specific association between a medical condition and a particular form of behavior. Whether this is due to the type of brain

lesion or, rather, to abnormal circulating metabolites is not known. It should also be added that, at least to some extent, the behavior is under environmental control (49), even though it is not basically environmentally determined.

These various findings on the associations between type of pathology and type of behavioral disturbance are not such as to give rise to any clearly formulated set of conclusions. However, some tentative suggestions may be made on hypotheses that need to be tested. First, the locus of the lesion seems least important with unilateral cortical injuries. Second, specific behavioral effects appear most striking with bilateral disorders involving both active physiological disturbance and subcortical as well as cortical damage. Third, insofar as there are locus of injury specificities they probably apply to brain systems rather than to some particular cortical gyrus.

■217

Age at Injury

A further issue that requires attention in terms of possible mechanisms involved in the genesis of psychiatric disorder is the child's age at the time of the brain injury. The matter was investigated in Chadwick, Shaffer, and associates' follow-up study of children with localized head injuries (12, 18) and also in our more recent prospective study of head injuries (7–9). In the former study, age at injury bore no relationship at all to the risk of psychiatric disorder and no consistent relationship with cognitive sequelae. In the latter study, too, there were no significant age effects, although there was a very slight suggestion that recovery may be marginally more rapid in the younger age groups.

Other investigations, however, have suggested the existence of important age differences in children's responses to brain injury. A review of the empirical findings does not allow any entirely satisfactory resolution of the conflicting claims and contradictory results (38, 40, 50). However, it seems reasonable to suppose that several entirely different processes are at work. On the one hand, various investigations have shown that very young infants tend to have more serious intellectual impairment following meningoencephalitis or therapeutic irradiation of the brain (5, 51). This finding does not contradict our own results on head injury because the worst prognosis mainly applies to the first 2 years of life and our samples included scarcely any children as young as that. The reason for this apparently greater vulnerability in early infancy is probably to be found at least in part in the general observations that immature organs are usually more susceptible to injury than mature ones and that organs tend to be most susceptible at the time of their most rapid growth—which in the case of the brain consists of the prenatal period and the first 2 years or so after birth.

On the other hand, there is also evidence that the

American Journal of Psychiatry, 1981, vol. 138, pp. 1533–1544

218▪

immature brain shows greater "plasticity" of functioning and, in particular, that there is greater potential for interhemispheric transfer of functions. This is most obvious in the studies showing that damage to the left hemisphere in infancy is much less likely to lead to permanent language impairment than similar lesions occurring in later childhood or adult life (5). More recent research findings suggest that the early claims for equipotentiality of the two hemispheres in infancy were overstated (52). Even in infancy there is substantial hemispheric specialization. Moreover, it is also evident that there are greater powers of recuperation after brain damage in adult life than is usually supposed (30, 40, 53). Nevertheless, it does seem that there is somewhat greater versatility of functioning in infancy and, in particular, that it is more readily possible for the right hemisphere to take over language functions. It should be noted, however, that the evidence mainly applies to interhemispheric effects and not to transfer of functions within one hemisphere. Accordingly, although the relevant empirical findings are lacking, it is likely that infants are just as vulnerable as older children to *bilateral* brain damage. Their relative invulnerability is likely to apply only to *unilateral* lesions.

It should be noted that the terms "plasticity" and "taking over" of functions imply a greater knowledge of the mechanisms involved than actually exists. In the first place, the extent of sparing of function varies with the site of the lesion and with the specific function being examined (54). Thus animal studies suggest that sparing often tends to be greater following cortical lesions than after subcortical damage (50). Similarly, in Byers and McLean's study (55), which showed that aphasias usually cleared up completely in children, not only did the hemiplegias remain permanently but also school performance was frequently markedly impaired. Second, "recovery" does not necessarily mean restoration of normal functions—subtle deficits often remain (56). Third, functional recovery may be a result of a variety of quite different processes, including 1) vicarious functioning of undamaged neural tissues (i.e., a part or a side of the brain deals with a function for which it would not ordinarily have responsibility), 2) behavioral substitution (i.e., undamaged systems become more efficient but do not alter their role), 3) functional reorganization (either through collateral sprouting or biochemical changes), 4) recovery of functioning impaired (but not destroyed) by vascular constriction, edema, or similar processes, 5) the beneficial effects of neuronal degeneration (as by the death of a neuron with an inhibitory function; an example of improved performance as a result of a second lesion is provided by the benefits in parkinsonism following a surgical lesion in the ventral lateral nucleus of the thalamus), and 6) the use of alternative strategies or "tricks" to circumvent handicaps (38, 50, 57). Fourth, it must be remembered that neuronal or

glial regrowth may lead to an interference with normal function as well as to improvements. The late onset of epilepsy can perhaps be considered as a case in point.

A third rather different consideration is that insofar as brain damage impairs *new* learning, it is likely to have greater practical effects in young children just because they have more new learning to do and less accumulated knowledge and established skills to rely on (58). This consideration means that any adequate testing of possible differences according to age at injury must differentiate between new learning and performance that relies in part on existing skills. Of course, this differentiation is a difficult one to make, but the point is that cognitive tasks may have a different meaning at different ages.

Fourth, insofar as age differences apply, they mainly concern differences between childhood, adulthood, and old age rather than differences *within* the childhood years.

It is obvious from this brief discussion of possible processes involved in the effects of age at injury that it would be premature to conclude that there are no such effects. In practice, there are often no sizable age differences in the psychological sequelae of brain injury, but this may be just because age affects different processes in contrasting ways.

Temperamental and Behavioral Features

In considering mechanisms involved in the genesis of psychiatric disorder, I have focused on various neurological features. However, I have already noted that the connections between brain damage and psychiatric disorder are often indirect. Accordingly, it is necessary to consider the possible importance of non-neurological variables in the development of emotional and behavioral disturbances in children suffering brain injury. Just three variables—behavioral characteristics, psychosocial adversity, and cognition—will be considered.

In our prospective study of children experiencing a severe head injury, my colleagues and I focused on disorders that began only after the accident, in order to maximize the chance that the disorders were directly caused by the injury (9). This meant that we excluded children who already showed psychiatric disturbance before their injury. However, even within the group without preexisting disorder it was possible to make a distinction between those without any behavioral abnormality and those with mild difficulties not sufficient to amount to a psychiatric diagnosis. The findings were striking in showing a strong relationship between the children's pre-injury behavior and their psychiatric state at the 1-year follow-up. Of the children with no behavioral difficulties before the accident, half were psychiatrically normal 1 year later, whereas this was so for *none* of those who showed mild behavior problems before the head injury. Pre-injury behavior was a strong predictor of children's psychiatric problems after severe head injury.

Psychosocial Adversity

Psychosocial adversity has also proved to be an important predictor of psychiatric outcome in all our studies of children with brain damage. In the original Isle of Wight studies of children with neuroepileptic conditions (5), psychiatric disorder was found to be more frequent in children from a "broken home" and in those whose mothers had had an emotional disturbance. Similarly, in Shaffer and associates' follow-up study of children with a localized head injury (18), psychiatric problems were much more frequent among children with a high score on an overall psychosocial adversity index, which combined items such as marital discord, parental mental disorder, and social disadvantage. In this connection, it should be noted that Backett and Johnston (59) found that children experiencing psychosocial adversity were also more likely to have road accidents and hence to suffer head injuries.

In our prospective study (7–9) we used a psychosocial adversity index similar to that used by Shaffer and associates (18). Before the accident, psychosocial adversity was associated with psychiatric disorder in both the study subjects and the control subjects in a closely comparable fashion. The rate of disorder in children with adversity was 20%–25%, whereas in those without adversity it was less than 7%. After the injury, persisting psychiatric disorders that had arisen de novo after the accident showed a similar association with psychosocial adversity. In the group of children with severe head injuries, the rate of psychiatric disorder was much increased even in the absence of psychosocial adversity, but it reached a peak in the children with both brain injury and psychosocial adversity. We may conclude that even in the presence of brain damage, psychosocial factors continue to play an important role in the genesis of psychiatric disorder.

Cognitive Factors

In the Isle of Wight studies of neuroepileptic conditions (5) and in the North London study of children with brain disorders associated with visible crippling (13), low IQ and reading difficulties were both associated with a higher risk of psychiatric disorder. In our prospective study of children with head injuries (8, 9), the associations between cognitive level and psychiatric disorder were much less marked and reached statistical significance only at the 4-month follow-up. Nevertheless, the pattern was similar in showing some association between psychiatric disorder and cognitive impairment. The mechanisms underlying this association are both complex and multiple and also ill-understood. The various alternative explanations have been considered more fully elsewhere (60, 61). But it is evident that intellectually less able children seem to be generally more vulnerable to psychiatric disturbance

and that one of the ways in which brain damage may increase psychiatric risk is through its role in predisposing to cognitive problems. The strength of this effect seems to vary across samples, but it constitutes one other mechanism to be taken into account.

As in an earlier review of the same topic (62), I must conclude that many mechanisms are operative in the associations between brain injury and psychiatric disorder. There is no doubt that brain damage substantially increases psychiatric risk. However, not only does it do so through a variety of different processes, but also psychosocial and temperamental influences must be considered alongside neurological mechanisms.

TYPES OF PSYCHIATRIC DISORDER ASSOCIATED WITH BRAIN DAMAGE

▪ 219

The question of the types of psychiatric disorder associated with brain trauma was examined in all our various studies of children with brain damage—with generally similar findings. In all the investigations, most children with psychiatric disorder showed the usual admixture of emotional and conduct disorders found in children without brain damage and clearly there was no stereotyped psychiatric syndrome (5, 62).

Of course, in spite of a broad similarity in diagnostic categories, it could still be that there were differences between children with and children without brain damage with respect to individual symptoms. This possibility was studied in the Isle of Wight survey (5) with consistently negative findings. Children with brain damage showed an excess of most types of symptoms, but when like was compared with like there was nothing characteristic about the symptoms.

It is important to recognize that our symptom assessments consisted of relatively gross ratings. There was a need for a comparable investigation using finer, more objective measures. This was provided in an independent study by Shaffer and associates (63) in which comparisons were made in a clinic sample according to the presence or absence of both conduct disorder and neurological abnormality. Actometers were used to measure limb movement in a free-play situation, a stabilimeter was used to assess the amount of wriggling when the child was seated during testing, and various special tests were carried out to assess impulsivity and attention.

The results showed that the behaviors supposed to be characteristic of brain damage were significantly more common in children with conduct disorders but showed no significant association with neurological abnormality. It seems that most of the features, such as impulsivity or hyperactivity, which are reputed to be indicators of brain damage, are in fact merely indicators of psychiatric disorder, regardless of the presence or absence of brain damage. The findings from other studies are generally similar. However, in a

American Journal of Psychiatry, 1981, vol. 138, pp. 1533–1544

study of a psychiatric clinic sample, Chess (64) found that perseveration was significantly more common in children with brain damage than in those without neurological impairment (unfortunately, it was not stated whether the groups were intellectually comparable).

Before concluding that there is no specificity to the behaviors associated with brain damage, however, we must recognize that all these studies suffered from a rather important limitation. Because none of them included a psychiatric assessment of the pre-injury state it was not possible to separate off the disorders specifically *caused* by the brain damage. Children with brain damage may develop psychiatric problems for reasons unconnected with the brain damage as well as for reasons directly associated with organic brain pathology. However, it was possible largely to overcome this limitation in our prospective study (8, 9) by picking out disorders that met three operational criteria: 1) the disorders occurred in children who experienced a head injury of sufficient severity that some form of brain dysfunction or damage could be regarded as likely (namely, injuries resulting in posttraumatic amnesia lasting at least 7 days), 2) the disorders arose *after* the head injury, and 3) they occurred in children who did *not* exhibit psychiatric disorder before the injury. These conditions could then be compared with psychiatric disorders known *not* to be due to brain injury because they occurred in control children with orthopedic injuries or because they had been present before the accident in children with head injuries.

These two groups were systematically compared according to psychiatric diagnoses (made by an independent rater who was blind to the child's group), detailed parental interview ratings of individual behavior, observations of the children's behavior during psychological testing, and teacher questionnaire ratings. All these separate comparisons showed that, in general, the emotional and behavioral problems attributable to head injury were closely similar to those known not to be due to head injury. The one exception to this overall pattern of negative findings concerns the marked and highly significant excess of socially inappropriate or socially disinhibited behavior in the group with disorders attributable to head injury. Indeed, there were five cases of disorder in which this constituted the predominant clinical feature—*all* were in the group of conditions attributable to head injury. These children were markedly outspoken and showed a general lack of regard for social convention. Frequently they made very personal remarks or asked embarrassing questions, and sometimes they undressed in social situations in which this would ordinarily be regarded as unacceptable behavior. Some of these disinhibited patterns of disorder also included forgetfulness, overtalkativeness, carelessness in personal hygiene and dress, and impulsiveness. It is obvious that these conditions resemble the so-called frontal

lobe syndrome seen in adults with brain damage. The adjective "so-called" is necessary because even in studies of adults with localized injuries there is far from a one-to-one association between these disinhibited behaviors and frontal lobe lesions (29).

These behaviors, however, were the only ones specifically attributable to brain injury. It was especially noteworthy, in view of hypotheses about hyperactivity and minimal brain dysfunction, that overactivity was *not* particularly linked with brain injury. Clearly, the presence of overactivity cannot be used as an indicator of brain damage. On the other hand, by the time of the 2¼-year follow-up there were two cases in which the disinhibited state, described above, changed its form and was then diagnosed as hyperkinetic syndrome. These constituted only a minority of cases with this diagnosis, but the possibility remains that there may be a small subvariety of the hyperkinetic syndrome which is attributable to brain damage—a possibility considered further in my companion paper (1). For the moment, let it suffice to conclude that, with the exception of social disinhibition (and possibly perseveration), no behavioral specificity attributable to brain damage has been identified.

TYPES OF PSYCHOLOGICAL DEFICIT ASSOCIATED WITH BRAIN DAMAGE

A parallel question with regard to cognitive sequelae must also be raised: to what extent are there varieties of psychological deficit specifically associated with brain damage? The topic has given rise to a large literature, and there have been many attempts to develop batteries of psychological tests with which to determine the presence of brain damage (65, 66). So far these attempts have been generally unsuccessful. Group differences between children with and without brain damage are frequently found, but there has been a lack of specificity as to the deficits associated with brain damage. There are many conceptual and practical difficulties involved in identifying cognitive features specific to brain injury. The most basic is that it requires the extremely dubious assumption that damage to one part of the brain will have consequences similar to those associated with damage to a quite different part. However, a further problem has stemmed from the difficulties of knowing when brain damage has occurred. When a child is paralyzed down one side the use of psychological tests to identify brain damage is redundant and unnecessary. The tests would be most useful when the clinical neurological examination is normal, but then there is the problem of a lack of any independent validation of brain damage.

One way around the latter difficulty is to study children who have a history of brain injury, which provides such validation even when the clinical neurological examination is normal. Just such a strategy was used in our prospective study of children with head injuries (8, 67). We followed two tactics. First, the course of cognitive recovery was used to identify children who had suffered intellectual impairment as a result of brain injury. That is, when scores increased markedly during the follow-up period ("markedly" was defined as an increase of a magnitude found in less than 5% of the group), it could be inferred that there must have been an initial deficit. By focusing on the psychological functions that showed this recovery phase it was possible to identify those features most susceptible to brain damage. The results showed that, on the whole, tests of visuospatial function were more affected by brain injury than tests of verbal skills. It was also found that tests involving *speed* of hand-eye coordination were most likely to be impaired following severe head injury. However, that was just about as far as one could take it with respect to specificity. A large battery of standardized and unstandardized tests was used to try to identify specific deficits. These included measures of paired associate learning, attentiveness and reaction time, impulsivity, distractibility, verbal fluency, immediate and delayed recall, manual dexterity, concentration over prolonged periods, and speed of information processing. Most of these showed deficits following head injury, but the pattern was not much different from that evident with the WISC performance subtests and there was no indication of any specific type of brain injury deficit.

The second research tactic focused on the possibility of subtle cognitive deficits in children *without* a persistent global intellectual impairment. The crucial feature in this analysis was to choose a group that had the dual characteristics of known brain injury but normal intelligence—the group for which tests of specific deficits are most needed. Such a group was obtained by taking children who met the triple criteria of 1) having suffered a severe head injury with a posttraumatic amnesia lasting at least 7 days, 2) having experienced cognitive recovery as shown by a gain of 24 performance IQ points over the first year after the injury, and 3) having an IQ score at the final 2¼-year follow-up within one standard deviation of the control group's mean. Only eight children met these rather stringent criteria; they were compared in detail with individually matched control subjects.

The results showed that by the time of the 1-year follow-up (when they no longer had any global intellectual deficit), the two groups had fairly similar psychological test findings. However, there was a slight tendency, sometimes accompanied by statistically significant differences, for the children with head injuries to show impairment in their speed of visuomotor and visuospatial functioning. Other studies, too, have found that Wechsler IQ tests are among the most sensitive indicators of brain damage and that highly specific cognitive deficits are unusual after widespread brain damage (68–71). We may conclude that it is possible for there to be subtle deficits on specific cognitive tests even when there is generally normal intelligence, but that such deficits tend to be neither common nor severe and, futhermore, that they do not seem to constitute any easily identifiable pattern.

CONCLUSIONS

The presence of brain damage or injury is associated with a markedly increased risk of both intellectual impairment and psychiatric disorder. Moreover, the evidence indicates that this association represents a *causal* influence of brain injury. Intellectual impairment is fairly directly associated with the overall severity of brain damage, especially with bilateral damage. However, many mechanisms, some direct and some indirect, are involved in the development of psychiatric disorder following brain injury. It, too, is somewhat more likely to occur after severe damage, but the "dose-response" relationship is neither as strong nor as consistent as that with intellectual impairment. The behavioral sequelae do not seem to be strongly influenced by the locus of injury, but that negative finding may be a consequence in part of a failure to take into account the nature of the underlying brain pathology.

Psychiatric disorder seems most likely to occur when there is abnormal neurophysiological activity; the type of activity may also be important, as indicated by the probably greater psychiatric risk associated with psychomotor seizures. The possible importance of the nature of the basic medical condition is suggested by the consistent association between infantile autism and some mental retardation syndromes and not others, and by the characteristic form of self-mutilation associated with Lesch-Nyhan's syndrome. The overall psychiatric and intellectual risks do not appear to be greatly affected by the child's age at the time of brain injury, but this negative finding may be the result of age having several different effects, which tend to counterbalance one another. Quite apart from these neurological considerations, the psychiatric consequences of brain injury are also very substantially influenced by the child's pre-injury behavior and by his psychosocial circumstances; cognitive factors, too, may play a part. Finally, in spite of claims to the contrary, there appear to be rather few specific cognitive or behavioral sequelae of brain injury. The association between brain damage and social disinhibition provides one of the few exceptions.

■ 221

REFERENCES

1. Rutter M: Syndromes attributed to "minimal brain dysfunction" in children. Am J Psychiatry (in press)
2. Crome L: The brain and mental retardation. Br Med J 1:897–904, 1960
3. Corbett J, Harris R, Taylor E, et al: Progressive disintegrative

American Journal of Psychiatry, 1981, vol. 138, pp. 1533–1544

psychosis in childhood. J Child Psychol Psychiatry 18:211–219, 1977

4. Still GF: Some abnormal psychical conditions in children. Lancet 1:1008–1012, 1077–1082, 1163–1168, 1902

5. Rutter M, Graham P, Yule W: A Neuropsychiatric Study in Childhood: Clinics in Developmental Medicine 35/36. London, William Heinemann Medical Books/SIMP, 1970

6. Annett M: Laterality of childhood hemiplegia and the growth of speech and intelligence. Cortex 9:4–33, 1973

7. Rutter M, Chadwick O, Shaffer D, et al: A prospective study of children with head injuries, I: design and methods. Psychol Med 10:633–645, 1980

8. Chadwick O, Rutter M, Brown G, et al: A prospective study of children with head injuries, II: cognitive sequelae. Psychol Med 11:49–61, 1981

9. Brown G, Chadwick O, Shaffer D, et al: A prospective study of children with head injuries in adulthood, III: psychiatric sequelae. Psychol Med 11:63–78, 1981

10. Brink JD, Garrett AL, Hale WR, et al: Recovery of motor and intellectual function in children sustaining severe head injuries. Dev Med Child Neurol 12:545–571, 1970

11. Heiskanen O, Kaste M: Late prognosis of severe brain injury in children. Dev Med Child Neurol 16:11–14, 1974

12. Chadwick O, Rutter M, Thompson J, et al: Intellectual performance and reading ability after localized head injury in childhood. J Child Psychol Psychiatry 22:117–139, 1981

13. Seidel UP, Chadwick OF, Rutter M: Psychological disorders in crippled children: a comparative study of children with and without brain damage. Dev Med Child Neurol 17:563–573, 1975

14. Rutter M: Epidemiological/longitudinal methods and causal research in child psychiatry. J Am Acad Child Psychiatry (in press)

15. Craft AW, Shaw DA, Cartlidge NE: Head injuries in children. Br Med J 4:200–203, 1972

16. Burton L: Vulnerable Children. New York, Schocken Books, 1968

17. Manheimer D, Mellinger GD: Personality characteristics of the child accident repeater. Child Dev 38:491–513, 1967

18. Shaffer D, Chadwick O, Rutter M: Psychiatric outcome of localized head injury in children, in Outcome of Severe Damage to the Central Nervous System: Ciba Foundation Symposium 34. Edited by Porter R, Fitzsimons DW. Amsterdam, Elsevier/Excerpta Medica/North-Holland, 1975

19. Guttmann E: Aphasia in children. Brain 65:205–219, 1942

20. Van Dongen HR, Loonen MCB: Factors related to prognosis of acquired aphasia in children. Cortex 13:131–136, 1977

21. Kertesz A, McCabe P: Recovery patterns and prognosis in aphasia. Brain 100:1–18, 1977

22. Sarno MT: The status of research in recovery from aphasia, in Recovery in Aphasia. Edited by Lebrun Y, Hoops R. Amsterdam, Swets and Zeitlinger, 1976

23. Smith E: Influence of site of impact on cognitive impairment persisting long after severe closed head injury. J Neurol Neurosurg Psychiatry 37:719–726, 1974

24. Löken AC: The pathologic-anatomical basis for late symptoms after brain injuries in adults. Acta Psychiatr Neurol Scand Suppl 137:30–42, 1959

25. Flor-Henry P: On certain aspects of the localization of the cerebral systems regulating and determining emotion. Biol Psychiatry 14:677–698, 1979

26. Lishman WA: Brain damage in relation to psychiatric disability after head injury. Br J Psychiatry 114:373–410, 1968

27. Lishman WA: Organic Psychiatry. London, Blackwell Scientific Publications, 1978

28. Ritvo ER, Ornitz EM, Walter RD, et al: Correlation of psychiatric diagnoses and EEG findings: a double-blind study of 184 hospitalized children. Am J Psychiatry 126:988–996, 1970

29. Stores G, Hart J, Piran N: Inattentiveness in schoolchildren with epilepsy. Epilepsia 19:169–175, 1978

30. Kershner JR, King AJ: Laterality of cognitive functions in achieving hemiplegic children. Percept Motor Skills 39:1283–1289, 1974

31. McFie J: Intellectual impairment in children with localized post-infantile cerebral lesions. J Neurol Neurosurg Psychiatry 24:361–365, 1961

32. McFie J: Brain injury in childhood and language development, in Language, Cognitive Deficits and Retardation. Edited by O'Connor N. Boston, Butterworths, 1975

33. Wedell K: Variations in perceptual ability among types of cerebral palsy. Cerebral Palsy Bulletin 2:149–157, 1960

34. Fedio P, Mirsky AF: Selective intellectual deficits in children with temporal lobe or centrencephalic epilepsy. Neuropsychologia 7:287–300, 1969

35. Stores G, Hart J: Reading skills of children with generalised or focal epilepsy attending ordinary school. Dev Med Child Neurol 18:705–716, 1976

36. Newcombe F: Missile Wounds of the Brain: A Study of Psychological Deficits. New York, Oxford University Press, 1969

37. Fitzhugh KB, Fitzhugh LC, Reitan RM: Wechsler-Bellevue comparisons in groups with "chronic" and "current" lateralized and diffuse brain lesions. J Consult Clin Psychol 26:306–310, 1962

38. Geschwind N: Late changes in the nervous system: an overview, in Plasticity and Recovery of Function in the Central Nervous System. Edited by Stein DG, Rosen JJ, Butters N. New York, Academic Press, 1974

39. Isaacson RL: The myth of recovery from early brain damage, in Aberrant Development in Infancy. Edited by Ellis NE. London, John Wiley & Sons, 1975

40. St James-Roberts J: Neurological plasticity, recovery from brain insult and child development, in Advances in Child Development and Behavior, vol 14. Edited by Reese HW, Lipsitt LP. New York, Academic Press, 1979

41. Falconer MM, Serafetinides EA: A follow-up study of surgery in temporal lobe epilepsy. J Neurol Neurosurg Psychiatry 26:154–165, 1963

42. James IP: Temporal lobectomy for psychomotor epilepsy. J Ment Sci 106:543–558, 1960

43. Griffith H, Davidson M: Long-term changes in intellect and behaviour after hemispherectomy. J Neurol Neurosurg Psychiatry 29:571–576, 1966

44. Kohn B, Dennis M: Patterns of hemispheric specialization after hemidecortication for infantile hemiplegia, in Hemispheric Disconnection and Cerebral Function. Edited by Kinsbourne M, Smith WL. Springfield, Ill, Charles C Thomas, 1974

45. Smith A, Sugar S: Development of above normal language and intelligence 21 years after left hemispherectomy. Neurology 25:813–818, 1975

46. Wing L, Gould J: Severe impairments of social interaction and associated anomalies in children: epidemiology and classification. J Autism Dev Disord 9:11–29, 1979

47. Rutter M: Psychiatry, in Mental Retardation: An Annual Review, III. Edited by Wortis J. New York, Grune & Stratton, 1971

48. Nyhan WL: Behavior in the Lesch-Nyhan syndrome. J Autism Child Schizo 6:235–252, 1976

49. Anderson L, Dancis J, Alpert M: Behavioral contingencies and self-mutilation in Lesch-Nyhan disease. J Consult Clin Psychol 46:529–536, 1978

50. Goldman PS: An alternative to developmental plasticity: heterology of CNS structures in infants and adults, in Plasticity and Recovery of Function in the Central Nervous System. Edited by Stein DG, Rosen JJ, Butters N. New York, Academic Press, 1974

51. Eiser C: Intellectual abilities among survivors of childhood leukemia as a function of CNS irradiation. Arch Dis Child 53:391–395, 1978

52. Witelson SF: Early hemisphere specialization and interhemisphere plasticity: an empirical and theoretical review, in Language Development and Neurological Theory. Edited by Segalowitz SJ, Gruber FA. New York, Academic Press, 1977

53. Luria AR: Traumatic Aphasia: The Syndromes, Psychology and Treatment. The Hague, Mouton, 1970

54. Nonneman AJ, Isaacson RL: Task dependent recovery after early brain damage. Behav Biol 8:143–172, 1973

55. Byers RK, McLean WT: Etiology and course of certain hemi-

222 ■

plegias with aphasia in childhood. Pediatrics 19:376–383, 1962

56. Dennis M, Whitaker HA: Hemispheric equipotentiality and language acquisition, in Language Development and Neurological Theory. Edited by Segalowitz SJ, Gruber FA. New York, Academic Press, 1977

57. Goldberger ME: Recovery of movement after CNS lesions in monkeys, in Plasticity and Recovery of Function in the Central Nervous System. Edited by Stein DG, Rosen JJ, Butters N. New York, Academic Press, 1974

58. Shaffer D, Bijur P, Chadwick OF, et al: Head injury and later reading disability. J Am Acad Child Psychiatry 19:592–610, 1980

59. Backett EM, Johnston AM: Social patterns of road accidents to children: some characteristics of vulnerable families. Br Med J 1:409–413, 1959

60. Rutter M, Madge N: Cycles of Disadvantage. London, William Heinemann Educational Books, 1976

61. Rutter M, Tizard J, Whitmore K (eds): Education, Health and Behaviour. New York, Robert Krieger Publishing, 1980

62. Rutter M: Brain damage syndromes in childhood: concepts and findings. J Child Psychol Psychiatry 18:1–21, 1977

63. Shaffer D, McNamara M, Pincus JH: Controlled observations on patterns of activity, attention and impulsivity in brain damaged and psychiatrically disturbed boys. Psychol Med 4:4–18, 1974

64. Chess S: Neurological dysfunction and childhood behavioral pathology. J Autism Child Schizo 2:299–311, 1972

65. Reitan RM, Boll TJ: Neuropsychological correlates of minimal brain dysfunction. Ann NY Acad Sci 205:65–88, 1973

66. Reitan RM, Heineman CE: Interactions of neurological deficits and emotional disturbance in children with learning disorders: methods for differential diagnosis, in Learning Disorders, vol 3. Edited by Hellmuth J. Seattle, Special Child Publications, 1968

67. Chadwick O, Rutter M, Shaffer D, et al: A prospective study of children with head injuries, IV: specific cognitive deficits. Journal of Clinical Neuropsychology 3:101–120, 1981

68. Reitan RM: Psychological effects of cerebral lesions in children of early school age, in Clinical Neuropsychology: Current Status and Applications. Edited by Reitan RM, Davison LA. New York, John Wiley & Sons, 1974

69. Boll TJ: Behavioral correlates of cerebral damage in children aged 9 through 14. Ibid

70. Klonoff H, Low M: Disordered brain function in young children and early adolescents: neuropsychological and electroencephalographic correlates. Ibid

71. Reed HBC, Reitan RM, Kløve H: Influence of cerebral lesions on psychological test performances of older children. J Consult Psychol 29:247–351, 1965

Journal of Child Psychology and Psychiatry, 1976, vol. 17, pp. 35–56

ADOLESCENT TURMOIL: FACT OR FICTION?*

MICHAEL RUTTER, PHILIP GRAHAM†, O. F. D. CHADWICK and W. YULE

Department of Child Psychiatry, Institute of Psychiatry,
De Crespigny Park, Denmark Hill, London SE5 8AF

INTRODUCTION

224∎

ALTHOUGH the period of adolescence has provided a constant source of fascination to adults, psychiatric and psychological writings on the topic are characterised more by confident assertion than by the presence of well based knowledge. The flavour of some of the most prevalent views on adolescence is best conveyed by a few quotations. Thus, Blos (1970) asserts (p. 11): "The more-or-less orderly course of development during latency is thrown into disarray with the child's entry into adolescence . . . adolescence cannot take its normal course without regression". Anna Freud (1958) writes: "Adolescence is by its nature an interruption of peaceful growth, and . . the upholding of a steady equilibrium during the adolescent process is in itself abnormal . . . adolescence resembles in appearance a variety of other emotional upsets and structural upheavals. The adolescent manifestations come close to symptom formation of the neurotic, psychotic or dissocial order and merge almost imperceptibly into . . . almost all the mental illnesses". Geleerd (1957) states: "Personally I would feel greater concern for the adolescent who causes no trouble and feels no disturbance". Eissler (1958) thinks of adolescence as predominantly "stormy and unpredictable behaviour marked by mood swings between elation and melancholy".

Psychiatrists and psychologists generally suppose that adolescence is a period of great psychological upheaval and disturbance. Furthermore, psychiatric disorders, which occur during this age period are often thought to be different from those in either childhood or adult life. Thus, Josselyn (1954) maintains that: "A typical adolescent may present a picture today of hysteria while the history indicates that a month ago his behaviour appeared typically impulsive". Eissler (1958) suggests the same variability and unpredictability when he states: ". . . (adolescent) psychopathology switches from one form to another, sometimes in the course of weeks or months, but also from one day to another. . . . The symptoms manifested by such patients may be neurotic at one time and almost psychotic at another. Then, sudden acts of delinquency may occur, only to be followed by a phase of perverted sexual activity".

These suppositions are reflected in psychiatrists' diagnostic habits, at least in the U.S.A. Among adolescents seen at outpatient clinics "transient situational

*Originally delivered by M. Rutter as the Chairman's Address to the Association for Child Psychology and Psychiatry, 13 February, 1974.

†Department of Psychological Medicine, Hospital for Sick Children, Great Ormond Street, London WC1.

Accepted manuscript received 7 November 1974

disorder" constituted much the commonest diagnostic category (Rosen *et al.*, 1965) and even among psychiatric inpatients the diagnosis was made in nearly a quarter of all adolescents (U.S. Department of Health, Education and Welfare, 1966).

Adolescence is the age-period when there is supposed to be an "identity crisis". As they achieve increasing autonomy and independence from their family of origin, youngsters struggle to achieve a sense of their own distinct personality. It is said that adolescents generally become increasingly estranged from their families and that parents complain that they can no longer "get through" to their children. Erikson (1955) has described identity formation as the main characteristic of adolescence. During this period of development the childhood identifications cease to be useful and a new configuration has to develop. The crisis at this point may lead to "role confusion" or "identity diffusion". He writes, ". . . in spite of the similarity of adolescent 'symptoms' and episodes to neurotic and psychotic symptoms and episodes, adolescence is not an affliction, but a *normative crisis,* i.e. a normal phase of increased conflict characterized by a seeming fluctuation in ego strength . . . what under prejudiced scrutiny may appear to be the onset of a neurosis, often is but an aggravated crisis which might prove to be self-liquidating and, in fact, contributive to the process of identity formation".

Social scientists have sometimes gone further in arguing that adolescents form a separate culture which has little in common with the rest of society. Coleman (1961), one of the most influential writers on this topic, states firmly (p. 3) that the adolescent: ". . . is 'cut off' from the rest of society, forced inward toward his own age group, made to carry out his whole social life with others his own age. With his fellows he comes to constitute a small society, one that has most of its important interactions *within* itself, and maintains only a few threads of connection with the outside adult society".

All these aspects of adolescence are "known" as part of our folklore but how far are they true? Is adolescent turmoil a fact or is it merely a picturesque fiction? In considering these questions let us first consider the source of these views. Adelson (1964) has argued that the mystique of adolescence is summarised by two caricatures: the "visionary–victim", a noble idealist betrayed, exploited or neglected by the adult world; and the "victimizer", leather-jacketed, cruel, sinister and amoral. He points out that the latter is based on the delinquents who hit the news headlines and who are prominent in films and novels, and that the former is based on the sensitive, articulate, intense, intelligent, estranged middle-class adolescent on whom the psychoanalytic theory of adolescence is almost exclusively based. Neither can be held to be representative of the ordinary teenager and generalizations based on clinical practice are very likely to be seriously misleading. Adelson suggests that epidemiological studies of the general population are required if you are to talk about the characteristics of the normal adolescent and that data should be preferred to personal opinions. All the quotations given above refer to clinical anecdote and opinion, with one exception—that of Coleman (1961). His statement about the separate culture of adolescence came from a book reporting interviews with a representative sample of over 7000 adolescents. It has the air of a definitive study but, as Jahoda and Warren (1965) have pointed out, much of his argument consists either of bald statements of assumption or appeals for agreement and the empirical

Journal of Child Psychology and Psychiatry, 1976, vol. 17, pp. 35–56

226 ▪

base is shaky. The Coleman study is much quoted as showing the existence of a separate youth culture, so it is appropriate to consider the evidence provided. For example, in order to assess the relative importance of parents and friends, the youngsters were asked "which . . . would be hardest for you to take—your parents' disapproval . . . or breaking with your friends?" (p. 5). As Epperson (1964) noted, *breaking* with someone and receiving *disapproval* differ in both emotional importance and likelihood of occurrence. In spite of this manifestly loaded question, over half the adolescents still said that parental disapproval counted for more than breaking with a friend. On the next page, Coleman (1961) states, ". . . those who 'set the standard' are more oriented than their followers to the adolescent culture itself. The consequences of this fact are important, for it means that those students who are highly regarded by others are themselves committed to the adolescent group, thus intensifying whatever inward forces the group already has". This supposedly important fact is based on a difference between 53·8 and 50·2%. Moreover, even in the group supposedly committed to youth culture a *majority* actually found parental disapproval harder to take than breaking with a friend. Later in the book (p. 139) much is made of adolescents' resistance to parental pressures but the figures show that some 70% would not join a school club if their parents disapproved. Further on still (p. 286) Coleman comments on the students' alienation from teachers. The table supporting the text shows that only 12·4% of students thought teachers were "not interested in teenagers".

More examples could be given but these are enough to indicate that in this emotionally loaded topic the actual data require careful examination before the conclusions based on those data are accepted. Needless to say, that also applies to the investigations reported in this paper.

Isle of Wight study

Nevertheless, in order to avoid the pitfalls of selective sampling and of personal opinion, the research findings are presented here in some detail and most emphasis is placed on epidemiological studies of the general population rather than on investigations of clinic patients. A variety of published studies are mentioned but most findings refer to the Isle of Wight study of 14–15-yr-olds. The methodology has been fully described previously (Rutter, Tizard and Whitmore, 1970; Graham and Rutter, 1973), but the main research strategy was as follows. Parents and teachers completed behavioural questionnaires for the total population of 2303 adolescents. From this overall group, two subsamples were chosen for individual study, (1) a random sample of the general population ($N = 200$), and (2) all the children with high, that is "deviant", scores on the questionnaires ($N = 304$)*. The children in both these groups were individually interviewed by psychiatrists (who did not know which subsample the child was in), and the parents and teachers of the youngsters were also interviewed using a standardized approach. On the basis of this detailed information an individual psychiatric diagnosis was made for each child who showed any disorder. As well as information relevant to psychiatric status, many systematic data were obtained about the adolescent's leisure activities and about patterns of

---

*This includes children selected because of contact with psychiatric services or the Juvenile Court during the previous year.

family life using methods developed by Rutter and Brown (Brown and Rutter, 1966; Rutter and Brown, 1966). The children also received psychological testing which included the short WISC (Wechsler, 1949), the Neale Analysis of Reading Ability (Neale, 1958), and the Vernon arithmetic–mathematics test (Vernon, 1949).

In addition to this cross-sectional survey, the study included a follow-up of all the children in the same age group who had been found to have psychiatric disorder at age 10 yr during the course of a previous epidemiological enquiry (Rutter, Tizard and Whitmore, 1970).

Alienation

So much for methodology. Let us now turn to the questions and to the findings. In doing this it is important to be clear just what are the hypotheses to be considered. First, we will take the concept of alienation, which suggests that during adolescence youngsters become increasingly estranged from their parents. A corollary of this is that the peer group comes to take precedence over the family as an influence on young people's behaviour. Coleman's (1961) study has already been mentioned in this connection and it has been suggested that, his claims notwithstanding, his data suggest that most adolescents are still considerably influenced by their parents. The relevant items seem to be; (1) that just over half the sample of American high school students felt that parental disapproval would be harder to take than breaking with a friend, (2) that most would follow parental suggestions regarding club membership, (3) that only a few felt that teachers were not interested in them and (4) that being accepted and liked by other students was rated as below average importance compared with pleasing parents, learning as much as possible at school, and living up to their religious ideals. In fact, the evidence provides few definitive findings. Also, although the findings suggest that parental influence is still high in adolescence, they say nothing about the quality of relationships or the closeness of ties.

Epperson's findings (1964), based on a much smaller survey of high school students, take the issue a little further in that he directly compared parental disapproval and friend's disapproval; 80% of adolescents said that parental disapproval would make them more unhappy than the disapproval of friends. Furthermore, secondary school students were if anything more concerned about parental approval than were younger children.

Douvan and Adelson (1966) were concerned with similar issues in their questionnaire survey of over three thousand American adolescents, mainly aged 14–16 yr. Most of the questions tapped attitudes and some of the findings were; (a) that of all other people parents were most often admired, (b) helping at home was the major source of self-esteem, (c) just over half said they had some part in rule-making at home, (d) most would be honest and trusting with their parents and (e) a quarter never had arguments with their parents. On the other hand, many had disagreements about clothing, dating, or being allowed to go out. Also four-fifths reported that they would like their parents to be less restrictive. About half stated that they thought friendship could be as close as family relationships. Douvan and Adelson conclude that, although inter-generation conflict exists, its importance has been much exaggerated. Normal adolescents share with their parents a common core of values

■227

Journal of Child Psychology and Psychiatry, 1976, vol. 17, pp. 35–56

in spite of sharp disagreements about matters of dress, hair length, pop music and how late they can stay out at night.

The findings from other studies are closely similar. For example, Meissner (1965), in another questionnaire survey of high school youngsters, found that about half thought their parents understood them, the great majority were satisfied and happy at home, and three-quarters generally approved of their parents' discipline. Nevertheless, about half thought their parents old-fashioned and although only a minority resisted parental discipline, the proportion was somewhat higher in late adolescence. Offer (1969) in a study of "modal" adolescents (in effect, the most normal third of the population) reported that most got on well with their parents and shared their values.

The Isle of Wight findings, which provide the only English data, are broadly in keeping with the American results.

TABLE 1. PARENT–CHILD ALIENATION AT 14 yr (GENERAL POPULATION SAMPLE)

	Boys ($n = 98$)	Girls ($n = 94$)
Parental account		
Altercation with parents (any)	17·6%	18·6%
Physical withdrawal of child (any)	12·1%	6·9%
Communication difficulties with child (any)	24·2%	9·3% *

* $\chi^2 = 5·93$; 1 $d.f.$; $p < 0·025$.

Table 1 shows some of the relevant findings from the parental interview. Parents were asked if they had any arguments with their adolescent children concerning when and where they went out, or about other activities. Only one in six parents in the randomly selected control group reported any altercations, although twice as many said they disapproved of their youngsters' clothing or hair styles and often prohibitions in these areas were enforced. The great majority of parents approved of their children's friends, and nearly all had discussed with their children what they might do when they left school.

In order to assess the extent to which the adolescents had become alienated or had withdrawn from their families, parents were first asked if their child tended to withdraw by going off to his room, or staying out of the house, or just not doing things with the rest of the family. This was termed "physical withdrawal" and as shown in Table 1 only a tiny minority of adolescents did so. We next asked if the parents had any difficulties "getting through" to their child and how much the youngster discussed with his parents how he was feeling and what were his plans. In the case of boys almost a quarter of the parents reported some emotional withdrawal or difficulty in communication, but in the great majority of cases this difficulty had always been present. In only 4% of cases had difficulties increased during adolescence. Communication difficulties were much less frequent with girls ($\chi^2 = 5·93$; 1 $d.f.$; $p < 0·025$).

Table 2 shows parent–child relationships as assessed from the interview with the adolescent. About two-thirds reported that they never disagreed with their parents about any of their activities and altercations were present in only a minority.

228 ∎

TABLE 2. PARENT–CHILD ALIENATION AT 14 yr (GENERAL POPULATION SAMPLE)

	Boys (n = 98)	Girls (n = 94)
Child's account		
Disagreements with parents (any)	32·3%	26·7%
Altercations with parents (any)	41·7%	30·2%
Criticism of mother (any)	27·1%	36·8%
Criticism of father (any)	31·6%	31·0%
Rejection of mother (any)	3·1%	2·3%
Rejection of father (any)	5·3%	9·2%
No outings with parents	42·7%	27·3%

Even in the minority who did have arguments, these were usually infrequent. All critical remarks concerning parents made at any time during the interview were noted, and only about a third of the adolescents made any criticisms at all. Frank rejection of parents was rarer still. Youngsters were asked about family outings and only a third or so reported that they never went out with their parents.

The findings of all the epidemiological studies are in general agreement. Alienation from parents is *not* common in 14-yr-olds, although it is probably more frequent by the late teens. Most young teenagers continue to be influenced by their parents and get on quite well with them. Most adolescents are *not* particularly critical of their parents and very few reject them. On the other hand, although still occurring in only half the group or less, petty disagreements about clothes, hair and going out are reasonably common. Some of these disagreements may get quite heated and many adolescents would like their parents to be less strict. Even so, most continue to share their parents' values on other things and respect the need for restrictions and control.

As these unexciting conclusions are so much at variance with some psychiatric opinion, we need to ask why there is this discrepancy. Figure 1 provides at least a partial answer.

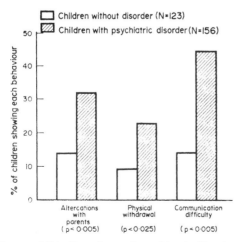

FIG. 1. Parent–child alienation and psychiatric disorder at 14 yr.

Journal of Child Psychology and Psychiatry, 1976, vol. 17, pp. 35–56

230 ■

This compares altercations, physical withdrawal and communication difficulties in the control group children who showed no psychiatric disorder and the total sample of children with some psychiatric condition. These indications of alienation were two or three times as frequent in the psychiatric group. Thus, opinions based on psychiatric patients are confirmed, in so much as alienation was found to be much more frequent in youngsters with psychiatric problems. Even so, alienation was found in less than half. However, here we have to remember that the Isle of Wight youngsters were not patients and other studies have shown that psychiatric clinic referral is related to stresses in the parent and in parent–child interaction as well as to disorder in the child (Shepherd *et al.*, 1971). In short, alienation is more common in adolescents with psychiatric disorder but also if there is alienation, clinic referral may be more likely other things being equal. In this way, clinic patients may be somewhat unrepresentative of youngsters with psychiatric disorder.

The next question concerns the meaning of the alienation, when it exists. Does it cause psychiatric disorder or is it a result of the child's problems? Before attempting to answer that question let us first consider the prevalence of inner turmoil and of psychiatric disorder in adolescence.

Inner turmoil

The assessment of inner turmoil presents many difficulties and questionnaire surveys are of negligible value in this connection. The Coleman (1961) interviews did not cover this area and the Offer (1969) study is non-contributory in that it excluded all adolescents with difficulties. Masterson (1967) reported that anxiety and depression were as common in ordinary adolescents as in his patient sample, which suggests considerable feelings of distress even in children without psychiatric disorder. That is the only relevant published study. So let us turn straight to the Isle of Wight findings from the psychiatric interview with the adolescent. A sample of results is given on Table 3.

The first four items refer to material reported at interview by the adolescent. Each youngster was asked if he sometimes felt miserable and unhappy to the extent that he was tearful or wanted to get away from it all. Nearly half reported some appreciable misery or depression and this was almost as common in boys as in girls. About a fifth said that they felt that what happened to them was less important than what happened to other people, that they didn't matter very much. Only a small minority admitted to any suicidal thoughts but a quarter said that they sometimes got the feeling that people were looking at them or talking about them or laughing at them.

TABLE 3. FINDINGS FROM PSYCHIATRIC INTERVIEW WITH ADOLESCENT
(GENERAL POPULATION SAMPLE)

	Boys (n = 96)	Girls (n = 88)
Reported misery	41·7%	47·7%
Self-depreciation	19·8%	23·0%
Suicidal ideas	7·3%	7·9%
Ideas of reference	28·1%	30·7%
Observed anxiety	19·8%	28·4%
Observed sadness	12·5%	14·8%

At the end of the interview, the psychiatrist had to note whether the youngster appeared anxious and whether he appeared sad or miserable. Interestingly, the proportion who looked sad was far less than the proportion who reported feelings of misery. Only about one in eight adolescents looked sad or miserable at interview.

The interview data refer to ratings made by psychiatrists on the basis of what the adolescents said to them. Accordingly, it is possible that the high proportion of youngsters said to be miserable and depressed might be due to psychiatrists placing undue weight on phenomena of little depth or meaning to the adolescents themselves. Some check on this is provided by the malaise inventory which is completed by the youngsters without any interpretation by psychiatrists. The findings are shown in Table 4.

■231

TABLE 4. INDIVIDUAL ITEMS ON THE MALAISE INVENTORY (GENERAL POPULATION SAMPLE)

	Boys (n = 96)	Girls (n = 87)	Mothers (n = 170)
Often feels miserable or depressed	20·8%	23·0%	14·3%
Usually has great difficulty in falling asleep or staying asleep	20·8%	17·2%	14·2%
Usually wakes unnecessarily early in the morning	22·9%	24·1%	10·0%

More than a fifth of the boys and girls reported that they felt miserable or depressed, and the same proportion reported great difficulties in sleeping, and waking unnecessarily early in the morning. Although these figures are considerably lower than those from the psychiatric interview, it is striking that they are substantially higher than the equivalent figures for mothers. In short, on the adolescents' own account more of them are depressed or miserable than is the case with their mothers (comparable data for fathers are not available).

There can be no doubt from these findings that many 14–15-yr-olds experience quite marked feelings of affective disturbance which could well be described as "inner turmoil". Although only a small minority appeared clinically depressed, many more reported feelings of misery which were often accompanied by self-depreciation and ideas of reference and occasionally even by suicidal thoughts. Of course, that still leaves half the group who did not experience such inner turmoil. But the findings show that inner experiences of misery and depreciation are very common.

The meaning of these feelings in terms of psychiatric disorder is another question, but before turning to that issue let us consider the prevalence of psychiatric disorder in adolescence.

Prevalence of psychiatric disorder

Apart from the Isle of Wight investigations, the only other studies to examine the prevalence of psychiatric disorder in adolescence are those by Krupinski *et al.* (1967), Henderson *et al.* (1971) and by Leslie (1974). Krupinski and his colleagues used medical students to interview all families in an Australian town in order to determine the prevalence of all forms of medical disability. Diagnoses were checked by supervisors and collateral inquiries were made when thought necessary. Some

Journal of Child Psychology and Psychiatry, 1976, vol. 17, pp. 35–56

10 per cent of children, 16 per cent of adolescents and 24 per cent of adults were diagnosed as showing some form of psychiatric disorder. The findings suggested a rate of disorder which increased during adolescence and early adult life, but as, unlike the other surveys, direct psychiatric assessments were not employed comparisons are problematic. Leslie (1974) examined 13–14-yr-old children in Blackburn, basing her diagnosis on interviews with parents and children and on questionnaires from teachers. The prevalence rate found was 21% in boys and 14% in girls. No comparisons with other age groups are possible from her figures. For this purpose, we need to turn to the Isle of Wight findings.

If we are to compare the rate of disorder at 14–15 yr with the rates at other ages, it is necessary to ensure that comparable methods of assessment are used at each age. In this connection we have data on three age-groups on the Isle of Wight— 10-yr-olds, 14–15-yr-olds, and adults (represented by the parents of children in both control groups). The same general strategy was employed in the case of the two groups of children but there were important differences in detail. In the first place, the child interviews were both longer and more thorough at age 14 yr than they had been at 10 yr. In the second place, we had interviews with teachers for the adolescents but only reports from teachers for the 10-yr-olds. Simply on the grounds that our assessments were more searching, we would expect to find more disorder at 14 yr than at 10 yr. With the adults, we had only one source of information— the interview with the mother which had to be used to assess disorder in both parents. In order to equate the methods of assessment as far as possible, only one source of information was used for each age group, in each case the best source available and comparisons were based on the appropriate control groups. The source of information was the parental interview for both groups of youngsters and for adults it was the maternal interview. The results are shown in Table 5.

It is clear that the prevalence of psychiatric disorder is roughly the same at all ages—namely just over 10%. The only group with an appreciably lower rate is that of adult men. In their case the figure may be somewhat of an underestimate because we had to use information from their wives rather than from the men themselves, or it could be truly lower. We have no satisfactory means of testing which is the correct explanation. However, whatever the explanation, the data provide no support for the view that psychiatric disorder is very much commoner during the mid-teens.

TABLE 5. PREVALENCE OF PSYCHIATRIC DISORDER BY AGE
(USING MAIN ACCOUNT)

	Ages		
	10 yr	14 yr	Adult (Parent)
Male	12·7%	13·2%	7·6%
	($n = 55$)	($n = 91$)	($n = 250$)
Female	10·9%	12·5%	11·9%
	($n = 46$)	($n = 88$)	($n = 270$)

In each case n refers to the total sample from the general population who were interviewed in order to determine the proportion with psychiatric disorder.

232 ■

It could be argued that we should have used the interview with the adolescent himself for this purpose. We did not because the evidence suggested that the parental measure was a better indicator of disorder. Nevertheless, we ought to see how this would affect the results. In the control group, 16·3% of adolescents were diagnosed as having psychiatric disorder on this basis. Therefore, on this measure, psychiatric problems were rather commoner in adolescence than they were in adult life. But caution should be used in drawing conclusions from this comparison as the interviews were different. The same applies to the comparison with 10-yr-olds.

Because of these methodological uncertainties, we need to look to other means of comparison. Let us turn to the teachers' questionnaires. We cannot use the teacher interview because it was undertaken only for the adolescents but the questionnaires were closely comparable at the two ages. At age 10–11 yr some 7% of the population obtain deviant scores (Rutter, Tizard and Whitmore, 1970), and at age 14–15 yr just over 6·5% do so. In short, on information from teachers, the rate of emotional and behavioural problems in adolescence is much the same as that at age 10–11 yr.

Another check is provided by scores on the self-completed health questionnaire which taps emotional and psychosomatic symptoms. This was not used with 10-yr-olds but it was with both adolescents and parents, for whom it has been shown to provide a reasonable indicator of psychiatric disorder. Among the 14–15-yr-old girls 17·2% had scores indicative of possible disorder whereas among the mothers 12·2% had similar scores. The comparable figures for boys and fathers were 10·4% and 3·8%. Accordingly, as judged on the basis of self-completed questionnaires, disorders appear rather more common in adolescence than in adult life.

The findings are largely negative so far, but we have used only separate pieces of information. In the original survey, the final estimate of prevalence was based on a two-stage procedure involving the screening of the total population by means of parents' and teachers' questionnaires and then individual diagnoses based on all available data. On this basis, we obtained a prevalence of 5·7% psychiatric disorder at age 10 yr. At 14–15 yr the figure was 7·7%, just a little higher.

Taking all these comparisons together, it may be concluded that psychiatric disorders occur at a fairly similar rate at age 14–15 yr and at age 10–11 yr, although the prevalence is probably rather higher in adolescence. Comparisons with adulthood are less certain as the findings differ according to which data are used. However, it seems that disorders may be somewhat more frequent in adolescence. It should be noted that psychiatric clinic referral rates are appreciably higher in adult life than in adolescence (Baldwin, 1968), although this difference may reflect referral practices rather than prevalence.

So far so good, but in these last comparisons there has been one missing step and it is that step which throws the whole issue into confusion once more. The missing step is the consideration of how many children with psychiatric disorder are missed by the screening procedures. At 14–15 yr, our data suggest that quite a few children are missed (Graham and Rutter, 1973). Indeed, if a correction is made on the basis of children not picked up on the screening procedures, the rate rises greatly—up to 21%. Unfortunately, the information at age 10 yr is not exactly comparable but the available data indicate that the proportion missed is very much smaller and hence the corrected prevalence is considerably lower (Rutter.

Journal of Child Psychology and Psychiatry, 1976, vol. 17, pp. 35–56

Tizard and Whitmore, 1970). As this one comparison runs counter to all the others we need to look very closely at what it means and search diligently for possible methodological artefacts.

The first point is where do all these extra children who missed the screening procedures come from? On which source of data is the psychiatric diagnosis based? The answer is that the single greatest source is the psychiatric interview with the adolescent himself. In fact no less than 28% are diagnosed *on this basis alone,* without supporting evidence from either the parent or teacher. As this picture is quite different to that in the group selected on the screening procedures, we need to consider whether the interview with the child is a valid and trustworthy indicator of psychiatric disorder.

234 ∎

TABLE 6. VALIDITY OF PSYCHIATRIC INTERVIEW WITH ADOLESCENT

	% with disorder on adolescent interview
Control group (n = 184)	16·3%
Psychiatric group (diagnosed on basis of information from parents/teachers) (n = 158)	48·7% *

* $\chi^2 = 51·78$; 1 *d.f.*; $p < 0·001$.

Table 6 shows the proportion of adolescents diagnosed as having psychiatric disorder (on the basis of the child interview) in two groups. The first group is the random control group where there was a rate of 16·3% and the second is the group of youngsters diagnosed as having psychiatric condition on the information from parents and teachers, where the rate was 48·7%. This provides convincing validation of the interview with the adolescent as a means of detecting disorder so that serious attention must be paid to its findings.

However, the fact remains that many youngsters who appear normal to parents and teachers are diagnosed as showing disorder on the adolescent interview. Thus, in the random control group *not* selected on either the parent or teacher questionnaire nearly one in five are nevertheless diagnosed as showing psychiatric disorder on the adolescent interview. Nearly all these disorders involved some type of emotional disturbance, often depression; and it was clear that the frequently expressed feelings of misery, self-depreciation and the ideas of reference, already noted when considering "inner turmoil", had been used to diagnose psychiatric disorder. Was this correct? No really satisfactory answer can be given to that question on the basis of existing data. Four points may be made, however. First, the data on impairment of functioning were less searching in the adolescent interview than in the parental interview, so that for this reason alone, less reliance can be placed on the diagnosis, if social impairment is required to be present (which it was on our criteria). Second, whether or not it is considered that they indicate psychiatric disorder, the feelings of affective disturbance were real enough. Regardless of what parents and teachers thought or noticed, the adolescents themselves experienced suffering. Thirdly, the proportion of youngsters who looked sad was much smaller than those who reported feeling miserable. This raises the question of whether the reported feelings meant clinical depression or whether they represented inner turmoil which is part of adolescent development rather than an indication of psychiatric disorder. Fourthly, the best test of the psychiatric meaning of these symptoms would be what happened to the youngsters' mental state over the next year or so after the interview. Did the feelings of misery develop into frank depression or some other disorder noticeable to others, *or did the feelings remain purely internal and not observable by other people?* No data on that point are available either from the Isle of Wight study or from other published investigations, but such a study would be most useful and informative.

In the absence of these data any conclusions about the true prevalence of psychiatric disorder in adolescence must remain rather tentative. However, putting the findings together as well as possible, it seems that overt socially handicapping psychiatric disorder is probably somewhat commoner in adolescence than in earlier childhood (and possibly more frequent than in adult life) but the age differences in prevalence are fairly small. But, in addition to these generally recognizable disorders there is a sizable group of adolescents, perhaps 10% of the general population, who suffer from marked internal feelings of misery and self-depreciation. These feelings are obviously important aspects of adolescence but their clinical significance in terms of overt handicapping disorder remains uncertain at present. In view of this uncertainty, from now on when referring to psychiatric disorder in adolescence attention will be confined to the 7·5% who were diagnosed on the basis of the two-stage procedure which involved both *general* population screening *and* individual interviews with parents, teachers and adolescents.

Types of psychiatric disorder in adolescence
It seems, then, that there is probably a slight rise in the rate of psychiatric disorder during early adolescence, but the increase is only moderate. The next issue is whether the disorders occurring in adolescence differ in *type* from those evident at age 10 yr. For the most part the disorders appear closely similar. At both ages there is the same mixture of emotional disorders and conduct disturbances with very few psychotic children. In fact at age 14 yr there were no clear cases of schizophrenia, although there was one boy with a disorder which might reflect the early signs of this condition. The findings emphase the rarity of psychosis in early adolescence.

However, there were two marked differences from the distribution of disorders at age 10 yr. First, depression was much commoner in adolescence. At 10 yr there were only 3 children with a depressive condition whereas at 14 yr there were 9, plus another 26 with an affective disorder involving both anxiety and depression. This difference indicates the beginning of a shift to an adult pattern of disorders, although there is not yet the marked female preponderance of neurotic disorders seen in adults. As shown by Shaffer's study (1974) this rise in affective disorders during adolescence is paralleled by a rise in the incidence of completed suicide. Secondly, at age 14 yr there were 15 cases of school refusal whereas there had been none at age 10 yr. In many cases the school refusal formed part of a more widespread anxiety state or affective disorder, but, in all, the reluctance to go to school constituted one of the main problems. The findings are in keeping with the clinical

■235

evidence that school refusal is most prevalent in early childhood and again in adolescence. In the younger children, the main problem is more in keeping with normal developmental patterns and the prognosis is usually very good. In contrast, school refusal in adolescents is more often part of a widespread psychiatric disorder and the prognosis is considerably worse (Rodriguez *et al.*, 1959). In short, although the psychiatric disorders shown at 14 yr are similar in many respects to those evident at age 10 yr, it is clear that the diagnostic pattern is different with respect to affective disorders and in this respect it is beginning to approximate the adult picture.

New disorders and persistent disorders

236 ■

We now need to turn to the question we started with, whether disorders arising for the first time in adolescence are in some way different from those arising in earlier childhood, and whether adolescent disorders are due in part to the troubles stemming from inner turmoil or alienation from parents. Let us start with the issue of whether the disorders are different. It will be recalled that, as well as the cross-sectional study at 14 yr, we had had a similar study at age 10 yr on the same children. By linking the two studies we were able to sort out the adolescents' disorders into those which were already evident at age 10 yr and those that began at some point between 10 and 14 yr. Table 7 shows how the group divided up.

TABLE 7. AGE OF ONSET IN ADOLESCENT PSYCHIATRIC DISORDERS

	Before 10 yr	After 10 yr	Total
Boys	43 (69·3%)	53 (56·4%)	96
Girls	19	41	60
Total	62	94	156
Sex ratio	2·3 : 1	1·3 : 1	

$\chi^2 = 2·13; 1 \ d.f.; N.S.$

There were 48 youngsters who had already shown handicapping psychiatric disorder at age 10 yr. In addition, there were a further 14 who had had deviant scores on the parents' or teachers' questionnaire at the same age, although a handicapping disorder was not diagnosed. These two groups were combined to make a single group of 62 adolescents who were already showing disorder at 10 yr. The remaining 94 children had given no indications of psychiatric problems at 10 yr, so the presumption is that their disorders began some time after that, during early adolescence. (For this comparison, of course, children leaving or coming to the Isle of Wight between 10 and 14 yr have been excluded.)

Thus, just over half the disorders constituted new conditions arising in adolescence and just under half were conditions persisting from earlier childhood. It should be noted that, compared with clinic studies, the proportion of new disorders is unusually high. Both Warren (1965) and Capes *et al.* (1971) found that among adolescent psychiatric patients the majority of disorders had their origins in early or middle childhood. In the Isle of Wight study there was no difference between those with new and those with persistent disorders in terms of the proportion who were seen by a psychiatrist during the last year (the figures were 15·5 and 17·5%). However, there was some difference in terms of those who had ever received psychiatric care, as would be expected on the basis of the duration of disorder. A third

(33·3%) of the persistent group had seen a psychiatrist compared with less than a fifth (19·0%) of the children with new disorders.

Let us now turn to the question of how the two groups of disorders differed. The first difference which is apparent is that there was a marked preponderance of boys among the persistent cases whereas in the new cases the sex ratio was nearer equal. In short, the disorders arising during adolescence are nearer to the adult pattern than those arising in earlier childhood. Interestingly, however, the diagnostic differences were small and statistically insignificant.

TABLE 8. SEVERITY OF PSYCHIATRIC DISORDER BY AGE OF ONSET

	New disorders	Persistent disorders
Mild	59 (62·8%)	32 (51·6%)
Moderate	29 (30·9%)	21 (33·9%)
Severe	6 (6·4%)	9 (14·5%)
Total	94	62

χ^2 for trends = 3·14; 1 $d.f.$; $N.S.$

Before turning to other differences it is necessary to check whether the two groups differed in terms of the severity of the disorder. This is shown in Table 8. There was a slight tendency for the most severe disorders to be found in the persistent group but the differences fell well short of statistical significance and overall the severity ratings were quite similar in the two groups.

In looking for differences between the groups, it is helpful to have some idea of what features differentiate between the children with psychiatric disorder and those without any psychiatric problems. These variables are summarized in the next two tables. First, there are a variety of cognitive or educational factors. As was the case with the younger children showing psychiatric disorder, there was a slight tendency for the psychiatric group to have a lower I.Q., and a marked tendency for them to have severe reading difficulties. They also had significantly lower arithmetic scores.

Again as with the younger children, psychiatric disorder was associated with various indicators of family pathology, such as break-up of the parent's marriage, the child going into care, marital discord, irritability between the parents, parental irritability towards the child, and mental disorder in the mother.

In addition, there were a number of items, not assessed at age 10 yr, which were associated with psychiatric disorder in adolescents. First, most of the items associated with parent–child alienation were more often found in the psychiatric group. More quarrelled with their parents, more showed physical withdrawal, more showed communication difficulties or emotional withdrawal, more of the parents disapproved of the adolescent's friends and fewer of the adolescents went out with their parents. Second, there was also a mixed group of items referring to the youngsters' leisure activities which were associated with psychiatric disorder. The significant items are just a few out of a large number of non-significant differences on leisure activities, so these few should not receive much emphasis.

These items will be used to look for possible differences between the youngsters with new disorders and those with disorders persisting from earlier childhood. Table

Journal of Child Psychology and Psychiatry, 1976, vol. 17, pp. 35–56

10 shows that there was no I.Q. difference, but the children with persistent disorders had much lower arithmetic scores ($t = 4\cdot30$; 144 $d.f.$; $p < 0\cdot01$).

The difference with respect to reading retardation was even greater, as shown in Table 10 and Figure 2. The children with new disorders had no more reading difficulties than did the general population ($3\cdot3$ vs $4\cdot1\%$). This was in marked

TABLE 9. ITEMS DIFFERENTIATING PSYCHIATRIC GROUP FROM CONTROLS

Low I.Q. Low arithmetic score Reading retardation	Cognitive/educational
Not living with natural parents Child been in care Marital discord Parental irritability Maternal psychiatric disorder	Family pathology
Altercations with parents Physical withdrawal Communication difficulties Parental disapproval of friends Does not go out with parents	Parent–child alienation
Goes to coffee bar Meets friends in public places Has paper round Smokes	Other

TABLE 10. FAMILY AND EDUCATIONAL VARIABLES AND TIME OF ONSET OF DISORDER

	New disorders (at age 14 yr) $n = 94$	Persistent disorders (10–14 yr) $n = 62$	Non-persistent disorders (after age 10 yr) $n = 45$
Not living with both natural parents	18·2%	37·3%**	25·5%
Poor marriage	20·8%	30·2%	18·9%
Child been in care	8·3%	32·8%***	8·7%†
Maternal psychiatric disorder	17·6%	30·2%	21·4%
Reading retardation (age 10 yr)	3·3%	14·3%*	11·1%
Reading retardation (age 14 yr)	2·2%	21·4%***	13·3%††
Mean I.Q.	105·0 ($s.d.$ = 17·14)	102·0 ($s.d.$ = 15·09)	102·3 ($s.d.$ = 20·60)
Mean arithmetic score	31·4 ($s.d.$ = 11·68)	23·3 ($s.d.$ = 10·82)	27·9 ($s.d.$ = 13.00)

Differences between new disorders and persistent disorders
　　* $p < 0\cdot05$
　　** $p < 0\cdot025$
　　*** $p < 0\cdot001$.
Differences between persistent disorders and non-persistent disorders
　　† $p < 0\cdot001$ ($\chi^2 = 7\cdot28$; 1 $d.f.$).
Differences between new disorders and non-persistent disorders
　　†† $p = 0\cdot015$ (Fisher's Exact test).

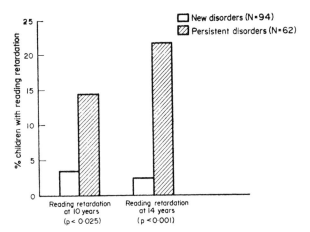

FIG. 2. Reading retardation and time of onset of psychiatric disorder.

contrast to the situation with respect to those with persistent disorders, many of whom (14·3%) were seriously retarded in reading. Interestingly the proportion who showed severe and specific reading retardation was even greater at 14 yr than it had been at age 10 yr. In short, the disorders persisting from earlier childhood were strongly and significantly associated with scholastic problems whereas this was not true at all with the disorders arising *de novo* during adolescence.

Figure 3 and Table 10 show a selection of the family variables associated with psychiatric problems. As is evident, in all cases family difficulties were much more strongly associated with the persistent cases than with the new cases. A third (32·8%) of the children with persistent disorders had been in care compared with only 8·3% of those with new disorders ($\chi^2 = 13·76$; 1 *d.f.*; $p < 0·001$). Almost two-fifths (37·3%) were not living with their two natural parents compared with less than a quarter (18·2%) of those with new conditions ($\chi^2 = 5·77$; 1 *d.f.*; $p < 0·025$). Maternal psychiatric disorder, irritability between parents and paternal irritability with the child were all nearly twice as common in the persistent group, although only the last difference reached statistical significance ($\chi^2 = 7·49$; 1 *d.f.*; $p < 0·01$).

A check was made to see if any of these differences were explicable in terms of diagnostic variation or difference in the severity of disorder. They were not. The differences remained even after the appropriate standardizations had been made.

In summary, as shown in Table 11, whereas persistent disorders at age 14 yr are strongly associated with various indices of family discord, parental difficulty and educational disadvantage (as were disorders at age 10 yr), these associations were much attenuated or non-existent in the case of psychiatric conditions arising for the first time during adolescence. The only association reaching statistical significance was that with marital disharmony.

However, it could be objected that the differences were explicable simply in terms of the different stages in the process of psychiatric disorder. The new disorders were recent whereas the persistent disorders were chronic. It is not possible to determine how far this constitutes an explanation but some check can be provided by a comparison with the 10-yr-old children who had *recovered* before 14 yr, as they,

Journal of Child Psychology and Psychiatry, 1976, vol. 17, pp. 35–56

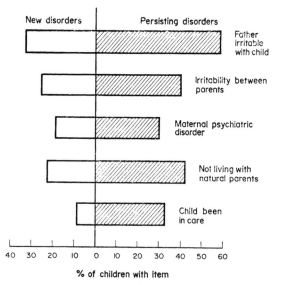

Fig. 3. Family variables and time of onset of disorder.

TABLE 11. FAMILY AND EDUCATIONAL VARIABLES AND DIFFERENCES FROM CONTROL GROUP

	Non-disordered controls ($n = 123$)	New disorders ($n = 94$)	Persistent disorders ($n = 62$)
Not living with both natural parents	14·9%	18·2%	37·3%**
Poor marriage	6·6%	20·8%**	30·2%***
Child been in care	3·3%	8·3%	32·8%
Maternal psychiatric disorder	9·5%	17·6%	30·2%**
Reading retardation (at age 10 yr)	4·1%	3·3%	14·3%*
Reading retardation (at age 14 yr)	3·3%	2·2%	21·4%***
Mean I.Q.	108·51	104·98	102·02**
	(*s.d.* = 14·32)	(*s.d.* = 17·14)	(*s.d.* = 15·09)
Mean arithmetic score	33·9	31·4	23·2***
	(*s.d.* = 11·24)	(*s.d.* = 11·68)	(*s.d.* = 10·82)

Differences from controls
* $p < 0.025$
** $p < 0.01$
*** $p < 0.001$.

too, constituted a group with relatively acute conditions. This comparison is complicated by the fact that the non-persistent disorders from age 10 yr differ somewhat in diagnosis from both the other groups, in being predominantly neurotic conditions. Accordingly, on these grounds alone a lesser association with family and educational variables would be expected. Nevertheless, the findings should be examined.

It is apparent from Table 10 that whereas reading retardation was associated with *both* the non-persistent and persistent disorders from age 10 yr, it was not associated with the disorders arising in adolescence. It may be firmly concluded that this is a difference associated with age of onset rather than with chronicity. However, the reverse is true with family variables. After controlling statistically for diagnostic differences between groups it was evident that the non-persistent group was closely similar to the new group in terms of family difficulties. Gross family pathology is mainly associated with chronic psychiatric disorders, but marital discord at parent–child alienation (see below) is found with both acute and chronic conditions.

Alienation and adolescent psychiatric disorder

We now need to turn to the possible importance of alienation from parents in the genesis of psychiatric disorder in adolescence. We have already seen that all the various measures of alienation are significantly associated with psychiatric problems. Altercations with parents, physical withdrawal and emotional withdrawal were all twice as common in the psychiatric group. But the question is: does alienation lead to disorder or does disorder lead to alienation? In order to answer that question we need to compare the disorders arising *de novo* in adolescence with those persisting from age 10 yr. The findings are shown in Table 12.

TABLE 12. PARENT–CHILD ALIENATION AND TIME OF ONSET OF DISORDER

	New disorders (n = 94)	Persistent disorders (n = 62)
Parental account		
Altercation with parents	28·0%	43·4%
Physical withdrawal	19·3%	29·1%
Emotional withdrawal	43·4%	43·6%
Child's account		
Altercation with parents	35·6%	41·8%
Rejection of mother	2·2%	8·2%
Rejection of father	9·0%	8·6%

No differences are statistically significant.

Alienation was found to be associated with *both* types of disorder, but on the whole it was somewhat more evident in the persistent group even after controlling for differences in the severity of disorder (although the differences fall short of statistical significance). At least in that group, alienation *arising in adolescence* could not have caused psychiatric disorder because the disorder long antedated the adolescent period. Either the association was the other way round, that is the alienation was part of or the *result*, not the cause, of psychiatric problems, or the alienation must have acted as a stress in the pre-adolescent years. Unfortunately the direction of association cannot be conclusively determined in the new group as we had no measure of alienation at age 10 yr. However, two findings militate *against* alienation arising during adolescence being a major causal factor. The first is that most parents said that the alienation began when the child was much younger; only in a very few cases did alienation increase during adolescence. Secondly, the finding that alienation was, if anything, more strong in the persistent disorders argues against alienation being a special causal factor in the new group.

It may be that alienation from parents in earlier childhood predisposes the child

Journal of Child Psychology and Psychiatry, 1976, vol. 17, pp. 35–56

to later disorder or it may be that the disorder leads to alienation, or both may be true. Nevertheless, it should not be assumed that the observed association between alienation and psychiatric disorder has the same meaning in the new disorders as it does in those persisting from early or middle childhood.

In the persistent group alienation probably stemmed from the psychiatric disorder in many cases. These children tended to come from disturbed homes in which parents showed psychiatric disorder, or there was severe marital discord, or the family had split up, and often the children had had periods "in care" as a result of the family difficulties. It seems that when marital discord is associated with gross family pathology, psychiatric disorder (if it occurs) is likely to develop in the children well before adolescence. In these cases alienation is probably just part of the general family disturbance.

The new disorders, in contrast, occurred in children from more stable families, although marital discord and alienation were also often present. As far as could be judged from parental reports, the alienation frequently began in earlier childhood *before* the onset of psychiatric disorder. In these cases alienation might well be a causal factor. The findings are in keeping with the hypothesis that deviant relationships and impaired communication patterns (i.e. alienation in the setting of marital discord) in families without severe disturbance may be factors in the development of psychiatric problems which do not become overt until the early or middle teens. On the other hand, our evidence suggests that alienation *arising for the first time* is *not* a common causal factor in either psychiatric group.

Does the same thing apply to "inner turmoil"? The findings are that misery, self-depreciation, suicidal ideas and ideas of reference occur with just the same frequency in the persistent disorders as in the new disorders. In short, if these are taken as reflections of "inner turmoil", "inner turmoil" is *no* more frequent in the children whose disorders have arisen *de novo* during adolescence.

The transience or persistence of adolescent disorders

Before attempting to summarize the findings, there is just one other set of data we have to consider and that refers to the prognosis of adolescent psychiatric conditions. An essential element in the concept of adolescent disorders, as a result of turmoil and alienation, is the supposition that the problems are variable in symptomatology, transient and benign. Is this borne out by the results of follow-up studies? We have no follow-up data on the Isle of Wight youngsters but data are available from several other studies such as those by Annesley (1961), Warren (1965), Masterson (1967) and Capes *et al.* (1971). As the findings from each are so closely similar they can be discussed together.

First, the question of symptom fluctuation. All the studies have shown that most disorders remain true to type and that symptom fluctuation is not a common feature. There is *no* reason to suppose that symptoms are more variable in adolescence than at any other age.

Secondly, the prognosis for adolescent psychiatric disorders does not appear to be any different (neither better or worse) from that for similar disorders in earlier childhood.

Thirdly, the prognosis varies markedly according to diagnosis. Psychoses have the worst outcome, neurotic conditions the best, with conduct disorders intermediate. This pattern is the same as that found in younger children.

These conclusions apply to the group of adolescent psychiatric disorders as a whole and not just to those whose problems arose *de novo* during adolescence. The evidence is not decisive but, so far as it goes, it suggests that their outlook is no different from the other. Warren (1965) found that the age of onset of the disorder did not influence the prognosis one way or the other. Capes *et al.* (1971) found that the prognosis was better for those whose first five years of life were reasonably trouble-free, but as nearly all of these had emotional disorders a good prognosis would have been expected on the basis of diagnosis alone. Neither Annesley (1961) nor Masterson (1967) presented their findings in a way which allows this comparison.

- 243

Generality of findings

The findings from the Isle of Wight study apply to 14–15-yr-old adolescents living in an area of small towns and villages. Whether the same apply to teenagers living in metropolitan or city areas remains uncertain. The level of psychiatric disorder among 10-yr-olds living in inner London is well above that found in Isle of Wight children of the same age (Rutter, 1973) and the same may be true at 14–15 yr. Nevertheless, the limited evidence from other investigations suggests that the *pattern* of findings from the present study may well be fairly general. Doubtless, the extent of parent–child alienation and the frequency of adolescent depression are influenced by socio-cultural factors, but how much so remains to be determined. It is also not known how far the pattern at age 18–19 yr differs from that in mid-adolescence. It is highly likely, however, that the situation will be much influenced by whether the young people are working and financially independent or whether they continue as students and remain dependent on their families.

CONCLUSIONS

The first conclusion is that although parent–child disagreements over items such as dress and hair length are fairly frequent, parent–child alienation is not a common feature at age 14 yr, unless the youngster is already showing psychiatric problems and even then it is present in only about half the group. We have no data concerning alienation during later adolescence but the findings from other studies suggest that it increases somewhat during the late teens but still remains a phenomenon confined to a minority, although possibly a substantial minority. The evidence is meagre and inconclusive but it may be that alienation and rebellion are most evident in those teenagers who, in spite of considerable maturity, remain economically or otherwise dependent on their parents (as would often be the case with respect to those in higher education).

Secondly, parents continue to have a substantial influence on their children right through adolescence. It is certainly true that peer group influences increase markedly during the teen-age period, but except in a minority of youngsters, they do *not* replace parental influences, although they sometimes rival them.

Thirdly, "inner turmoil" as represented by feelings of misery, self-depreciation and ideas of reference are quite common in 14-yr-olds. These feelings cause appreciable personal suffering but often they are unnoticed by adults. It remains uncertain how far these feelings constitute indicators or portents of psychiatric disorder.

Fourthly, psychiatric conditions are probably a little commoner during adolescence than during middle childhood but the difference is not a very great one and most adolescents do *not* show psychiatric disorder. On the other hand, the *pattern* of disorders shows a substantial shift in terms of the increased prevalence of both depression and school refusal.

Fifthly, many adolescent psychiatric problems arise in early childhood so that if prevention is to be attempted it must take place long before the child reaches his teens.

Sixthly, parent–child alienation arising in adolescence is probably not a very common *cause* of psychiatric disorder, in adolescence, although it is commonly *associated* with disorder. Alienation arising in earlier childhood, however, may be aetiologically important.

Seventhly, conditions arising for the first time during adolescence differ in certain important respects from those which persist from earlier childhood. The new conditions are more commonly found in girls, they are *un*associated with educational difficulties, and adverse family factors are less often found than in the early onset conditions.

Lastly, the prognosis for adolescent psychiatric disorders seems to be much more dependent upon diagnosis than upon the age of onset. Although the evidence is limited, there is no indication that disorders arising in adolescence have any different prognosis from those which arise in younger children.

Adolescent turmoil is a fact, not a fiction, but its psychiatric importance has probably been over-estimated in the past. Certainly it would be most *unwise* to assume that adolescents will "grow out" of their problems to a greater extent than do younger children.

SUMMARY

The concept of adolescent turmoil is considered in the context of findings from a total population epidemiological study of Isle of Wight 14–15-yr-olds. It is concluded that parent–child alienation is not a common feature unless the adolescents are already showing psychiatric problems. Inner turmoil, however, as represented by feelings of misery and self-depreciation is quite frequent. Psychiatric conditions are only slightly commoner during adolescence than in middle childhood but the pattern of disorders changes in terms of an increase in depression and school refusal. Many adolescent psychiatric problems arise in early childhood but conditions arising for the first time during adolescence differ in important respect from those with an earlier onset.

Acknowledgements—We are grateful to Professor J. Tizard (co-director of the project with M. R.) and Mr. L. Rigley who were jointly concerned with the organisation and planning of the Isle of Wight studies, and to our many colleagues who participated in the interviewing and testing. The project was supported by grants from the Nuffield Foundation and the Social Science Research Council.

REFERENCES

ADELSON, J. (1964) The mystique of adolescence. *Psychiat.* **27**, 1–5.
ANNESLEY, P. T. (1961) Psychiatric illness in adolescence: presentation and prognosis. *J. ment. Sci.* **107**, 268–278.

BALDWIN, J. A. (1968) Psychiatric illness from birth to maturity: an epidemiological study. *Acta psychiat. Scand.* **44,** 313–333.

BLOS, P. (1970) *The Young Adolescent: Clinical Studies.* Collier–Macmillan, London.

BROWN, G. W. and RUTTER, M. (1966) The measurement of family activities and relationships: a methodological study. *Human Relations* **19,** 241–263.

CAPES, M., GOULD, E. and TOWNSEND, M. (1971) *Stress in Youth.* Oxford University Press, London.

COLEMAN, J. S. (1961) *The Adolescent Society.* Collier–Macmillan, London.

DOUVAN, E. and ADELSON, J. (1966) *The Adolescent Experience.* Wiley, New York.

EISSLER, K. R. (1958) Notes on problems of technique in the psychoanalytic treatment of adolescents. *Psychoanal. Stud. Child* **13,** 223–254.

EPPERSON, D. C. (1964) A re-assessment of indices of parental influence in "The Adolescent Society". *Am. Sociol. Rev.* **29,** 93–96.

ERIKSON, E. H. (1955) The problem of ego identity. *J. Am. Psychoanal. Assoc.* **4,** 56–121.

FREUD, A. (1952) Adolescence. *Psychoanal. Stud. Child* **13,** 255–278.

GELEERD, E. R. (1961) Some aspects of ego vicissitudes in adolescence. *J. Am. Psychoanal. Ass.* **9,** 394–405.

GRAHAM, P. and RUTTER, M. (1973) Psychiatric disorder in the young adolescent: a follow-up study. *Proc. R. Soc. Med.* **66,** 1226–1229.

HENDERSON, A. S., KRUPINSKI, J. and STOLLER, A. (1971) Epidemiological aspects of adolescent psychiatry. In *Modern Perspectives in Adolescent Psychiatry* (Edited by HOWELLS, J. G.). Oliver & Boyd, Edinburgh, pp. 183–208.

JAHODA, M. and WARREN, N. (1965) The myths of youth. *Sociol. Education* **38,** 138–149.

JOSSELYN, I. M. (1954) The ego in adolescence. *Am. J. Orthopsychiat.* **24,** 223–237.

KRUPINSKI, J., BAIKIE, A. G., STOLLER, A., GRAVES, J., O'DAY, D. M. and POLKE, P. (1967) Community mental health survey of Heyfield, Victoria. *Med. J. Aust.* **1,** 1204–1211.

LESLIE, S. A. (1974) Psychiatric disorders in the young adolescents of an industrial town. *Br. J. Psychiat.* **125,** 113–124.

MASTERSON, J. F. (1967) *The Psychiatric Dilemma of Adolescence.* Churchill, London.

MEISSNER, W. W. (1965) Parental interaction of the adolescent boy. *J. genet. Psychol.* **107,** 225–233.

NEALE, M. D. (1958) *Neale Analysis of Reading Ability Manual.* Macmillan, London.

OFFER, D. (1969) *The Psychological World of the Teenager.* Basic Books, London.

RODRIGUEZ, A., RODRIGUEZ, M. and EISENBERG, L. (1959) The outcome of school phobia in a follow-up study based on 41 cases. *Am. J. Psychiat.* **116,** 540–544.

ROSEN, B. M., BAHN, A. K., SHELLOW, R. and BOWER, E. M. (1965) Adolescent patients served in outpatient psychiatric clinics. *Am. J. publ. Health* **55,** 1563–1577.

RUTTER, M. (1973) Why are London children so disturbed? *Proc. R. Soc. Med.* **66,** 1221–1225.

RUTTER, M. and BROWN, G. W. (1966) The reliability and validity of measures of family life and relationships in families containing a psychiatric patient. *Social Psychiat.* **1,** 38–53.

RUTTER, M., TIZARD, J. and WHITMORE, K. (Editors) (1970) *Education, Health and Behaviour.* Longmans, London.

SHAFFER, D. (1974) Suicide in childhood and early adolescence. *J. Child Psychol. Psychiat.* **15,** 275–292.

SHEPHERD, M., OPPENHEIM, B. and MITCHELL, S. (1971) *Childhood Behaviour and Mental Health.* University of London Press, London.

U.S. DEPARTMENT OF HEALTH, EDUCATION AND WELFARE (1966) *Patients in Mental Hospitals.* Public Service Publication No. 1818. Chevy Chase, M.D.

VERNON, P. E. (1949) *Graded Arithmetic–Mathematic Test.* University of London Press, London.

WARREN, W. (1965) A study of psychiatric in-patients and the outcome six or more years later—II. The follow-up study. *J. Child Psychol. Psychiat.* **6,** 141–160.

WECHSLER, D. (1949) *Wechsler Intelligence Scale for Children.* Psychological Corporation, New York.

245

Part V
Psychosocial risks

Child Development, 1979, vol. 50, pp. 283–305

Maternal Deprivation, 1972–1978: New Findings, New Concepts, New Approaches

Michael Rutter

Institute of Psychiatry, London

RUTTER, MICHAEL. *Maternal Deprivation, 1972–1978: New Findings, New Concepts, New Approaches.* CHILD DEVELOPMENT, 1979, **50**, 283–305. Research since 1972 in the field of "maternal deprivation" is critically reviewed. The results are used to reassess briefly the formulations proposed in 1972 and to discuss more fully the meaning and practical implications of fresh findings on new or recently revived topics. These include the development of social relationships and the process of bonding, critical periods of development, the links between childhood experiences and parenting behavior, influences on parenting, and the possible reasons why so many children do not succumb to deprivation or disadvantage.

■249

In some respects the reference to "maternal deprivation" in the title of this paper is a misnomer: the main focus is not on either mothers or deprivation in the sense of loss. Nevertheless, the title is appropriate because it emphasizes how much recent research owes to the pioneers who established the concept over a quarter of a century ago (cf. Bowlby 1951; Goldfarb 1955; Spitz 1946).

When the topic was reviewed in 1972 (Rutter 1972), it was pointed out that Bowlby's claim that early-life experiences may have serious and lasting effects on development, which was controversial in 1951, was so no longer. There was much good evidence in support. However, the same evidence had also shown that the term "maternal deprivation" covered a most heterogeneous range of experiences and outcomes due to quite disparate mechanisms.

In many ways the suggestions about possible mechanisms made in the 1972 review were no more than restatements of ideas already apparent in Bowlby's (1951) World Health Organization report or in Ainsworth's (1962) thoughtful reappraisal of the topic a decade later. But there were a few crucial differences (Rutter 1972, 1974), some of which proved more controversial than expected.

First, it was argued that the original emphasis on the supposedly deleterious effects of separation *as such* were incorrect (Rutter 1971, 1972, in press-b). Antisocial disorders were linked with broken homes not because of the separation involved but, rather, because of the discord and disharmony which led to the break. Affectionless psychopathy was due not to the breaking of relationships but, rather, to the initial failure to form bonds. Intellectual retardation was due to lack of appropriate experiences and not to separations.

Second, there was disagreement with Bowlby's views on the supposedly special importance of the mother. In particular, it was suggested that the evidence did not support the notion that the child's main bond with the mother differed in kind and in quality from all his other bonds.

Third, the review indicated that "the most important recent development in 'maternal deprivation' research has been the emphasis on individual differences in children's responses to 'deprivation'" (Rutter 1972, p. 127). All investigations had shown that many children are not damaged by deprivation, and it was argued that exploration of the reasons for their apparent invulnerability should prove a particularly fruitful field for study.

In this paper there is a brief mention of how far the 1972 formulations have proved valid, but a greater emphasis is placed on some of the new concepts and ideas which have come to the forefront more recently.

Syndromes

It is appropriate to begin with a consideration of the four principal syndromes and the mechanisms proposed for their causation.

Child Development, 1979, vol. 50, pp. 283–305

Acute distress syndrome.—First, there is the acute distress reaction shown by many young children admitted to hospitals or residential nurseries. In 1972, most weight was placed on the work of Hinde and of the Robertsons in concluding that the syndrome was due to some kind of interference with attachment behavior and not primarily to separation as such. Their work is still the most important and relevant to this issue.

Briefly, the Robertsons (1971) found that young children separated from their parents but cared for in a family (rather than institutional) setting, although they were influenced by the separation, did not show the same acute distress reaction exhibited by children admitted to hospitals or residential nurseries. Hinde and his colleagues (Hinde & McGinnis 1977) investigated separation experiences in young rhesus monkeys and found that much of the infants' emotional disturbance following reunion with the mother stemmed from tensions in the mother-infant relationship. The strong inference from both sets of studies is that separation, although a crucial precipitant, is not the essential causal agent in the distress syndrome. On the other hand, there is much evidence to link the syndrome with the process of attachment and bonding (see Rutter 1972, in press–a, in press–b). Probably the distress is associated with some kind of interference with attachment behavior, either because separation happens to disrupt an existing bond (note that separation and bond disruption are not synonymous) or because conditions during separation fail to facilitate attachment behavior.

Conduct disorders.—The second syndrome to consider is that of conduct disorders or antisocial problems. Earlier work (Rutter 1971) had shown that conduct disorders were strongly associated with family discord and disharmony even where there had been no break or separation. Furthermore, whereas parental divorce was strongly linked with delinquency, parental death was not. Thus, it appeared that the key variable was disturbed interpersonal relationships, rather than separation.

Further research during recent years has consistently confirmed these findings. For example, several recent general-population epidemiological studies (Rutter, Cox, Tupling, Berger, & Yule 1975; West & Farrington 1973, 1977) have all shown important links between marital discord and disorders of conduct in the children. Moreover, Power, Ash, Schoenberg, and Sorey (1974) found that, among boys who had already made a court appearance for de-

linquency, those from intact homes with severe and persistent family problems were more likely to become recidivist than those from broken homes (or from intact homes without serious problems). Lambert, Essen, and Head (1977), using longitudinal data, showed that most of the behavioral disturbance found in children removed from their homes into the care of the local authority preceded the removal. The separation may have added to the stresses, but it was not the prime cause of the children's problems. Hetherington, Cox, and Cox (Note 1) found that, during the transition period of family disequilibrium and reorganization following divorce, children's problems may be exacerbated. However, improvement then tends to follow, and 2 years after divorce the children showed significantly less disturbance than those remaining in intact homes with continuing marital conflict.

It seems quite clear that family discord and disharmony are indeed the damaging factors, with separations largely incidental. Of course, that still leaves open the question of why and how disturbed interpersonal relationships lead to conduct disorders. Also, it should be emphasized that family discord is only one of many causal influences for delinquency (Rutter & Madge 1976; West & Farrington 1973, 1977).

Intellectual retardation.—Intellectual retardation is the third syndrome to be discussed. In the 1972 review it was suggested that perceptual and linguistic experiences played the main environmental role in the development of intelligence and that personal mothering (although important for other aspects of development) was largely irrelevant for cognitive growth.

The role of mothering and of interpersonal relationships can be assessed by examining the intellectual development of children reared in environments which are deviant in these respects. Barbara Tizard's important studies of children reared in institutions from infancy and followed to age 8 have shown them to be of normal intelligence (Tizard & Joseph 1970; Tizard & Rees 1974). Their mean WISC full-scale IQ was 99, compared with 110 in the general-population family-reared control group (Tizard & Hodges 1978). This was so despite the fact that they had experienced some 50–80 parent surrogates, with quite appalling discontinuities in parent-child relationships. As discussed below, this had ill effects on their psychosocial development, but it did not appreciably retard their intellectual growth. Penny Dixon's findings (Note 2) on larger samples are closely comparable. She, too, has studied children reared in institutions from the first year of life. At 5–8 years they showed various social problems, but they were of normal intelligence. Their mean WISC full-scale IQ was 108, compared with 106 in a comparable group of foster children and 116 in a general-population control group.

It is evident that normal levels of functioning on standard IQ tests are usually attained by children reared in environments which lack personal mothering but which nevertheless provide experiences which are adequate in other respects. There is the clear implication that continuities in family relationships do not have the central role in intellectual development that they do in social development (see below). To an important extent, intellectual growth and social growth have their main influences from rather different sources.[1]

The evidence for the view that perceptual and linguistic experiences do influence intellectual development comes from both natural and contrived experiments. For example, Dennis (1973) showed that a shift from a poor institutional environment in Lebanon to an adoptive home was associated with a marked gain in IQ. Heber and Garber (Garber & Heber 1977; Heber & Garber 1975; Heber, Note 3; Heber, Garber, Harrington, Hoffman, & Falender, Note 4) have demonstrated marked intellectual gains, compared with controls, in socially disadvantaged black children given a very intensive educational intervention program (see also Bronfenbrenner, Note 5). It is also relevant that Scarr and Weinberg (1976) found that black children reared by white parents have a mean IQ some 15 points above black children reared in their own homes.

Caldwell and her colleagues (Bradley & Caldwell 1976; Elardo, Bradley, & Caldwell 1975) have shown that systematic measures of home stimulation are related to children's IQ scores at age 3; Clarke-Stewart (1973) found that maternal attention was correlated with changes in children's developmental quotient; and McCall, Appelbaum, and Hogarty (1973) have concluded that parental behavior is related to IQ in later childhood. Furthermore,

Tizard, Cooperman, Joseph, and Tizard (1972) have shown significant (but low) correlations between institutional children's experiences and their language comprehension.

It would be wrong to exaggerate the strength of any of these findings. All the relationships are quite modest, and many are insignificant (Fisch, Bilek, Deinard, & Chang 1976). Nevertheless, there is evidence that learning experiences in and outside the home influence cognitive development. We do not yet know precisely what mechanisms are involved. However, it is clear that the sheer amount of stimulation is irrelevant (some of the most disadvantaging environments are full of noise—with shouting and the blare of the radio at full blast). Rather, the quality and meaningfulness of active experiences (especially conversational interchange) seem crucial.

Affectionless psychopathy.—The fourth syndrome, affectionless psychopathy, has been the subject of very little direct research in the last 6 years, and hence there is nothing to add to the 1972 review in terms of findings on the syndrome itself. On the other hand, there have been important advances in knowledge on the development of social relationships and on the abnormalities of bonding thought to underlie the syndrome. These warrant some detailed discussion.

Development of Social Relationships

Bowlby (1969, 1973) has put forward a theory of attachment in which early bonding to the mother is seen as the essential precursor of later social relationships. There is now abundant evidence that infants usually develop an attachment to a specific person some time around 6–12 months of age. Also, something is known of the factors most likely to foster the development of attachments (see Ainsworth 1973 and Rutter 1979). A baby's tendency to seek attachments is increased by anxiety and fear and also by illness and fatigue (Bowlby 1969; Maccoby & Masters 1970). Attachments are probably particularly likely to develop to the person who brings comfort at such times. However, the way a parent responds to the infant is also important. Attachments are most

[1] Even so, it would be absurd to regard intellectual development as something which is independent of personal relationships or isolated from the emotional and social life of the child. The same studies of institutional children show them to have poor task involvement in the classroom (see below), and this is very likely to affect their learning and some aspects of their later cognitive growth even if it does not have much impact on their overall IQ scores. Similarly, Matas, Arend, and Sroufe (1978) showed continuities between measures of attachment and of problem-solving style but not between attachment and Bayley scores at 2 years.

Child Development, 1979, vol. 50, pp. 283–305

252 ∎

likely to develop to people who actively interact with the baby and who are responsive to the baby's cues (see Ainsworth 1973). Moreover, these same parental qualities seem to predispose to secure rather than anxious attachments (Blehar, Lieberman, & Ainsworth 1977). As Ainsworth suggested, sensitive responsiveness seems to be the one quality in any interaction most likely to foster secure personal bonding.

These rather general conclusions would be accepted by most workers, but five areas of controversy and uncertainty remain: the concept of "sensitive responsiveness," Bowlby's (1969) notion of monotropy, the distinctions to be made within the overall group of attachment behaviors, early bonding and later social relationships, and the process by which attachments develop.

Sensitive responsiveness.—The concept of *sensitive responsiveness* reflects the general shift of view from parenting as doing things to the baby to parenting as a process of reciprocal interaction—an active dialogue between parent and child (see Lewis & Rosenblum 1974). For example, Brazelton and his colleagues (Brazelton, Tronick, Adamson, Als, & Weise 1975) have examined the rhythms and patterns involved in face-to-face interaction in the neonatal period; Condon and Sander (1974) and Stern (Stern, Jaffe, Beebe, & Bennett 1975) have done the same with early communication; and Dunn (1975) has investigated the longitudinal development of styles of mothering in the first years of life. Brown and Bateman (1978) showed that mothers responded differently to premature than to full-term babies. The premature infants were less active and responsive, and it seemed that as a consequence the mothers became more active and more likely to initiate interactions. Clarke-Stewart's findings (1973, Note 6) from her cross-lagged correlational analysis of longitudinal data suggested not only a two-way interaction, in which parents both influenced and were influenced by their children, but also a reciprocal relationship which changed in balance and characteristics as the children grew older.

Everyone is agreed that parenting involves reciprocity and sensitivity to the baby's cues and signals, but study of this sequential process had proved extremely difficult. Ainsworth, Bell, and Stayton (1974) found that rapid responses to the baby's crying were effective in reducing the amount of crying both immediately and later in the first year of life (Bell & Ainsworth 1972). On the other hand, there are problems

in the interpretation of these results (Gewirtz & Boyd 1978), and the findings from other studies have been quite different (Etzel & Gewirtz 1967; Sander 1969; Sander, Stechler, Burns, & Julia 1970) in showing that rapid responses may increase babies' crying and in showing weak correlations between measures of responsiveness in the neonatal period and in later infancy (Dunn 1975). Babies' cries are of several quite different kinds (Wasz-Höckert, Lind, Vuorenkoski, Partanen, & Valanne 1968; Wolff 1969), and it may be that it is the parent's ability to discriminate between these and to respond appropriately which is important.

Clearly, we have some way to go before we have either adequate concepts or adequate measures of what is meant by sensitive responsiveness. However, it is likely that it involves not only the discrimination between different cues provided by the baby but, in addition, the giving of appropriate differentiating responses, the ability to get pleasure from the baby's reciprocity, and the initiation of interactions.

Monotropy.—All studies have shown that most children develop multiple attachments. However, there is continuing controversy on whether these attachments all have the same meaning. Bowlby (1969) has suggested that there is an innate bias for a child to attach himself especially to one figure and that this main attachment differs in kind from those to other subsidiary figures. However, this statement involves two rather different propositions, one of which is supported by the evidence and one of which is not. The first proposition is that the several attachments are not of equal strength and are not freely interchangeable. This is well supported by the findings from several studies which show that there is a persisting hierarchy among attachments, with some continuing to be stronger than others (Ainsworth 1967; Schaffer & Emerson 1964). Even in institutions, children tend to have their "favorite" adult, to whom they will go in preference to others (Stevens, Note 7).

The second proposition is that the first or main attachment differs in kind from all other subsidiary ones. Most research findings suggest that this is not the case. The proposition may be tested in two different ways. First, it may be determined whether the function or effects of all attachments are similar in quality even though they differ in intensity. The evidence indicates that they are. Attachment may be shown by protest or distress if the attached person leaves the child, by reduction of anxiety and increase of exploration in a strange situation when the attached person is present, and by following or the seeking of closeness (see below). Each of these qualities has been shown for attachments to sibs (Heinicke & Westheimer 1965), to peers (Kissel 1965; Schwartz 1972), to fathers (Cohen & Campos 1974; Lamb 1977a, 1977b; Spelke, Zelazo, Kagan, & Kotelchuck 1973), to adult caretakers in a nursery (Arsenian 1943), and to inanimate objects (Harlow & Zimmermann 1959; Mason & Berkson 1975; Passman 1977; Passman & Weisberg 1975), as well as to mothers (Ainsworth 1967; Ainsworth & Wittig 1969; Corter 1973; Cox & Campbell 1968; Maccoby & Feldman 1972; Morgan & Ricciuti 1969; Stayton, Ainsworth, & Main 1973; Tracy, Lamb, & Ainsworth 1976). It is also crucial that these attachment responses to other persons occur even in children who have developed bonds with their mothers. However, the responses do not occur with strangers.

Second, the proposition may be tested by determining if the difference in intensity of attachment between the person at the top of the hierarchy and the person second in the hierarchy is greater than that between the second and third persons. Stevens (Note 7) found that in most cases it was not (although in some it was). It may be concluded that multiple attachments tend to have rather similar functions in spite of a persisting hierarchy among them. Of course, it is not suggested that all relationships are similar in quality and function. The evidence that this is not the case is more fully discussed later in this paper. However, Bowlby's argument is that the child's relationship with mother differs from other relationships specifically with respect to its attachment qualities, and the evidence indicates that this is not so.

Attachment behaviors.—In early writings on attachment there tended to be an implicit assumption that it was a unitary concept. However, it is now clear that this is not so (Coates, Anderson, & Hartup 1972; Rosenthal 1973; Stayton & Ainsworth 1973). Attachment is not a personality trait but, rather, a construct (Sroufe & Waters 1977) which involves several different features. Probably at least two distinctions need to be made. First, there is the difference between attachment behavior and persisting bonds. Infants show a general tendency to seek attachments to other people (Robertson & Robertson 1971). However, the concept of bonding implies selective attachment (Cohen 1974) which persists over time even during a period of no contact with the person with whom bonds exist. The importance of this distinction

was shown in the Harlow experiments with rhesus monkeys. Infants reared in social isolation clung to inanimate models (so-called cloth mothers) and rushed back to them when threatened or frightened, as by a blast of air in their faces (Harlow 1958; Harlow & Zimmermann 1959). The behavior clearly indicates attachment. However, follow-up studies have indicated that these early attachments to inanimate objects did not lead to normal social relationships in adult life, as peer or parent attachments usually do (Harlow & Harlow 1969; Ruppenthal, Arling, Harlow, Sackett, & Suomi 1976). The difference between human attachment behavior and bonding is shown by Tizard and Rees's (1975) findings regarding institutional children. Four-year-old children reared in institutions showed more clinging and following behavior than family-reared children, but they were also less likely to show selective bonding or deep relationships. The findings may mean that the processes involved are different or, more likely, that the nature of the attached object's response to the infant will influence the quality of the relationship formed and hence its function in relation to later development.

The second distinction is between secure and insecure bonding (Stayton & Ainsworth 1973). One of the characteristics of bonding is that it enables children to feel secure in strange situations. The apparent "purpose" of bonding is to give the child security of relationships in order that it may stop clinging and following and in that sense become detached. Thus, Stayton and Ainsworth (1973) found that the children of sensitive responsive mothers showed more positive greeting on reunion and more following behavior (suggesting stronger attachments) than the children of insensitive unresponsive mothers, but they showed less crying on separation, which suggested that they had a more "secure" attachment. Children who are securely attached to one parent are likely also to be securely attached to the other, but there is sufficient variability in a child's relationships with his two parents to suggest that to an appreciable extent the quality of security is specific to the relationship (Lamb, in press–b). It is also relevant that Hinde and Spencer-Booth (1970) showed that infant rhesus monkeys who exhibited most distress after separation were those who had experienced most rejection by their mothers and for whom there was the most tension in the infant-mother relationship.

One further issue is how far the concept of attachment encompasses all positive social interactions in young children. The evidence

■253

Child Development, 1979, vol. 50, pp. 283–305

suggests that it does not. In particular, the effects of anxiety sharply differentiate attachment from other forms of social interaction; whereas social play is inhibited by anxiety, attachment is intensified. Thus, Lamb (1977a) found that when a child was with his parents the entrance of a stranger inhibited playful interactions but intensified attachment behavior. Children may prefer to play with peers (Eckerman, Whatley, & Katz 1975) or a stranger (Ross & Goldman 1977) but will nevertheless prefer to go to a parent for comfort. The same applies to rhesus monkeys (Patterson, Bonvillian, Reynolds, & Maccoby 1975). Similarly, in an unfamiliar situation infants are much more likely to follow their mother than a stranger when both leave the room by different doors (Corter 1973). Following and the seeking of proximity are characteristic of attachment, and both tend to increase at times of stress. It should be noted that this differential reaction to anxiety is not a consequence of parents being more skilled at providing comfort at times of stress. Harlow and his colleagues showed that infant monkeys clung tightly even to cloth models which repeatedly punished them with a blast of compressed air (Rosenblum & Harlow 1963) or to deprived mothers who severely abused them (Seay, Alexander, & Harlow 1964). Anxiety seems to increase attachment regardless of the response of the attachment object. Systematic data are lacking for humans, but the same seems to apply (Bowlby 1969).

Play and attachment clearly overlap greatly, but they exhibit rather different qualities (Hartup 1979, in press). The ways children play together (Heathers 1955) and the ways they interact with a stranger (Ross & Goldman 1977) are rather different from their style of interaction with parents. Clinging or hugging one another is rarely seen in peer play except in the unusual circumstances of rearing in the absence of parents (Freud & Dann 1951). The same applies to monkey interactions with peers (Harlow 1969; Harlow & Harlow 1972). If there are no parents, peer relationships may serve as a fair substitute in providing attachments, but in these circumstances fully adequate social development may be more difficult to achieve (Ruppenthal et al. 1976; Goldberger, Note 8).

Lamb's studies (in press–a) also indicate that father-child interactions differ in some respects from mother-child interactions. Fathers tend to spend less time in caretaking but are more likely to engage in physically stimulating and unpredictable play, which is often pre-

ferred by infants. Somewhat comparable findings have been reported for rhesus monkeys (Suomi 1977).

Taken together, the findings suggest that any one relationship may involve both attachment and playful interactions. On the whole the former is most characteristic of parent-child relationships and the latter is most characteristic of peer relationships, but there is overlap. Clearly, it is useful conceptually to separate the two types of interactions. However, it remains uncertain how far they are linked and, in particular, how far early bonding is necessary for the optimal development of later playful interaction (see below).

Further research is necessary to sort out the various dimensions of social interaction. However, it may be that attachment behaviors are most readily differentiated from play by the amount of close physical contact in attachment and by its tendency to increase (rather than decrease) at times of fear. Within the overall concept of attachment, specific bonding is probably best differentiated from general attachment behavior by the presence of selectivity in relationships which persist over time and place. The strength of bonding may be best determined by the degree of reduction of distress in a frightening situation when the bonded person is present. The security of bonding, on the other hand, may perhaps be assessed by the relative lack of distress following separation or by the extent of moving away from the bonded person in a strange situation (of course, obviously, this measurement would have to control for strength of bonding).

Early bonding and later social relationships.—The next issue regarding the development of social relationships concerns the sequelae of early bonding. It has usually been thought that early selective bonds provide the basis for later social development (Bowlby 1969; Rutter 1978a), but there has been an extreme paucity of evidence on whether this is actually the case. Two recent British studies by Barbara Tizard (Tizard 1977; Tizard & Hodges 1978) and by Penny Dixon (Dixon, Note 2) have provided crucial data which begin to fill that important gap in our knowledge. Both have followed samples of children reared in institutions with multiple caretakers.

Tizard (Tizard & Rees 1975; Tizard & Tizard 1971) found that at 2 years institution-reared children were both more clinging and more diffuse in their attachments than children brought up in ordinary families. At 4 years, the institutional children were still more clinging and less likely to have deep attachments, and, in addition, they now tended to be overly friendly with strangers and attention seeking. These findings are very much in keeping with other studies of institutional children.

What is new is the followthrough to age 8 (Tizard 1977; Tizard & Hodges 1978). Less than half of the institutional children were said to be closely attached to their housemothers, and still they tended to seek affection more than other children. However, the differences at school were even more striking. Compared with controls, the institutional children were more attention seeking, restless, disobedient, and unpopular.

Dixon (Note 2) also studied the school behavior of children reared in institutions from the first year of life. Her interview and questionnaire findings were closely comparable to those obtained by Tizard. Again, the institution-reared children showed more disruptive and attention-seeking behavior, fighting with other children and not being liked by them. It is just possible that both sets of findings could be artifacts of parental and teacher preconceptions of what institutional children should be like. However, Dixon (Note 2) also made systematic time-sampled observations in the classroom which confirmed the interview and questionnaire data and ruled out the possibility of a rating artifact. The institution children showed more approach to both teachers and other children, but their social interactions were less successful in the sense that they were more likely to behave in unacceptable ways, calling out in class and disregarding teachers' directions. Furthermore, the institution children showed more off-task behavior in the classroom.

It seems probable that this inept social behavior at school was a consequence of the children's relative lack of selective bonding in infancy (due in turn to a pattern of upbringing in which each child experienced as many as 50–80 caretakers). On the other hand, it could be suggested that the social difficulties were a result of genetic endowment. However, this seems unlikely in view of Dixon's (Note 2) finding that children born to similarly disadvantaged biological parents who were personally fostered from infancy were much less likely to exhibit social and emotional problems.

Tizard's results are important in showing continuities between excessive clinging and more diffuse attachment behavior in infancy,

attention seeking and indiscriminate friendliness at age 4 years, and impaired relationships with adults and other children in middle childhood. It is interesting that disturbed relationships are also associated with abnormalities in task involvement—indicating the social as well as the cognitive components of assigned work. Note that in both studies the children were of normal intelligence.

It appears that early bonding is linked with later social development, although the form of the disorder in relationships alters as the child grows older. Of course, many questions remain. For example, it is uncertain whether the children lack fundamental social qualities or, rather, whether they have merely learned patterns of interaction which are adaptive in the institution but maladaptive in other settings. Similarly, it is uncertain how far the difficulties at 8 years mean that there is likely to be impaired personality functioning in adulthood. Further longitudinal or follow-up studies are required to answer that question.

Process of bonding.—The fifth area of controversy concerns the process by which attachments and bonds develop (Cairns 1977; Corter 1974; Gewirtz 1972; Rajeki, Lamb, & Obmascher, in press; Rutter 1979). The topic has attracted the attention and interest of many theorists, and there is a wide variety of quite disparate explanations of attachment behavior (see Rajeki, Lamb, & Obmascher [in press] for a good summary and appraisal). Some, although historically important, no longer warrant serious attention in view of the mass of findings inconsistent with the theory. Thus, Lorenz's (1937/1970) original view of imprinting has had to be greatly modified in the light of research data; Freud's (1946) notion that object relations develop on the basis of feeding and Dollard and Miller's (1950) view of attachment as the result of secondary reinforcement are both inconsistent with the findings showing the irrelevance of feeding and physical caretaking; Schneirla's (1965) epigenetic model lacks empirical support; and Scott's (1971) concept that attachment develops as a response to separation is out of keeping with research findings.

Bowlby (1969) and Ainsworth (1973) have both suggested that infants are born with a biological propensity to behave in ways which promote proximity and contact with their mother figure. According to their views, attachment then develops as a consequence of parental responsiveness to these innate behaviors during a sensitive period in the first years of life. In this

■ 255

Child Development, 1979, vol. 50, pp. 283–305

way, attachment is seen as a specific phenomenon which differs qualitatively from dependency.

Gewirtz (1961, 1972 [in which see esp. his article "Attachment, Dependence, and a Distinction in Terms of Stimulus Control"]), in contrast, argues that both develop as a result of differential reinforcement, the difference being simply that positive stimulus control is restricted to a particular person (rather than to a class of objects) in the case of attachment. Cairns (1966), on the other hand, proposes a contiguity conditioning process which does not rely on any rewarding properties of the attached object. In his view, attachment occurs because a proximate relationship with a salient object predisposes to conditioning. Hoffman and Ratner (1973) suggest a somewhat different form of conditioning model, and Salzen (1978), Sears (1972), and Solomon and Corbit (1974) posit a more central role for the child's emotional state.

Theorists are agreed on several crucial issues. First, the process of bonding obviously involves a reciprocal interaction between infant and parent in which both play an active role (see, e.g., Bowlby 1969; Cairns 1977; Gewirtz & Boyd 1976). Second, maturational as well as environmental factors are important in determining when bonding occurs (see Cairns 1972, 1977; Schaffer 1971). Thus, the development of selective attachment necessarily presupposes that the child can differentiate between people and has a repertoire of social signals and responses. However, while this is a necessary condition it is not a sufficient one, as bonding does not occur until some weeks or months later and may be even further delayed if the environment lacks adequate social opportunities. Third, attachment clearly develops as a result of some form of social learning. Moreover, differential reinforcement manifestly plays an important role in determining the patterning of social interactions (Hinde & Stevenson-Hinde 1976).

Dispute mainly centers on the question of how far bonding is a process which is qualitatively distinct from other forms of social learning and on the nature and importance of possible innate propensities. Five key observations demand explanation, and together these pose problems for all of the theories. First, there is the secure-base effect—the fact that the presence of an attachment object makes it more likely that the infant will move away and explore (Cox & Campbell 1968; Morgan & Ricciuti 1969; Rheingold & Eckerman 1973). Ains-

worth and Bowlby's ethological model accounts best for the phenomenon, but it is not at all clear from their theory why inanimate objects should serve this purpose. The various learning theories can only account for the behavior by making several assumptions that do not arise directly from the theories.

Second, there is the consistent observation that attachment still develops in the face of maltreatment and severe punishment (Harlow & Harlow 1971; Kovach & Hess 1963; Seay, Alexander, & Harlow 1964). Ethological theory correctly predicts that stress should enhance attachment behavior, but Bowlby's (1969) and Lamb's (1978) emphasis on the importance of an "appropriate" parental response does not seem to fit easily with the findings. Cairns's contiguity conditioning theory is in keeping, but it is difficult to see how Gewirtz's reinforcement model could satisfactorily account for the observations.

Third, there is the observation that attachments develop to inanimate objects (Harlow & Zimmermann 1959; Mason & Berkson 1975; Passman 1977; Passman & Weisberg 1975). In this instance, the monkey data and human observations seem to be somewhat in conflict. Socially isolated monkeys readily develop attachments to cloth surrogates, but it has been found that institutional children (who show impaired human attachments) do not. Indeed, it seems that institutional children are less likely than family-reared children to be attached to blankets and cuddly toys. On the Bowlby-Ainsworth theory, it is easy to see how strongly attached children might "generalize" their attachments to inanimate objects. On the other hand, if there is a strong biological propensity to seek attachments (as they suggest), it is not at all clear why institutional children do not use cuddly blankets when they lack adequate human bonds. Of course, it might be suggested that the inanimate objects gain their bonding properties through association with the mother (in learning-theory terms) or because of their symbolic link with the mother (in psychodynamic terms). This might explain the occurrence in normal children and its lack in institutional children, but it does not account for the animal observations, or for the fact that many normal children do not become attached to inanimate objects, or for the observation that autistic children (who lack attachments to their parents) show attachments to (usually nonsoft) inanimate objects (Marchant, Howlin, Yule, & Rutter 1974). It may be that the mechanisms involved in these different cases are different, but, so far, the observations are not well explained by any of the theories.

Fourth, it is necessary to account for the finding that whereas anxiety inhibits play it intensifies attachment. This is exactly what the Bowlby-Ainsworth theory predicts. The phenomenon in normal individuals is also readily explicable in social-learning terms in view of the very different responses elicited by infants in the two situations. On the other hand, it is less obvious in reinforcement terms why the attachment effect should apply to inanimate objects.

Fifth, there are the observations which suggest that not all forms of attachment are equivalent. In particular, it is necessary to explain why the monkey attachments to cloth surrogates do not lead to normal social relationships in the way that parent and (to a lesser extent) peer attachments usually do. The distinction between secure and insecure attachment has also to be accounted for. In both instances the nature of the attached object's response to the infant seems crucial. Social learning provides an adequate explanation as part of most of the main theories, but the findings are out of keeping with a mechanistic imprinting view.

It may be concluded that none of the theories fully accounts for all the phenomena and that theoretical closure is not yet possible. The widespread occurrence of attachment in many animal species certainly suggests some kind of biological propensity, as the ethological theory argues. Also, as suggested by almost all theories, social learning plays a major role in the process of bonding and in determining the characteristics of the parent-child relationship. However, several crucial questions have still to receive satisfactory answers.

Critical Periods

The next issue which has come to notice again in the last 6 years is that of critical periods and the crucial importance (or otherwise) of the early years. In an important recent book on the topic, Alan Clarke and Ann Clarke (1976) have argued that the whole of development is important and that the early years are no more formative than any others. This view has been vigorously attacked (Pringle 1976), and it is appropriate to review the evidence briefly. It is a large topic, and I will confine attention to just two aspects of development—intelligence and socialization.

In both cases the main arguments in favor of the critical nature of the early years are that (1) many disorders have their roots in early childhood, (2) therapeutic interventions in later childhood have usually been rather unsuccessful in the case of persistent disorders, and (3) the correlation (for IQ or personality measures) with adult status rises rapidly during the first half of childhood, with much less change in the second half.

All three arguments are unsatisfactory (Rutter 1974). In the first place, critical periods can only be studied when there are major environmental changes. Psychosocial disadvantages tend to be very persistent, and the continuities in development will necessarily be influenced by continuities in deprivation. In the second place, the effects of environmental change at age 2, after 2 years of deprivation, and environmental change at age 12, after 12 years of deprivation, are not at all comparable. In no way do comparisons of these effects provide a test of critical periods. In the third place, therapeutic interventions in later childhood mostly consist of talking about adapting to disadvantage—only very rarely do they actually involve complete changes of environment. Little is to be gained by considering such arguments. Instead, we have to focus on direct investigations of environmental change at different ages.

Intellectual development.—The first question with respect to intellectual and language development is whether an environment which improves only in middle or later childhood leads to major gains. The evidence is unequivocal that it does. This is most dramatically shown by the achievement of normal intelligence in severely deprived children who have been rescued from their appalling circumstances only at the age of 6 or 7 years (Davis 1947; Koluchova 1972, 1976). Thus, in the Koluchova twins an IQ in the 40s at age 7 increased to 100 at age 14. Dennis (1973) found an increase of some 30 points in Lebanese orphans moved from a poor to a better institution at age 6; and Kagan (1976) found differences held to imply considerable cognitive gains between 4 and 8 years of age in his Guatemalan study. Even later improvements were shown by Genie, who was not removed from her appallingly deprived environment until age 13 (Curtiss 1977). When discovered she was incontinent, without language, and able to walk only with difficulty, and she had a nonverbal mental age of less than 5 years.

■257

Child Development, 1979, vol. 50, pp. 283–305

Four years later Genie still had many problems, but she was talking in phrases and had a nonverbal mental age of 11 years. Less dramatically, Swedish studies have shown that continued schooling in late adolescence also leads to IQ gains (Harnqvist 1968; Husen 1951). It is quite clear that major environmental improvements in middle childhood can lead to substantial increases in IQ.

The second question is whether good experiences in the early years can protect children from the ill effects of later disadvantages. The evidence suggests that they cannot. Thus, educational enrichment programs in the preschool years lead to only limited or temporary benefits if the children continue in a disadvantaged environment. Furthermore, as Fogelman and Goldstein (1976) showed, children whose families go down the social scale during their middle school years fall in IQ.

The third question is whether environmental improvements in early childhood have a greater effect than similar improvements in later childhood. The evidence on this point is limited, but it suggests that they may. Thus, Dennis (1973), Goldfarb (1943), and Tizard and Hodges (1978) have all found that later-adopted children had lower IQs than children adopted in infancy. It is difficult to rule out biases due to selective placement, but it seems that the IQ gains for children adopted in middle childhood were less than for those adopted when younger. It should be appreciated that this does not necessarily indicate a real age difference in environmental effects on intellectual growth. First, the duration of deprivation is not comparable. By definition, the late-adopted children had been deprived for longer, and the lesser gains could simply be a function of that fact. Second, the amount and character of parent-child interaction in middle childhood is very different from that in the preschool years. It may be that the lesser intellectual gains in older late-adopted children were simply due to the fact that they had less opportunity for interacting with their parents.

The issues are by no means entirely resolved. However, what is clear is that children's intellectual development is sensitive to environmental change in both later and earlier childhood. Whether the early years have more effect remains uncertain, but if they do it is only a relative difference and not a qualitative distinction due to a critical period of development.

Socialization.—Much the same questions apply to social development. Again there is good evidence from studies of late-adopted children that environmental improvement in middle or later childhood leads to marked social and behavioral improvement (see Kadushin 1970; Rathbun, Di Virgilio, & Waldfogel 1958; Rathbun, McLaughlin, Bennett, & Garland 1965; Tizard & Hodges 1978). We have shown the same in our studies of children from severely disturbed homes who later experience a more harmonious family environment (Rutter 1971, in press–a).

Clearly, too, a good home in the early years does not prevent damage from psychosocial stresses later. This is shown, for example, by the links between bereavement or other losses in adult life and depression (Brown, Bhrolchain, & Harris 1975; Parkes 1964). Psychosocial development is influenced by environmental changes at any stage in the child's life.

Three key questions remain. First, there is the issue of whether, in general, environmental effects are greater in the early years than in later childhood. Actually, this is not a very sensible question, as the answer is likely to depend on the kinds of stresses invloved. Clearly, there are age effects with some. For example, young children are much more likely to respond adversely to hospital admission (see Rutter 1972). However, it is very dubious whether this applies generally. Thus, immediate grief reactions following bereavement are more common in adolescence (Rutter 1966).

The second question is whether certain experiences have to occur in the early years for normal development to proceed. The most likely candidate for this critical-period notion is the initial formation of selective attachments. Unfortunately, the evidence is meager, but the best data are provided by Tizard and Hodges's (1978) study of late-adopted children. Two main findings emerge from their work. First, even children adopted after the age of 4 years usually developed deep relationships with their adoptive parents. As this was so for children who had not been closely attached to anyone while they were in the institution, it is evident that first bonds can develop as late as 4–6 years. Second, however, and in spite of this, the late-adopted children showed the same social and attentional problems in school as those who had remained in the institutions. It may be that, although attachments can still develop after infancy, fully normal social development is nevertheless dependent on early bonding. As the children are only 8 years old, it is still too early to know whether this is so. However, the evidence is consistent with the possibility of a sensitive period for optimal early socialization.

The third question is whether acute and transient stresses in early childhood can have long-lasting effects on psychological development. Douglas's (1975) findings from the British National Survey raised this possibility with respect to hospital admission. However, both his study and that of Quinton and Rutter (1976) showed no long-term sequelae following single hospital admissions of less than a week. This link with later disorder in both studies applied to multiple or recurrent admissions. The findings have important practical implications, but their theoretical interpretation is made more difficult by the fact that recurrent admission is often associated with chronic psychosocial disadvantage. It may be concluded that single isolated stresses in early life only rarely lead to long-term disorder, that multiple acute stresses more often do so, and that long-term damage is most likely when multiple acute stresses arise against a background of chronic disadvantage.

Intergenerational Cycles

One issue, not discussed at all in the 1972 review, which has come into recent prominence is that of intergenerational cycles of disadvantage—that is, whether deprivation in one generation can lead to problems in the next. The topic is an immense one, and, as it has recently been extensively reviewed (Rutter & Madge 1976), it will not be discussed here.

Childhood experiences and parenting behavior.—However, one special category requires mention: the connections between experiences during childhood and parenting behavior during adult life. Several studies (see Rutter & Madge 1976) have shown that people who were brought up in unhappy or disrupted homes are more likely to have illegitimate children, to become teenage mothers, to make unhappy marriages, and to divorce. Thus, Illsley and Thompson (1961), in their study of 3,000 Aberdeen women having their first baby, found that those who had themselves been illegitimate or whose parents had divorced or separated were twice as likely as other women to have an illegitimate child or a prenuptial conception. Crellin, Pringle, and West (1971) noted much the same in the National Child Development Study. Moreover, a variety of studies (Gurin, Veroff, & Feld 1960; Jonsson 1967; Langer & Michael 1963; Waller & Hill 1951) have shown

that people whose parents were unhappily married are more likely themselves to show poor marital adjustment or to have marriages which end in divorce. Meier's (1965, 1966) follow-up study of former foster children indicated rates of marriage breakdown several times those in the general population.

Furthermore, a variety of investigations (see Spinetta & Rigler 1972) have found that parents who batter their children tend to have had a seriously disturbed upbringing themselves, often associated with neglect, rejection, or violence. This has been demonstrated in studies from a variety of countries, including England (e.g., Gibbens & Walker 1956; Scott 1973; Smith 1975), Ireland (Lukianowicz 1971), and the United States of America (Parke & Collmer 1975; Steele & Pollock 1968). The links are quite strong in that at least half and probably some three-quarters of battering parents have experienced an unhappy, rejecting, cruel, or violent upbringing. Even so, a substantial minority do not have this adverse background, and a few seem to have had quite unexceptionable childhoods. Also, it is necessary to recognize that the links are far stronger looking back than they are looking forward. That is to say, although more battering parents come from unhappy, affectionless, and sometimes violent homes, it is likely that only a tiny minority of youngsters from such homes go on to abuse their children physically. Moreover, in that many battering parents show abnormalities of personality or emotional disorder, it remains uncertain how far the links concern these general problems and how far they concern specific difficulties in parenting. Clearly there are important links between childhood experiences and parenting behavior, although further research is required to determine both the strength of the associations and the mechanisms involved.

Three studies should be mentioned in this connection. Frommer and O'Shea (1973a, 1937b) were the first workers to relate childhood experiences to direct measurement of patterns of parental care during the infancy period. They found that women reared in disrupted homes were more likely to prop up their 2-month-old babies to feed themselves, and more of the deprived mothers became pregnant again during the year after delivery. Wolkind, Hall, and Pawlby (1977) have also studied the parenting patterns of women from broken families using interview measures together with sophisticated techniques for observing mother-child interaction. They found that these women who had had disadvantaged childhoods interacted

■259

Child Development, 1979, vol. 50, pp. 283–305

less with their 4-month-old infants and were less likely to see them as individuals in their own right.

Quinton's (Note 9) studies have focused more specifically on the nature of the childhood experiences likely to lead to difficulties in parenting. He compared the backgrounds of parents who have had a child taken into care for the second time with those of a general-population sample of similar social status. Far more of the fathers and mothers with children in care had had multiple chronic adverse experiences in childhood—often associated with overt psychiatric problems. However, it was not just a matter of stresses in childhood. The parents with children in care, unlike the controls, had failed to move out of stress situations. Two factors seemed crucial—they bore children in their teens and they married (or cohabited with) someone from a similarly disadvantaged background. The findings point to the need to study the factors which determine how parents bring up their children.

Parenting

For years clinicians have been urging parents to deal with their children in this way or that, but very little attention has been paid to the issue of what influences parental behavior. Five main variables have now come to the fore. First, as already mentioned, there is the important factor of the parents' own childhood experiences. Second, as the elegant studies of Klaus, Kennell, Leiderman, and their colleagues (see Kennell, Trause, & Klaus 1975; Klaus, Jerauld, Kreger, McAlpine, Steffa, & Kennell 1972; Leiderman & Seashore 1975) have demonstrated, events in the postnatal period may be influential. It has been found that mothers who are separated from their babies in the neonatal period are less confident and less competent in some aspects of mothering during the subsequent months. Early physical contact seemed to foster closer physical relationships and increased communication later. However, the findings are contradictory regarding the persistence of these effects. Rather long-lasting changes in mother-infant interaction were found by Klaus and Kennell in their groups of socially disadvantaged mothers. On the other hand, the effects were much more transitory in the studies by Leiderman and Seashore (1975) and Whiten (1977). It seems unlikely that these events in

the neonatal period have an inevitable lasting impact on mother-child relationships, but if early stresses are combined with persisting disadvantage the damage may be enduring.

It has been suggested that these early days after birth constitute a sensitive period for the development of maternal attachment (Hales, Lozoff, Sosa, & Kennell 1977; Kennell et al. 1975).[2] Data are so far lacking to test this hypothesis, but at first sight it seems implausible—if only because adoptive parents usually develop close relationships with their children in spite of lack of neonatal contact. Of course, that in no way diminishes the need to allow parents to have close contact with their newborn children, but it does raise queries about the mechanisms involved. It may be that the damage comes from the effect of being denied access (rather than just not having contact), of the fears engendered by having a baby placed in special care, and of restraints placed by a hospital environment on spontaneous interactions.

The third influence on parenting comes from the child himself, as Richard Bell has emphasized (Bell 1968, 1971, 1974). There is now considerable evidence that how adults speak to children is affected by the verbal skills of the children with whom they interact (Pratt, Bumstead, & Raynes 1976; Siegel & Harkins 1963; Snow & Ferguson 1977; Spradlin & Rosenberg 1964; Gardner, Note 10). Osofsky and O'Connell (1972) showed that experimental manipulation of children's dependency altered parental behavior. Neonatal characteristics have also been found to influence parental responses (Brown & Bateman 1978; Levy 1958; Osofsky & Danzger 1974). The sex of the infant, too, may be important. Thus, socially isolated monkeys tend to become rejecting and indifferent mothers, but they are much more likely to physically abuse male infants (Ruppenthal et al. 1976).

The fourth influence on parenting is the very experience of bringing up children. Several studies (Clausen 1966; Hilton 1967; Lasko 1954; Rothbart 1971) have shown that parents respond differently to their second child than they do to their firstborn. With their second child they tend to be more relaxed, more consistent, and less punitive. Even more remarkable are the Harlow studies of rhesus monkeys subjected to appalling social isolation in early life. When adult they showed grossly abnormal sex-

---

[2] These findings have often been considered in terms of the implication for parent-infant bonding or attachment. There may be such implications, but so far the studies have not included any specific measures of bonding or selective attachment.

ual behavior and were rejecting or indifferent parents of their firstborn. However, some became more maternal during the postpartum period and were much better mothers of their second and subsequent babies (Harlow & Suomi 1971). It appears that later experiences with young monkeys can do something to ameliorate the damage done by early social isolation (Novak & Harlow 1975; Suomi, Harlow, & Novak 1974).

The fifth influence on parenting is the wider social environment. In general-population studies of families of 10-year-old children, Rutter and Quinton (1977) found that marital discord and maternal depression were much more common among working-class women living in inner-city areas. The particular strains of child rearing for women of low social status have been well demonstrated by Brown and his colleagues (Brown et al. 1975). It remains unclear why inner-city life should inflict such stresses on families and on parenting, but it is evident that the wider social environment does indeed have an important impact.

Invulnerability

The final issue to be discussed in this paper is that of invulnerability, or why children do not succumb to deprivation or disadvantage.

All studies of deprived or disadvantaged children have noted wide variations in response. Even with the most terrible homes and the most stressful experiences, some individuals come through unscathed and seem to have a stable, healthy personality development (Rutter, in press-a). This is an old and well-established observation, but it is only in the last few years that we have begun to meet the challenge and ask why. What is different about the children who rise above the tide of disadvantage? What are the protective factors? What are the ameliorating circumstances? At the moment, very few answers to these questions are available. However, there has been a recent upsurge of interest in the problem, and over the next decade this is likely to be a major growth area in the field of research into deprivation. Here there is space to consider modifying variables in relation to only one aspect of the subject. Family discord and disharmony have been selected, as data are available from a series of epidemiological studies. Protective factors may be considered under five headings: multiplicity of stresses, changed circumstances, factors in the child, factors in the family, and factors outside the home.

Multiplicity of stresses.—The first very striking finding is that single isolated chronic stresses carry no appreciable psychiatric risk. In a general-population study of families of 10-year-olds, Rutter, Yule, Quinton, Rowlands, Yule, and Berger (1975) identified six family variables (including marital discord), all of which were strongly and significantly associated with child psychiatric disorder. Then families which had one, but only one, of these risk factors were separated out. None of these risk factors, when they occurred in isolation, was associated with disorder in the children; the risk was no higher than that for children without any family stresses. However, when any two stresses occurred together, the risk went up no less than fourfold. With three and four concurrent stresses, the risk went up several times further still. It is clear that the combination of chronic stresses provided very much more than an additive effect. There was an interactive effect such that the risk which attended several concurrent stresses was much more than the sum of the effects of the stresses considered individually. Brown et al. (1975) found much the same for vulnerability factors and depression in adults.

This effect by which the presence of one stress potentiates the damage caused by another has been noted in several other circumstances. For example, it was found that children from a chronically deprived home background were more likely to be adversely affected by recurrent admission to hospital (Quinton & Rutter 1976). The same applies to the interaction of biological and social factors. Thus, over a decade ago, Drillien (1964) noticed that the effect of low birth weight on intelligence was most marked in children who also had the added disadvantage of poor social circumstances. Sameroff and Chandler (1975) have emphasized the same interactive effect with more recent data. This was also shown in the follow-up study of Kauai children (Werner, Bierman, & French 1971; Werner & Smith 1977).

However, it is important to appreciate that there are also transactional effects, whereby one stress (biological or social) actually increases the likelihood of occurrence of others. Thus, children from deprived homes were twice as likely to have recurrent admissions to hospital (Quinton & Rutter 1976). The presence of chronic stresses increased the rate of occurrence of multiple acute stresses. This is an important issue, considered further below.

Change in circumstances.—The next issue

■261

Child Development, 1979, vol. 50, pp. 283–305

concerns the effect of a change in family circumstances. To what extent are children better off if family stresses diminish or cease? The benefits of an improved environment in middle or late childhood were noted when discussing critical periods. The matter has been examined by studying children who had been separated from their parents in early childhood as a result of family discord or family problems (Rutter 1971, in press–a). Within this group of children, all of whom had experienced severe early stresses, those who were still in homes characterized by discord and disharmony were compared with those for whom things had improved and who were now in harmonious, happy homes. It was evident that disorders were very much less frequent when discord had ceased. A change for the better in family circumstances was associated with a marked reduction in psychiatric risk for the child.

Factors in the child.—Factors in the child which are known to be important in modifying responses to deprivation or disadvantage include the child's sex, temperament, and genetic background.

It is well known that males are more vulnerable than females to all manner of physical stresses and hazards (see Rutter 1970). It now appears that to some extent this male weakness also applies to psychosocial stresses. This is most obvious with respect to family discord and disharmony, which consistently have been found to have a greater association with conduct disorders in boys (Rutter 1970; Wolkind & Rutter 1973). However, this greater vulnerability of the male does not apply to all forms of deprivation or disadvantage. Thus, it has not been found with an institutional upbringing (Wolkind 1974). It should also be noted that the presence of overt brain damage seems to equalize vulnerability between boys and girls (Rutter 1977a; Rutter, Graham, & Yule 1970).

The child's temperament is also important. Using interview measurement techniques based on the Thomas, Chess, and Birch (1968; Thomas, Birch, Chess, Hertzig, & Korn 1963) approach, it has been found that children who showed the features of low regularity, low malleability, negative mood, and low fastidiousness were the ones most likely to develop a psychiatric disorder (Graham, Rutter, & George 1973). The presence of at least two of these adverse temperamental features increased the psychiatric risk during the next 4 years threefold. Part of the reason why temperamental adversity put the child at increased risk was to

be found in the transactional effect with parental criticism (Rutter 1978b). Children with adverse temperamental features were twice as likely as other children to be the target of parental criticism. Thus, in discordant and quarrelsome homes a child's temperament protected him or put him at risk by virtue of its influence on parent-child interaction. Even when there was marked disharmony in the home, the temperamentally easy child tended to escape much of the flak.

Third, there may be a heredity-environment interaction. This was suggested by the finding that the effects of marital discord on the child were most marked when the parent had a life-long personality disorder (Rutter 1971). However, genetic and nongenetic factors are better differentiated by adoption studies. For example, Hutchings and Mednick (1974), using a cross-fostering design, showed that criminality in children was most common when both the biological and the adoptive fathers had a crime record. The rate was increased to a lesser extent if only the biological father was criminal but not at all if only the adoptive father was. The implication is that genetic factors make a child more vulnerable to adverse environmental influences which have little impact on children who are not genetically susceptible. Crowe's (1974) data showed the same. Of course, as with all these leads on factors leading to vulnerability or invulnerability, the findings need to be replicated (particularly as the findings are based on small numbers, with some of the differences falling short of statistical significance). However, all the pointers at the moment are in the direction of a fluid view of development in which hereditary and environmental influences not only interact but also alter each other in transactional fashion as growth proceeds (see Rutter 1976).

At the moment, information is lacking on the value of children's coping skills in relation to family discord. However, the possibility that these may be important is raised by the finding from Stacey, Dearden, Pill, and Robinson (1970) that children who had had brief, graded, happy separation experiences were less likely than other children to be disturbed by hospital admission. Certainly, research attention needs to be paid to the possibility of learned coping skills which may help protect a child against the stresses of a depriving or disadvantaged environment.

Factors in the family.—Up to now almost all investigations of the family have concentrated on what goes wrong, and almost no attention has been paid to positive or protective effects. However, there are a few leads. It has been found (Rutter 1971, 1978a) that a good relationship with one parent serves to protect children brought up in an otherwise discordant, unhappy home. Children with one good relationship were less likely to develop conduct disorders than other children in similar homes whose relationships with both parents were poor. The few relevant findings from other studies are also consistent with the protective effect of a good relationship with a parental figure (Pringle & Bossio 1960; Pringle & Clifford 1962; Conway, Note 11; Wolkind, Note 12). However, a recent prospective study of children's behavior during the 2 years following parental divorce (Hetherington, Cox, & Cox, Note 1) has indicated that the relationship must be both a particularly good one and also one with a parent currently living with the child in order for there to be a significant buffering effect. Robins, West, and Herjanic (1975) found that black children living in broken homes of low social status were less likely to drop out of school if brought up by grandparents. In these circumstances, the extended family appeared to provide continuity and support in an otherwise unstable situation. Wilson (1974) also noted that careful supervision of children in multiple-problem families was associated with a reduced risk of delinquency.

At the moment these findings provide no more than a few scattered pointers. The mechanisms involved are ill understood and, in any case, are probably varied. What is important, however, is that even in the worst family circumstances it appears that a few "good" factors can do much to balance the serious maladaptive and disruptive influences.

Factors outside the home.—Last, there are protective factors outside the home. First, there is the impact of schooling. In our London studies we found that some schools were much more successful than others in helping children to develop normally without emotional or behavioral problems (Rutter 1977b; Rutter, Maughan, Mortimore, Ouston, & Smith, in press; Rutter, Yule, Quinton, Rowlands, Yule, & Berger 1975). Children from disadvantaged and discordant homes were less likely to develop problems if they attended better-functioning schools. For obvious reasons, this protective effect was most marked in relation to children's behavior at school. However, it did seem that, to some extent, good experiences at school could mitigate stresses experienced within the home.

A variety of other investigations in other areas have similarly indicated that there are major differences between schools in rates of absenteeism, behavioral disturbance, delinquency, and even employment after leaving schooling (see Rutter et al., in press). Moreover, it has been shown that these differences are not artifacts of selective intake; they do indeed reflect a school influence. However, a well-functioning school is not primarily a matter of buildings, size, or finance (see Rutter & Madge 1976). Rather, it is something about the school as a social institution. It appears that the crucial features include setting appropriately high expectations, good group management, effective feedback to the children with ample use of praise, the setting of good models of behavior by the teachers, pleasant working conditions, and giving pupils positions of trust and responsibility (Rutter et al., in press).

As far as other factors outside the home are concerned, the most obvious is the area in which families live. Much higher rates of psychiatric disorder have been found among families living in inner-city areas than among those living in small towns or in the countryside (Rutter, Cox, Tupling, Berger, & Yule 1975). This finding has been recently replicated in Oslo (Lavik 1977). It is important now to identify what stresses are involved in living in inner-city areas. However, it is at least as important to identify what makes some cities relatively free of these stress effects. Several investigations have found industrial towns and cities with quite low rates of disorder (Johnson, in press; Rutter 1967). We need to find out what makes them different.

In summary, on this topic of why children do not succumb to deprivation, it is beginning to be clear that ameliorating or protective factors can do much to aid normal development even in the worst circumstances. So far, knowledge on these factors is extremely limited, but if it could be increased it is likely that it would have very substantial policy, preventive, and therapeutic implications.

Conclusions

In conclusion, the last 6 years have seen the continuing accumulation of evidence showing the importance of deprivation and disadvantage as influences on children's psychological development. Bowlby's (1951) original arguments on that score have been amply confirmed. However, as in 1972, it is now very clear that deprivation involves a most heterogenous group

■263

Child Development, 1979, vol. 50, pp. 283–305

of adversities which operate through several quite different psychological mechanisms. Thus, insofar as deprivation is a causal factor, the acute distress syndrome sometimes shown after admission to hospital or to a residential nursery is probably due in large part to an interference with attachment behavior; intellectual retardation is a function of a lack of adequate meaningful experiences; conduct disorders are in part a response to family discord and disturbed interpersonal relationships, and affectionless psychopathy may be a consequence of abnormal early bonding. New research has confirmed that, although an important stress, separation is not the crucial factor in most varieties of deprivation. Investigations have also demonstrated the importance of a child's relationship with people other than his mother. Most important of all, there has been the repeated finding that many children are not damaged by deprivation.

The old issue of critical periods of development and the crucial importance of the early years has been reopened and reexamined. The evidence is unequivocal that experiences at all ages have an impact. However, it may be that the first few years do have a special importance for bond formation and social development.

New issues have also come to the fore in the last 6 years. Those which are particularly likely to continue to influence our thinking and our practical policies are: first, a focus on the reciprocal nature of parent-child interaction and on the process by which parent-child relationships develop; second, a concern with the links between childhood experiences and parenting behavior; third, an appreciation of the importance of factors outside the home (both in terms of ecological influences on family functioning and the crucial impact of experiences at school on child development); and fourth, an attempt to study invulnerability and the factors which protect children and enable them to develop normally in spite of stress and disadvantage. The issue of maternal deprivation continues to be a source of fruitful new findings, new concepts, and new approaches.

Reference Notes

1. Hetherington, E. M.; Cox, M.; & Cox, R. Family interaction and the social, emotional and cognitive development of children following divorce. Paper presented at the Symposium on the Family: Setting Priorities, Washington, D.C., May 17–20, 1978.
2. Dixon, P. Paper in preparation, 1978.
3. Heber, R. Rehabilitation of families at risk for mental retardation: a progress report. Madison, Wis.: Rahabilitation Research and Training Center in Mental Retardation, 1971.
4. Heber, R.; Garber, H.; Harrington, S.; Hoffman, C.; & Falender, C. Rehabilitation of families at risk for mental retardation: December progress report. Madison: University of Wisconsin, 1972.
5. Bronfenbrenner, U. Is early intervention effective? A report on the longitudinal evaluations of pre-school programs. Bethesda, Md.: Office of Child Development, U.S. Department of Health, Education, and Welfare, 1974.
6. Clarke-Stewart, K. A. The father's impact on mother and child. Paper presented to the Society for Research in Child Development, New Orleans, March 1977.
7. Stevens, A. Attachment and polymatric rearing: a study of attachment formation, separation anxiety and fear of strangers in infants reared by multiple mothering in an institutional setting. Unpublished D.M. thesis, Oxford University, 1975.
8. Goldberger, A. Follow up notes on the children from Bulldog Bank. Unpublished manuscript, 1972. (Available from Hampstead Child Therapy Clinic, London.)
9. Quinton, D. Paper in preparation, 1978.
10. Gardner, J. Three aspects of childhood autism: mother-child interactions, autonomic responsivity, and cognitive functioning. Unpublished Ph.D. thesis, University of Leicester, 1977.
11. Conway, E. S. The institutional care of children: a case history. Unpublished Ph.D. thesis, University of London, 1957.
12. Wolkind, S. N. Children in care: a psychiatric study. Unpublished M.D. thesis, University of London, 1971.

References

Ainsworth, M. D. S. The effects of maternal deprivation: a review of findings and controversy in the context of research strategy. In *Deprivation of maternal care: a reassessment of its effects.* (Public Health Papers, No. 14.) Geneva: World Health Organization, 1962.

Ainsworth, M. D. S. *Infancy in Uganda: infant care and the growth of attachment.* Baltimore: Johns Hopkins Press, 1967.

Ainsworth, M. D. S. The development of infant-mother attachment. In B. M. Caldwell & H. N. Ricciuti (Eds.), *Review of child development research.* Vol. **3.** Chicago: University of Chicago Press, 1973.

Ainsworth, M. D. S.; Bell, S. M.; & Stayton, D. J. Infant-mother attachment and social develop-

264■

ment: socialization as a product of reciprocal responsiveness to signals. In M. P. M. Richards (Ed.), *The integration of a child into a social world*. Cambridge: Cambridge University Press, 1974.

Ainsworth, M. D. S., & Wittig, B. A. Attachment and exploratory behaviour of one year olds in a strange situation. In B. M. Foss (Ed.), *Determinants of infant behaviour*. Vol. 4. London: Methuen, 1969.

Arsenian, J. M. Young children in an insecure situation. *Journal of Abnormal and Social Psychology*, 1943, **38**, 225–249.

Bell, R. Q. A reinterpretation of the direction of effects in studies of socialization. *Psychological Review*, 1968, **75**, 81–95.

Bell, R. Q. Stimulus control of parent or caretaker behavior by offspring. *Developmental Psychology*, 1971, **4**, 63–72.

Bell, R. Q. Contributions of human infants to care giving and social interaction. In Lewis & Rosenblum 1974.

Bell, S. M., & Ainsworth, M. D. S. Infant crying and and maternal responsiveness. *Child Development*, 1972, **43**, 1171–1190.

Blehar, M. C.; Lieberman, A. F.; & Ainsworth, M. D. S. Early face-to-face interaction and its relation to later infant-mother attachment. *Child Development*, 1977, **48**, 182–194.

Bowlby, J. *Maternal care and mental health*. Geneva: World Health Organization, 1951.

Bowlby, J. *Attachment and loss*. Vol. **1**. *Attachment*. London: Hogarth, 1969.

Bowlby, J. *Attachment and loss*. Vol. **2**. *Separation, anxiety and anger*. London: Hogarth, 1973.

Bradley, R. H., & Caldwell, B. M. Early home environment and changes in mental test performance in children from 6 to 36 months. *Developmental Psychology*, 1976, **12**, 93–97.

Brazelton, T. B.; Tronick, E.; Adamson, L.; Als, H.; & Weise, S. Early mother-infant reciprocity. In R. Porter & M. O'Connor (Eds.), *Parent-infant interaction*. (CIBA Foundation Symposium 33, new series.) Amsterdam: Associated Scientific Publishers, 1975.

Brown, G. W.; Bhrolchain, M. N.; & Harris, T. Social class and psychiatric disturbance among women in an urban population. *Sociology*, 1975, **9**, 225–254.

Brown, J. V., & Bateman, R. Relationships of human mothers with their infants during the first year of life: effects of prematurity. In R. W. Bell & W. P. Smotherman (Eds.), *Maternal influences and early behavior*. Holliswood, N.Y.: Spectrum, 1978.

Cairns, R. B. Development, maintenance, and extinction of social attachment behavior in sheep.

Journal of Comparative Physiology and Psychology, 1966, **62**, 298–306.

Cairns, R. B. Attachment and dependency: a psychobiological and social learning synthesis. In Gewirtz 1972.

Cairns, R. B. Beyond social attachment: the dynamics of interactional development. In T. Alloway, P. Pliner, & L. Krames (Eds.), *Advances in the study of communication and affect*. Vol. **3**. New York: Plenum, 1977.

Clarke, A. M., & Clarke, A. D. B. (Eds.). *Early experience: myth and evidence*. London: Open Books, 1976.

Clarke-Stewart, K. A. Interactions between mothers and their young children: characteristics and consequences. *Monographs of the Society for Research in Child Development*, 1973, **38**(6–7, Serial No. 153).

Clausen, J. A. Family structure, socialization and personality. In L. W. Hoffman & M. Hoffman (Eds.), *Review of child development research*. Vol. **2**. New York: Russell Sage, 1966.

Coates, B.; Anderson, E. P.; & Hartup, W. W. Interrelations in the attachment behavior of human infants. *Developmental Psychology*, 1972, **6**, 218–230.

Cohen, L. J. The operational definition of human attachment. *Psychological Bulletin*, 1974, **81**, 107–217.

Cohen, L. J., & Campos, J. J. Father, mother and stranger as elicitors of attachment behaviors in infancy. *Developmental Psychology*, 1974, **10**, 146–154.

Condon, W. S., & Sander, L. W. Speech: interactional participation and language acquisition. *Science*, 1974, **183**, 99–101.

Corter, C. Infant attachment. In B. Foss (Ed.), *New perspectives in child devlopment*. Harmondsworth, Middlesex: Penguin, 1974.

Corter, C. M. A comparison of the mother's and a stranger's control over the behavior of infants. *Child Development*, 1973, **44**, 705–713.

Cox, F. N., & Campbell, D. Young children in a new situation with and without their mothers. *Child Development*, 1968, **39**, 123–131.

Crellin, E.; Pringle, M. L. K.; & West, P. *Born illegitimate: social and educational implications*. Slough, Buckinghamshire: NFER, 1971.

Crowe, R. R. An adoption study of antisocial personality. *Archives of General Psychiatry*, 1974, **31**, 785–791.

Curtiss, S. *Genie: a psycholinguistic study of a modern-day "wild child."* New York: Academic Press, 1977.

Davis, K. Final note on a case of extreme isolation. *American Journal of Sociology*, 1947, **52**, 432–437.

265

Dennis, W. *Children of the creche*. New York: Appleton-Century-Crofts, 1973.

Dollard, J., & Miller, N. E. *Personality and psychotherapy*. New York: McGraw-Hill, 1950.

Douglas, J. W. B. Early hospital admissions and later disturbances of behaviour and learning. *Developmental Medicine and Child Neurology*, 1975, **17**, 456–480.

Drillien, C. M. *Growth and development of the prematurely born infant*. London: Livingstone, 1964.

Dunn, J. Consistency and change in styles of mothering. In R. Porter & M. O'Connor (Eds.), *Parent-infant interaction*. (CIBA Foundation Symposium 33, new series.) Amsterdam: Associated Scientific Publishers, 1975.

Eckerman, C. O.; Whatley, J. L.; & Katz, S. L. Growth of social play with peers during the second year of life. *Developmental Psychology*, 1975, **11**, 42–49.

Elardo, R.; Bradley, R. H.; & Caldwell, B. M. The relation of infants' home environment to mental test performance from six to thirty-six months: a longitudinal analysis. *Child Development*, 1975, **46**, 71–76.

Etzel, B. C., & Gewirtz, J. L. Experimental modification of caretaker-maintained high rate operant crying in a 6- and a 20-week infant (Infans tyrannotearus): extinction of crying with reinforcement of eye contact and smiling. *Journal of Experimental Child Psychology*, 1967, **5**, 303–313.

Fisch, R. O.; Bilek, M. K.; Deinard, A. S.; & Chang, P.-N. Growth, behavioral psychologic measurements of adopted children: the influences of genetic and socioeconomic factors in a prospective study. *Journal of Pediatrics*, 1976, **89**, 494–500.

Fogelman, K. R., & Goldstein, H. Social factors associated with changes in educational attainment between 7 and 11 years of age. *Educational Studies*, 1976, **2**, 95–109.

Freud, A. *The psycho-analytical treatment of children*. London: Imago, 1946.

Freud, A., & Dann, S. An experiment in group upbringing. *Psychoanalytic Study of the Child*, 1951, **6**, 127–168.

Frommer, E. A., & O'Shea, G. Antenatal identification of women liable to have problems in managing their infants. *British Journal of Psychiatry*, 1973, **123**, 149–156. (a)

Frommer, E. A., & O'Shea, G. The importance of childhood experience in relation to problems of marriage and family-building. *British Journal of Psychiatry*, 1973, **123**, 157–160. (b)

Garber, H., & Heber, F. R. The Milwaukee Project: indications of the effectiveness of early intervention in preventing mental retardation. In P. Mittler (Ed.), *Research to practice in mental retardation. Vol. 1. Care and intervention*. Baltimore: University Park, 1977.

Gewirtz, J. L. A learning analysis of the effects of normal stimulation, privation and deprivation on the acquisition of social motivation and attachment. In B. M. Foss (Ed.), *Determinants of infant behaviour*. London: Methuen, 1961.

Gewirtz, J. L. (Ed.). *Attachment and dependency*. Washington, D.C.: Winston, 1972.

Gewirtz, J. L., & Boyd, E. F. Mother-infant interaction and its study. In H. W. Reese (Ed.), *Advances in child development and behavior*. Vol. **11**. New York: Academic Press, 1976.

Gewirtz, J. L., & Boyd, E. F. Does maternal responding imply reduced infant crying? A critique of the 1972 Bell and Ainsworth report. *Child Development*, 1978, **48**, 1200–1207.

Gibbens, T. C. N., & Walker, A. *Cruel parents: case studies of prisoners convicted of violence towards children*. London: Institute for the Study and Treatment of Delinquency, 1956.

Goldfarb, W. The effects of early institutional care on adolescent personality. *Journal of Experimental Education*, 1943, **12**, 106–129.

Goldfarb, W. Emotional and intellectual consequences of psychologic deprivation in infancy: a revaluation. In P. H. Hoch & J. Zubin (Eds.), *Psychopathology of childhood*. New York: Grune & Stratton, 1955.

Graham, P.; Rutter, M.; & George, S. Temperamental characteristics as predictors of behavior disorders in children. *American Journal of Orthopsychiatry*, 1973, **43**, 328–339.

Gurin, G.; Veroff, J.; & Feld, S. *Americans and their mental health: a nationwide interview survey*. New York: Basic, 1960.

Hales, D. J.; Lozoff, B.; Sosa, R.; & Kennell, J. H. Defining the limits of the maternal sensitive period. *Developmental Medicine and Child Neurology*, 1977, **19**, 454–461.

Harlow, H. F. The nature of love. *American Psychologist*, 1958, **13**, 673–685.

Harlow, H. F. Age-mate or peer affectional systems. In D. S. Lehrman, R. A. Hinde, & E. Shaw (Eds.), *Advances in the study of behavior*. Vol. **2**. New York: Academic Press, 1969.

Harlow, H. F., & Harlow, M. K. Effects of various mother-infant relationships on rhesus monkey behaviours. In B. M. Foss (Ed.), *Determinants of infant behaviour*. Vol. **4**. London: Methuen, 1969.

Harlow, H. F., & Harlow, M. K. Psychopathology in monkeys. In H. D. Kimmel (Ed.), *Experimental psychopathology*. New York: Academic Press, 1971.

Harlow, H. F., & Harlow, M. K. The affectional systems. In A. Schrier, H. F. Harlow, & F. Stoll-

266 ∎

nitz (Eds.), *Behavior in non-human primates.* Vol. **2.** New York: Academic Press, 1972.

Harlow, H. F., & Suomi, S. J. Social recovery by isolation-reared monkeys. *Proceedings of the National Academy of Science,* 1971, **68,** 1534–1538.

Harlow, H. F., & Zimmermann, R. R. Affectional responses in the infant monkey. *Science,* 1959, **130,** 421–432.

Harnqvist, K. Relative changes in intelligence from 13 to 18. *Scandinavian Journal of Psychology,* 1968, **9,** 50–82.

Hartup, W. W. Two social worlds: family relations and peer relations. In Rutter 1979.

Hartup, W. W. Peer relations and the growth of social competence. In M. W. Kent & J. E. Rolf (Eds.), *The primary prevention of psychopathology.* Vol. **3.** *Promoting social competence and coping in children.* Hanover, N.H.: University Press of New England, in press.

Heathers, G. Emotional dependence and independence in nursery school play. *Journal of Genetic Psychology,* 1955, **87,** 37–57.

Heber, R., & Garber, H. Progress report II: an experiment in the prevention of cultural-familial retardation. In D. A. A. Primrose (Ed.), *Proceedings of the Third Congress of the International Association for the Scientific Study of Mental Deficiency.* Warsaw: Polish Medical Publishers, 1975.

Heinicke, C. M., & Westheimer, I. J. *Brief separations.* London: Longman, 1965.

Hilton, I. Differences in the behavior of mothers toward first and later-born children. *Journal of Personality and Social Psychology,* 1967, **7,** 282–290.

Hinde, R. A., & McGinnis, L. Some factors influencing the effect of temporary mother-infant separation: some experiments with rhesus monkeys. *Psychological Medicine,* 1977, **7,** 197–212.

Hinde, R. A., & Spencer-Booth, Y. Individual differences in the responses of rhesus monkeys to a period of separation from their mothers. *Journal of Child Psychology and Psychiatry,* 1970, **11,** 159–176.

Hinde, R. A., & Stevenson-Hinde, J. Towards understanding relationships: dynamic stability. In P. P. G. Bateson & R. A. Hinde (Eds.), *Growing points in ethology.* Cambridge: Cambridge University Press, 1976.

Hoffman, H. S., & Ratner, A. M. A reinforcement model of imprinting: implications for socialisation in monkeys and men. *Psychological Review,* 1973, **80,** 527–544.

Husen, T. The influence of schooling upon IQ. *Theoria,* 1951, **17,** 61–68.

Hutchings, B., & Mednick, S. A. Registered criminality in the adoptive and biological parents of registered male adoptees. In S. A. Mednick, F. Schulsinger, J. Higgins, & B. Bell (Eds.), *Genetics, environment and psychopathology.* Amsterdam: North-Holland, 1974.

Illsley, R., & Thompson, B. Women from broken homes. *Sociological Review,* 1961, **9,** 27–54.

Johnson, M. C. Social adjustment of junior school children in a South Wales town. *Journal of Child Psychology and Psychiatry,* in press.

Jonsson, G. Delinquent boys, their parents and grandparents. *Acta Psychiatric Scandinavica,* 1967, **43,** Suppl. 195.

Kadushin, A. *Adopting older children.* New York: Columbia University Press, 1970.

Kagan, J. Resilience and continuity in psychological development. In Clarke & Clarke 1976.

Kennell, J.; Trause, M. A.; & Klaus, M. H. Evidence for a sensitive period in the human mother. In R. Porter & M. O'Connor (Eds.), *Parent-infant interaction.* (CIBA Foundation Symposium 33, new series.) Amsterdam: Associated Scientific Publishers, 1975.

Kissel, S. Stress-reducing properties of social stimuli. *Journal of Personality and Social Psychology,* 1965, **2,** 378–384.

Klaus, M.; Jerauld, R.; Kreger, N.; McAlpine, W.; Steffa, M.; & Kennell, J. Maternal attachment—importance of the first post-partum days. *New England Journal of Medicine,* 1972, **286,** 460–463.

Koluchova, J. Severe deprivation in twins: a case study. *Journal of Child Psychology and Psychiatry,* 1972, **13,** 107–114.

Koluchova, J. The further development of twins after severe and prolonged deprivation: a second report. *Journal of Child Psychology and Psychiatry,* 1976, **17,** 181–188.

Kovach, J. K., & Hess, E. H. Imprinting: effects of painful stimulation on the following response. *Journal of Comparative and Physiological Psychology,* 1963, **56,** 461–464.

Lamb, M. E. The development of mother-infant and father-infant attachments in the second year of life. *Developmental Psychology,* 1977, **13,** 637–648. (a)

Lamb, M. E. Father-infant and mother-infant interaction in the first year of life. *Child Development,* 1977, **48,** 167–181. (b)

Lamb, M. E. Social interaction in infancy and the development of personality. In M. E. Lamb (Ed.), *Social and personality development.* New York: Holt, Rinehart & Winston, 1978.

Lamb, M. E. Father-infant relationships: their nature and importance. *Youth and Society,* in press. (a)

Lamb, M. E. Qualitative aspects of mother- and father-infant attachments. *Infant Behavior and Development,* in press. (b)

268 ▪

Lambert, L.; Essen, J.; & Head, J. Variations in behaviour ratings of children who have been in care. *Journal of Child Psychology and Psychiatry*, 1977, **18**, 335–346.

Langner, T. S., & Michael, S. T. *Life stress and mental health*. London: Collier-Macmillan, 1963.

Lasko, J. K. Parent behavior toward first and second children. *Genetic Psychology Monographs*, 1954, **49**, 96–137.

Lavik, N. Urban-rural differences in rates of disorder. In P. J. Graham (Ed.), *Epidemiological approaches in child psychiatry*. London: Academic Press, 1977.

Leiderman, P. H., & Seashore, M. J. Mother-infant neonatal separation: some delayed consequences. In R. Porter & M. O'Connor (Eds.), *Parent-infant interaction*. (CIBA Foundation Symposium 33, new series.) Amsterdam: Associated Scientific Publishers, 1975.

Levy, D. M. *Behavioral analysis: analysis of clinical observations of behavior as applied to mother-newborn relationships*. Springfield, Ill.: Charles C. Thomas, 1958.

Lewis, M., & Rosenblum, L. A. (Eds.). *The effect of the infant on its caregiver*. New York: Wiley, 1974.

Lorenz, K. [The establishment of the instinct concept. In *Studies in Animal and Human Behaviour*. Vol. 1.] (R. Martin, Trans.). London: Methuen, 1970. (Originally published 1937.)

Lukianowicz, N. Battered children. *Psychiatria Clinica (Basel)*, 1971, **4**, 257–280.

McCall, R. B.; Appelbaum, M. I.; & Hogarty, P. S. Developmental changes in mental performance. *Monographs of the Society for Research in Child Development*, 1973, **38**(3, Serial No. 150).

Maccoby, E. E., & Feldman, S. S. Mother-attachment and stranger reactions in the third year of life. *Monographs of the Society for Research in Child Development*, 1972, **37**(1, Serial No. 146).

Maccoby, E. E., & Masters, J. C. Attachment and dependency. In P. H. Mussen (Ed.), *Carmichael's manual of child psychology* (3d ed.). New York: Wiley, 1970.

Marchant, R.; Howlin, P.; Yule, W.; & Rutter, M. Graded change in the treatment of the behaviour of autistic children. *Journal of Child Psychology and Psychiatry*, 1974, **15**, 221–228.

Mason, W. A., & Berkson, G. Effects of maternal motility on the development of rocking and other behaviors in rhesus monkeys: a study with artificial mothers. *Developmental Psychobiology*, 1975, **8**, 197–211.

Matas, L.; Arend, R. A.; & Sroufe, L. A. Continuity of adaptation in the second year: the relationship between quality of attachment and later competence. *Child Development*, 1978, **49**, 547–556.

Meier, E. G. Current circumstances of former foster children. *Child Welfare*, 1965, **44**, 196.

Meier, E. G. Adults who were foster children. *Children*, 1966, **13**, 16–22.

Morgan, G. A., & Ricciuti, H. N. Infants' responses to strangers during the first year. In B. M. Foss (Ed.), *Determinants of infant behaviour*. Vol. **4**. London: Methuen, 1969.

Novak, M. A., & Harlow, H. F. Social recovery of monkeys isolated for the first year of life, I: Rehabilitation and therapy. *Developmental Psychology*, 1975, **11**, 453–465.

Osofsky, J. D., & Danzger, B. Relationships between neonatal characteristics and mother-infant interaction. *Developmental Psychology*, 1974, **10**, 124–130.

Osofsky, J. D., & O'Connell, E. J. Parent-child interaction: daughters' effects upon mothers' and fathers' behaviors. *Developmental Psychology*, 1972, **7**, 157–168.

Parke, R. D., & Collmer, C. W. Child abuse: an interdisciplinary analysis. In E. M. Hetherington (Ed.), *Review of child development research*. Vol. **5**. Chicago: University of Chicago Press, 1975.

Parkes, C. M. Recent bereavement as a cause of mental illness. *British Journal of Psychiatry*, 1964, **118**, 275–288.

Passman, R. H. Providing attachment objects to facilitate learning and reduce distress: effects of mothers and security blankets. *Developmental Psychology*, 1977, **13**, 25–28.

Passman, R. H., & Weisberg, P. Mothers and blankets as agents for promoting play and exploration by young children in a novel environment: the effects of social and nonsocial objects. *Developmental Psychology*, 1975, **11**, 170–177.

Patterson, F. G.; Bonvillian, J. D.; Reynolds, P. C.; & Maccoby, E. E. Mother and peer attachment under conditions of fear in rhesus monkeys (macaca mulatta). *Primates*, 1975, **16**, 75–81.

Power, M. J.; Ash, P. M.; Schoenberg, E.; & Sorey, E. C. Delinquency and the family. *British Journal of Social Work*, 1974, **4**, 13–38.

Pratt, M. W.; Bumstead, D. C.; & Raynes, N. V. Attendant staff speech to the institutionalized retarded: language use as a measure of the quality of care. *Journal of Child Psychology and Psychiatry*, 1976, **17**, 133–144.

Pringle, M. L. K. Rights of adults or needs of children? *Times Educational Supplement*, July 23, 1976.

Pringle, M. L. K., & Bossio, V. Early prolonged separations and emotional adjustment. *Journal of Child Psychology and Psychiatry*, 1960, **1**, 37–48.

Pringle, M. L. K., & Clifford, L. Conditions associated with emotional maladjustment among children in care. *Educational Review*, 1962, **14**, 112–123.

Quinton, D., & Rutter, M. Early hospital admissions and later disturbances of behaviour: an attempted replication of Douglas' findings. *Developmental Medicine and Child Neurology*, 1976, **18**, 447–459.

Rajeki, D. W.; Lamb, M. E.; & Obmascher, P. Toward a general theory of infantile attachment: a comparative review of aspects of the social bond. *Behavioral and Brain Sciences*, in press.

Rathbun, C.; Di Virgilio, L.; & Waldfogel, S. The restitutive process in children following radical separation from family and culture. *American Journal of Orthopsychiatry*, 1958, **28**, 408–415.

Rathbun, C.; McLaughlin H.; Bennett, O.; & Garland, J. A. Later adjustment of children following radical separation from family and culture. *American Journal of Orthopsychiatry*, 1965, **35**, 604–609.

Rheingold, H. L., & Eckerman, C. O. Fear of the stranger: a critical examination. In H. W. Reese (Ed.), *Advances in child development and behavior*. Vol. **8**. New York: Academic Press, 1973.

Robertson, J., & Robertson, J. Young children in brief separations: a fresh look. *Psychoanalytic Study of the Child*, 1971, **26**, 264–315.

Robins, L. N.; West, P. A.; & Herjanic, B. L. Arrests and delinquency in two generations: a study of black urban families and their children. *Journal of Child Psychology and Psychiatry*, 1975, **16**, 125–140.

Rosenblum, L. A., & Harlow, H. F. Approach-avoidance conflict in the mother surrogate situation. *Psychological Reports*, 1963, **12**, 83–85.

Rosenthal, M. K. Attachment and mother-infant interaction: some research impasses and a suggested change in orientation. *Journal of Child Psychology and Psychiatry*, 1973, **14**, 201–207.

Ross, H. S., & Goldman, B. D. Establishing new social relations in infancy. In T. Alloway, P. Pliner, & L. Krames (Eds.), *Advances in the study of communication and affect*. Vol. **3**. *Attachment behavior*. New York: Plenum, 1977.

Rothbart, M. K. Birth order and mother-child interaction in an achievement situation. *Journal of Personality and Social Psychology*, 1971, **17**, 113–120.

Ruppenthal, G. C.; Arling, G. L.; Harlow, H. F.; Sackett, G. P.; & Suomi, S. J. A 10-year perspective of motherless-mother monkey behavior. *Journal of Abnormal Psychology*, 1976, **85**, 341–349.

Rutter, M. *Children of sick parents: an environmental and psychiatric study* (Institute of Psychiatry Maudsley Monograph No. 16). London: Oxford University Press, 1966.

Rutter, M. A children's behaviour questionnaire for completion by teachers: preliminary findings. *Journal of Child Psychology and Psychiatry*, 1967, **8**, 1–11.

Rutter, M. Sex differences in children's responses to family stress. In E. J. Anthony & C. Koupernik (Eds.), *The child in his family*. New York: Wiley, 1970.

Rutter, M. Parent-child separation: psychological effects on the children. *Journal of Child Psychology and Psychiatry*, 1971, **12**, 233–260.

Rutter, M. *Maternal deprivation reassessed*. Harmondsworth, Middlesex: Penguin, 1972.

Rutter, M. Dimensions of parenthood: some myths and some suggestions. In Department of Health and Social Security Report, *The family in society: dimensions of parenthood*. London: HMSO, 1974.

Rutter, M. *Helping troubled children*. New York: Plenum, 1976.

Rutter, M. Brain damage syndromes in childhood: concepts and findings. *Journal of Child Psychology and Psychiatry*, 1977, **18**, 1–21. (a)

Rutter, M. Prospective studies to investigate behavioral change. In J. S. Strauss, H. M. Babigian, & M. Roff (Eds.), *The origins and course of psychopathology*. New York: Plenum, 1977. (b)

Rutter, M. Early sources of security and competence. In J. S. Bruner & A. Garton (Eds.), *Human growth and development*. London: Oxford University Press, 1978. (a)

Rutter, M. Family, area and school influences in the genesis of conduct disorders. In L. Hersov, M. Berger, & D. Shaffer (Eds.), *Aggression and antisocial behaviour in childhood and adolescence*. (Journal of Child Psychology and Psychiatry Book Series, No. 1). Oxford: Pergamon, 1978. (b)

Rutter, M. Attachment and the development of social relationships. In M. Rutter (Ed.), *Scientific foundations of developmental psychiatry*. London: Heinemann Medical, 1979.

Rutter, M. Protective factors in children's responses to stress and disadvantage. In M. W. Kent & J. E. Rolf (Eds.), *Primary prevention of psychopathology*. Vol. **3**. *Promoting social competence and coping in children*. Hanover, N.H.: University Press of New England, in press. (a)

Rutter, M. Separation experiences: a new look at an old topic. *Journal of Pediatrics*, in press. (b)

Rutter, M.; Cox, A.; Tupling, C.; Berger, M.; & Yule, W. Attainment and adjustment in two geographical areas, I: The prevalence of psychiatric disorder. *British Journal of Psychiatry*, 1975, **126**, 493–509.

Child Development, 1979, vol. 50, pp. 283–305

Rutter, M.; Graham, P.; & Yule, W. *A neuropsychiatric study in childhood.* (Clinics in Developmental Medicine, Nos. 35–36.) London: Spastics International Medical Publishers/Heinemann, 1970.

Rutter, M., & Madge, N. *Cycles of disadvantage: a review of research.* London: Heinemann, 1976.

Rutter, M.; Maughan, B.; Mortimore, P.; Ouston, J.; & Smith, A. *Secondary schools and their effects on children: 15,000 hours.* London: Open Books, 1979.

Rutter, M., & Quinton, D. Psychiatric disorder—ecological factors and concepts of causation. In H. McGurk (Ed.), *Ecological factors in human development.* Amsterdam: North-Holland, 1977.

Rutter, M.; Yule, B.; Quinton, D.; Rowlands, O.; Yule, W.; & Berger, M. Attainment and adjustment in two geographical areas, III: Some factors accounting for area differences. *British Journal of Psychiatry*, 1975, **126**, 520–533.

Salzen, E. A. Social attachment and a sense of security: a review. *Social Science Information*, 1978, **17**, 555–627.

Sameroff, A. J., & Chandler, M. J. Reproductive risk and the continuum of caretaking casualty. In F. D. Horowitz (Ed.), *Review of child development research.* Vol. **4.** Chicago: University of Chicago Press, 1975.

Sander, L. W. Comments on regulation and organisation in the early infant-caretaker system. In R. J. Robinson (Ed.), *Brain and early behaviour.* London: Academic Press, 1969.

Sander, L. W.; Stechler, G.; Burns, P.; & Julia, H. Early mother-infant interaction and twenty-four-hour patterns of activity and sleep. *Journal of the American Academy of Child Psychiatry*, 1970, **9**, 103–123.

Scarr, S., & Weinberg, R. A. IQ test performance of black children adopted by white families. *American Psychologist*, 1976, **31**, 726–739.

Schaffer, H. R . *The growth of sociability.* Harmondsworth, Middlesex: Penguin, 1971.

Schaffer, H. R., & Emerson, P. E. The development of social attachments in infancy. *Monograph of the Society for Research in Child Development*, 1964, **29**(3, Serial No. 94).

Schneirla, T. A. Aspects of stimulation and organization in approach/withdrawal processes underlying vertebrate behavioral development. In D. S. Lehrman, R. A. Hinde, & E. Shaw (Eds.), *Advances in the study of behavior.* Vol. **1.** New York and London: Academic Press, 1965.

Schwartz, J. Effects of peer familiarity on the behaviour of preschoolers in a novel situation. *Journal of Personality and Social Psychology*, 1972, **24**, 276–285.

Scott, J. P. Attachment and separation in dog and man: theoretical propositions. In H. R. Schaffer (Ed.), *The origins of human social relations.* London: Academic Press, 1971.

Scott, P. D. Fatal battered baby cases. *Medicine, Science and the Law*, 1973, **13**, 197–206.

Sears, R. R. Attachment, dependency and frustration. In Gewirtz 1972.

Seay, B.; Alexander, B. K.; & Harlow, H. F. Maternal behavior of socially deprived rhesus monkeys. *Journal of Abnormal Social Psychology*, 1964, **69**, 345–354.

Siegel, G. M., & Harkins, J. P. Verbal behavior of adults in two conditions with institutionalized retarded children. *Journal of Speech and Hearing Disorders*, 1963, **10**, 39–47. (Monograph)

Smith, S. M. *The battered child syndrome.* London: Butterworth, 1975.

Snow, C. E., & Ferguson, C. A. (Eds.), *Talking to children: language input and acquisition.* London: Cambridge University Press, 1977.

Solomon, R. L., & Corbit, J. D. An opponent-process theory of motivation, I: Temporal dynamics of affect. *Psychological Review*, 1974, **81**, 119–145.

Spelke, E.; Zelazo, P.; Kagan, J.; & Kotelchuck, M. Father interaction and separation protest. *Developmental Psychology*, 1973, **9**, 83–90.

Spinetta, J. J., & Rigler, D. The child-abusing parent: a psychological review. *Psychological Bulletin*, 1972, **77**, 296–304.

Spitz, R. A. Anaclitic depression. *Psychoanalytic Study of the Child*, 1946, **2**, 313–342.

Spradlin, J. E., & Rosenberg, S. Complexity of adult verbal behavior in a dyadic situation with retarded children. *Journal of Abnormal Social Psychology*, 1964, **68**, 694–698.

Sroufe, L. A., & Waters, E. Attachment as an organizational construct. *Child Development*, 1977, **48**, 1184–1199.

Stacey, M.; Dearden, R.; Pill, R.; & Robinson, D. *Hospitals, children and their families: the report of a pilot study.* London: Routledge & Kegan Paul, 1970.

Stayton, D. J., & Ainsworth, M. D. S. Individual differences in infant responses to brief, everyday separations as related to other infant and maternal behaviors. *Developmental Psychology*, 1973, **9**, 226–235.

Stayton, D. J.; Ainsworth, M. D. S.; & Main, M. B. Development of separation behavior in the first year of life: protest, following, and greeting. *Developmental Psychology*, 1973, **9**, 213–225.

Steele, B. F., & Pollock, C. B. A psychiatric study of parents who abuse infants and small children. In R. E. Helfer & C. H. Kempe (Eds.), *The battered child.* Chicago: University of Chicago Press, 1968.

Stern, D.; Jaffe, J.; Beebe, B.; & Bennett, S. L.

Vocalising in unison and in alternation: two modes of communication within the mother-infant dyad. *Annals of the New York Academy of Sciences*, 1975, **263**, 89–100.

Suomi, S. J. Adult male-infant interactions among monkeys living in nuclear families. *Child Development*, 1977, **48**, 1255–1270.

Suomi, S. J.; Harlow, H. F.; & Novak, M. A. Reversal of social deficits produced by isolation rearing in monkeys. *Journal of Human Evolution*, 1974, **3**, 527–534.

Thomas, A.; Birch, H. G.; Chess, S.; Hertzig, M. E.; & Korn, S. *Behavioral individuality in early childhood*. New York: New York University Press, 1963.

Thomas, A.; Chess, S.; & Birch, H. G. *Temperament and behaviour disorders in children*. New York: New York University Press, 1968.

Tizard, B. *Adoption: a second chance*. London: Open Books, 1977.

Tizard, B.; Cooperman, O.; Joseph, A.; & Tizard, J. Environmental effects on language development: a study of young children in long-stay residential nurseries. *Child Development*, 1972, **43**, 337–358.

Tizard, B., & Hodges, J. The effect of early institutional rearing on the development of eight-year-old children. *Journal of Child Psychology and Psychiatry*, 1978, **19**, 99–118.

Tizard, B., & Joseph, A. Cognitive development of young children in residential care: a study of children aged 24 months. *Journal of Child Psychology and Psychiatry*, 1970, **11**, 177–186.

Tizard, B., & Rees, J. A comparison of the effects of adoption, restoration to the natural mother, and continued institutionalization on the cognitive development of four-year-old children. *Child Development*, 1974, **45**, 92–99.

Tizard, B., & Rees, J. The effect of early institutional rearing on the behaviour problems and affectional relationships of four-year-old children. *Journal of Child Psychology and Psychiatry*, 1975, **16**, 61–74.

Tizard, J., & Tizard, B. The social development of two year old children in residential nurseries. In H. E. Schaffer (Ed.), *The origins of human social relations*. London: Academic Press, 1971.

Tracy, R. L.; Lamb, M. E.; & Ainsworth, M. D. S. Infant approach behavior as related to attachment. *Child Development*, 1976, **47**, 571–578.

Waller, W. W., & Hill, R. *The family: a dynamic interpretation*. New York: Dryden, 1951.

Wasz-Höckert, O.; Lind, J.; Vuorenkoski, V.; Partanen T.; & Valanne, E. *The infant cry: a spectrographic and auditory analysis*. (Clinics in Developmental Medicine, No. 29.) London: Heinemann/Spastics International Medical Publishers, 1968.

Werner, E. E.; Bierman, J. M.; & French, F. E. *The children of Kauai*. Honolulu: University of Hawaii Press, 1971.

Werner, E. E., & Smith, R. S. *Kauai's children come of age*. Honolulu: University of Hawaii Press, 1977.

West, D. J., & Farrington, D. P. *Who becomes delinquent?* London: Heinemann Educational, 1973.

West, D. J., & Farrington, D. P. *The delinquent way of life*. London: Heinemann Educational, 1977.

Whiten, A. Assessing the effects of perinatal events on the success of the mother-infant relationship. In H. R. Schaffer (Ed.), *Studies in mother-infant interaction*. London: Academic Press, 1977.

Wilson, H. Parenting in poverty. *British Journal of Social Work*, 1974, **4**, 241–254.

Wolff, P. H. The natural history of crying and other vocalisations in early infancy. In B. M. Foss (Ed.), *Determinants of infant behaviour*. Vol. **4**. London: Methuen, 1969.

Wolkind, S.; Hall, F.; & Pawlby, S. Individual differences in mothering behaviour: a combined epidemiological and observational approach. In P. J. Graham (Ed.), *Epidemiological approaches in child psychiatry*. London: Academic Press, 1977.

Wolkind, S., & Rutter, M. Children who have been "in care"—an epidemiological study. *Journal of Child Psychology and Psychiatry*, 1973, **14**, 97–105.

Wolkind, S. N. The components of "affectionless psychopathy" in institutionalised children. *Journal of Child Psychology and Psychiatry*, 1974, **15**, 215–220.

■271

Journal of Child Psychology and Psychiatry, 1985, vol. 26, pp. 683–704

FAMILY AND SCHOOL INFLUENCES ON COGNITIVE DEVELOPMENT

MICHAEL RUTTER

Institute of Psychiatry, London

272 ∎

Abstract—Family and school influences on cognitive development are reviewed in terms of the empirical research findings on (i) variations within the ordinary environment; (ii) family intervention studies; (iii) the effects of abnormal environments; (iv) extreme environmental conditions; (v) variations within the ordinary school environment; and (vi) preschool and school intervention studies. It is concluded that environmental effects on IQ are relatively modest within the normal range of environments, but that the effects of markedly disadvantageous circumstances are very substantial. Cognitive development is influenced both by direct effects on cognition and by indirect effects through alterations in self-concept, aspirations, attitudes to learning and styles of interaction with other people.

Keywords: Cognitive development, family influences, school effect, compulsory education

INTRODUCTION

FEW TOPICS have given rise to such prolonged controversy as that concerning the relative importance of genetic and environmental influences on intelligence. One might suppose that the immense literature on this issue would provide a wealth of data on the ways in which psychosocial factors serve to influence cognitive development. Unfortunately it does not. That is because most of the arguments have concerned estimates of the relative strength of genetic and environmental forces rather than *how* the latter operate.

It is not necessary here to discuss the findings on the heritability of intelligence as they have been reviewed extensively on many previous occasions (see, for example, Jencks, Smith, Acland, Bane, Cohen, Gintis, Heyns & Michelson, 1973; Rutter & Madge, 1976; Scarr, 1981; Vernon, 1979). Although there have been extreme claims that there are only minor environmental effects (Munsinger, 1975) or near-zero genetic effects (Kamin, 1974), the evidence clearly indicates that both genetic and non-genetic factors are influential. There is little point in arguing further on the precise level of heritability both because heritability estimates are necessarily population-specific (being affected by the extent of genetic and environmental variations) and because such estimates refer to population *variance* rather than population *level*. It is likely that a move from a severely disadvantaged to a more

Requests for reprints to: Prof. M. Rutter, Department of Child and Adolescent Psychiatry, Institute of Psychiatry, Denmark Hill, London SE5 8AF, U.K.

Accepted manuscript received 25 *February* 1985

normal environment may result in a substantial elevation in IQ level without making much difference to genetic contributions to within-population variance (Scarr, 1981).

A further important consideration concerns the effect of genetic-environment covariation and the likelihood that to an important extent genotypic differences serve to create different environments (Scarr & McCartney, 1983). In other words, parents or teachers treat children differently both because the children themselves are different and because of the adult's own genetically determined propensities. Not only is the environment not statistically independent of genetic influences, but also people tend to make their own environments. That probability creates two important methodological issues. First, in the analysis of psychosocial influences it is crucial to take into account the possibility that the supposed psychosocial effects were in fact genetically determined. Second, it is necessary to differentiate between psychosocial influences that impinge similarly on all children in the same family and those that affect each child differently [i.e. shared and non-shared environmental influences; Rowe and Plomin (1981)].

The bulk of the literature on genetic and environmental effects on cognition has been restricted to findings in IQ scores. In contrast, this paper is concerned with cognitive performance as more broadly defined to include scholastic and other attainments. The reasons for doing so are three-fold. First, IQ tests tap performance just as do tests of reading or mathematics; they differ only in that they assess a much wider range of cognitive skills that are less likely to have been the subject of direct teaching at school (Vernon, 1970). Second, many psychosocial factors tend to influence both general and specific aspects of cognitive performance in broadly comparable ways. Third, neither intelligence nor scholastic attainment are unitary skills, so that in both cases it is necessary to search for possibly different types of influence on different elements of those skills. It should not be assumed that all psychosocial influences operate in the same way. In particular, with both IQ and scholastic attainment tests it is necessary to differentiate between effects on cognitive capacity (i.e. the level of *competence*) and effects on cognitive performance (i.e. the *use* of skills).

It may be that environmental factors are more influential on variance in scholastic attainment than in IQ (Jensen, 1973), although that is not certain (Scarr & Kidd, 1983), but that possibility will not be examined here. Also, almost by definition, direct teaching will have a greater impact on accomplishments in school-taught subjects than on IQ, but such teaching effects will not be discussed. Rather, the concern is for the most general aspects of cognitive growth and performance, with special attention to developmental issues. The main focus is on three key questions— *which* aspects of the psychosocial environment have the strongest effects on cognitive growth and performance; *how* the effects are mediated, that is what processes are involved; and to what *extent* the effects are seen across the range of ordinary environments and to what extent are they restricted to extremes of disadvantage.

In general it is clear that the kinds of environmental influences that have the greatest impact on social behaviour are very different from those with the most effect on cognition (Rutter, 1981, 1985; Rutter & Madge, 1976). Thus, family discord is a potent factor in relation to the development of conduct disorders but it is of less relevance for cognitive development. Similarly, even a good institutional upbringing predisposes to disruptive and maladaptive social behaviour but has less impact on

■273

intelligence. Bereavement predisposes to emotional disturbance but it does not impede cognitive development to the same degree. Nevertheless, it would be absurd completely to separate social relationships and cognitive development. Accordingly, in the review of evidence, some attention will be paid to the extent to which the two may be linked with respect to the influence of psychosocial variables.

FAMILY INFLUENCES

Family influences are most conveniently considered in terms of the separate findings regarding the effects of variations in the ordinary environment, of planned interventions, of abnormal environments, and of extreme environmental conditions.

Variations within the ordinary environment

Most of the literature examines psychosocial effects on cognitive development in terms of the performance of socially disadvantaged groups (Birch & Gussow, 1970), of correlations between IQ and social class (e.g. Douglas, 1964), or of correlations between IQ and child-rearing variables within samples of children reared by their biological parents (Wachs & Gruen, 1982). However, it is clear that all three approaches confound genetic and environmental influences. To study the latter it is necessary to control the former or to choose circumstances in which they are unlikely to operate. Three main strategies may be employed for this purpose: (1) the study of ordinal position effects; (2) the study of family influences after statistically partialling out the effects of parental IQ; and (3) the study of parental effects within an adopted sample.

Ordinal position. There are several problems associated with the examination of ordinal position effects but there seems no doubt that eldest or only children tend to show slightly higher scholastic achievement and verbal intelligence levels than later born ones (see Rutter & Madge, 1976). The difference is small but in within-family comparisons it involves a 3½ point difference between first born and fifth born children (Records, McKeown & Edwards, 1969). The processes by which this effect is brought about are not known with any certainty but parents do tend to interact differently with their first born than with subsequent children. In general, they do more things with, and are more pressuring with, the first child (Gottfried, 1984; Rutter, 1981). Thus Davie, Hutt, Vincent and Mason (1984) in an observational study found that parents interacted or talked more with their first borns; conversely, youngest children spent more time playing and talking with other children but, compared with eldest children, they were more likely to be followers rather than initiators. It is plausible, although not demonstrated, that these interactional differences may have had an influence on the children's cognitive development. In passing, it should be noted that the ordinal position effects for socio-emotional behaviour are rather different. Whereas eldest children may be at a slight advantage intellectually they are at a slight disadvantage socio-emotionally. Eldest children tend to be more aggressive, less cheerful (Davie *et al.*, 1984), more socially assertive (Snow, Jacklin & Maccoby, 1981) and more liable to show emotional disorder (Rutter, Tizard & Whitmore, 1970).

Parent–child interaction, controlling for parental IQ. Ideally, to control for genetic factors when searching for environmentally mediated family influences, the effects of

274∎

both paternal and maternal IQ should be partialled out. No study has managed to accomplish this but partial control has been achieved in several investigations by taking into account maternal IQ or education, or, less satisfactorily, socio-economic status (Gottfried, 1984). In all cases the family environment–child IQ correlations were reduced after controlling for IQ, but the extent of the reduction varied greatly across studies. In some (Longstreth, Davies, Carter, Flint, Owen, Rickert & Taylor, 1981) the introduction of maternal IQ reduced the home environment effect to insigificant levels whereas in others it resulted in only a minor reduction (see several chapters in Gottfried, 1984). However, there is general agreement that, whatever the extent of the reduction in home environment effects, it does not seem to alter the overall pattern of variables associated with children's cognitive performance.

Because of variations in sampling and measures across studies, it is not possible to derive firm conclusions about the specifics of family influences. However, certain inferences may be drawn. First, the amount of the variance accounted for by overall home environment variables is typically quite low—with corrected correlations generally in the 0.15–0.35 range. Second, the effects tend to be greater with IQ at 3–5 years than with developmental quotients in the first 2 years. Third, family measures at 2 years and older tend to have greater effects than similar measures in infancy. This may be especially the case after correction for parental IQ (Yeates, McPhee, Campbell & Ramey, 1983). In other words, the very early family environment seems less influential than that experienced at the toddler age period and later; that is so whether correlations are with contemporaneous or later cognitive measures.

Fourth, whereas no one type of parent–child interaction stands out above all others as of critical importance, the relevant features include: avoidance of noise-confusion (meaning a background of high intensity sound that is either not discriminable or not meaningful to the child), the provision of a variety of activities and experiences, ample parent–child play and conversation, responsivity to the child's verbal and non-verbal signals, parental nurturance, teaching of specific skills, and opportunities for the child to explore and to try out new skills and activities (Gottfried, 1984; Wachs & Gruen, 1982). It is evident that the traditional notion that it is 'stimulation' that promotes cognitive growth is seriously misleading. Although varied and interesting parent–child interactions are beneficial, a high level of noise is not. Moreover, it seems that the crucial feature is not so much the parental 'input' in a stimulus sense as the reciprocity of the interactions, the variety and meaningfulness of their content, and the active role taken by the child. Nevertheless, this does *not* amount to a non-involved passive parental style in which the children are left to discover everything for themselves; both a degree of structure and considerable direct teaching seem to be desirable.

Fifthly, although it seems reasonable to suppose that differences in the children's characteristics might make them responsive to different sorts of home environment, the matter has been so little explored (with the exception of sex differences) that no conclusions are possible. However, there is some weak indication that children's needs may change with age. For example, Wachs and Gruen (1982) argued that physical contact was important only before 6 months of age, that conversation and responsiveness to the child's non-verbal signals become important during the second year of life, that responsiveness to the child's talk increases in relevance in the third year and that the variety of contacts with a range of other adults (and an avoidance of noise-confusion) increase in relevance after 3 years of age. Bradley and Caldwell's (1984) findings at age 7 years from their longitudinal study suggested that by the time children reach school maternal responsivity is less important but parental encouragement and the availability of a range of play materials and of experiences remain salient.

Finally, there is some indication that the effects on verbal intelligence may possibly be greater than those on non-verbal intelligence; and that effects on scholastic attainment may be greater than those on IQ. However, the evidence on these points is less than adequate.

Adopted children. Early studies of families with both biological and adopted children (see Bouchard & McGue, 1981; Rutter & Madge, 1976) showed that the correlations for IQ between biological children and their parents were about twice as high as those between adopted children and their adopting parents (*ca.* 0.34 vs 0.19). More recent studies have added substantially to this body of evidence. Scarr and Weinberg (1983) in a study of transracial adoptions found correlations of 0.43 vs 0.29, and in a study of adolescents an even greater disparity with an adoptive mid-parent–child correlation of only 0.14. Horn's (1983) findings from the Texas adoption project showed much the same (0.28 vs 0.15). Both sets of studies also produced the parallel finding that adopted children's IQ scores correlated more highly with those of their biological parents who did not raise them than those of their adoptive parents who did raise them but who did not share their genes. There is a clear inference that part of the parental effects on children's intelligence is genetic rather than environmental; however, some environmental effect is also suggested. Plomin and De Fries (1983) in the Colorado Adoption Project sought to assess environmental effects more directly by using the Caldwell and Bradley HOME interview-cum-observation assessment of the home environment. In line with the biological family findings discussed above, the HOME scores showed little correlation with Bayley developmental scores at age 1 year but there were significant correlations at 2 years: 0.22 for the adoptive families and 0.39 for the control families (the variance on the HOME inventory being similar in the two groups). Interestingly, the adoptive and control groups did not differ in the level of correlation between the HOME scores at 1 and the Bayley scores at 2, suggesting that genetic factors may not be involved in the predictive ability of HOME, at least up to the age of 2 years.

It may be concluded that the three different types of study of variations in the ordinary home environment are in fairly good agreement, and hence provide reasonable guidelines regarding family influences that may be influential for cognitive development. However, the family measures account for a rather small proportion of population variance and most of the results apply to very young children. The ordinal position data stand out in showing comparable effects throughout the course of development; however, they reflect within—rather than between—family differences. The findings on age differences in home environment effects are inconclusive. Horn's (1983) data showed a possibly reduced genetic effect for children over 10 years but no comparable increase of family environment effects. Scarr and Weinberg's (1983) data on adolescent sibling correlations suggested that shared familial influences decreased with age. Possibly shared family environment effects are most marked in early childhood, with both non-shared family effects and outside the home influences greater in adolescence. However, that hypothesis is speculative and requires systematic testing.

Family intervention studies

There have been a wide range of family interventions designed to influence children's cognitive development but the findings can be considered most conveniently in terms of the degree of change entailed.

Adoption. The most complete family change is that brought about by adoption. The effects of adoption have been considered already in terms of family effects *within* adopted groups. However, because of deliberate policies in the selection of adoptive parents the range of home environments within such groups is relatively favoured. A rather different use of the adopted child research strategy is to compare the mean *level* of adopted children's intelligence and scholastic attainment with that expected on the basis of the characteristics of their biological parents.

Skodak and Skeels (1949) were the first to use this approach—showing that children born to mothers of below average IQ when adopted in homes somewhat above the average had a mean IQ of 106 compared with the mean of 86 for their biological mothers and an estimated 90–95 that might have been expected if they had been reared by their biological parents. There are important criticisms to be made of Skeels' later research (Longstreth, 1981) but although they do not invalidate this observation, there are still major problems stemming from the fact that the early versions of the Binet had both means and standard deviations that varied greatly from age to age (Clarke, 1982).

More recently, Scarr and Weinberg's (1976) study of socially classified black children, most of whom were born as a result of interracial matings, adopted by white families of high socioeconomic status provided better data that showed a similar effect. The adopted black children had a mean IQ of 106, somewhat above the white general population mean (although a little below the mean of 111 for white adopted children), and more than a standard deviation above that expected on the basis of their biological parentage. The adopted black children's scholastic attainments were also slightly above population norms.

Horn's (1983) data from the Texas adoption project showed the same. Although the children's IQ *correlated* more strongly with those of their biological mothers than those of their adoptive mothers, the mean IQ of the children (111.5) was actually *closer* to that of their adoptive mothers (112.4) than to that of their biological mothers (108.4) [see Walker and Emory (in press) for a discussion of this point].

Lastly there are the important findings from the Shiff, Duyme, Dumaret and Tomkiewicz (1982) study. Thirty-two children born to biological parents both of whom were unskilled workers were abandoned at birth and adopted by families spanning the top 13% of the socio-professional scale. The effects of this change in social situation were assessed by comparing the children's IQs with those of their biological half-sibs (*n* = 20) reared by the biological parents (109 vs 95) and with those of general population studies of children of unskilled workers (mean IQ = 95) and of upper middle class parents (mean IQ = 110). Although the sample size is small, in many ways these data provide the strongest evidence of an environmental enhance-

■277

ment of IQ through the adoption into socially favoured homes of children from a socially disadvantaged background.

Inevitably there are limitations in these data. Ideally there should be measures of the biological parents' IQs (these were available for mothers in the Horn project but other investigators have had to rely on years of education); and a comparison between the adopted children and their biological siblings reared by their biological parents (partially available in the Schiffé study) would be even more informative. Nevertheless, the findings indicate a rather strong effect on intelligence and scholastic attainments of a *major* change of environment from social disadvantage to above average social circumstances. The rather small effect of environmental variations within the adopted sample may indicate that environmental effects are greater with respect to the removal of adversity than to normal variations within the range of acceptable environments; however, also, this may reflect the lack of sufficiently discriminating measures within the normal range.

There has been some discussion in the literature of the possibility that environmental effects on intellectual development are greater during the preschool years than they are in later childhood (see Clarke & Clarke, 1976; Clarke, 1984; Rutter, 1981). The main evidence in support of this suggestion comes from the observation that the IQ scores of later adopted children tend to be slightly lower than those of children adopted in infancy (see Dennis, 1973). The finding is interesting but there are three reasons why it does not point unequivocally to a greater effect of the early family environment. First, it is difficult entirely to rule out the possibility of biases due to selective placement. Second, the durations of disadvantageous environmental circumstances are not comparable; by definition the late adopted children have experienced more prolonged disadvantage. Thirdly, the amount and character of parent–child interaction in middle childhood is very different from that in infancy. It may be that the lesser intellectual gains of older late-adopted children simply reflect their lesser opportunities for intensive interaction with their adoptive parents. It should be added that the differences in cognitive outcome between early and late adopted children are small, and that late adopted children perform relatively well educationally (Triseliotis & Russell, 1985).

Milwaukee project. During the last two decades there have been many varied preschool interventions. With the exception of the Parent Child Development Centers (see below) most have placed their main emphasis on some form of out of the home education. However, beginning with Gray's pioneering Early Training project (Gray, Ramsey & Kalus, 1982; Klaus & Gray, 1968), a number included work with parents as an integral part of the programme. In a few cases this feature, combined with the pervasiveness of the interventions, suggests that they should be considered in some senses as family interventions. The most intensive and extensive programme undertaken so far is that provided by the Milwaukee project (Garber & Heber, 1977, 1982; Heber, Harrington, Hoffman & Falender, 1972). The mothers in the experimental programme were given home management and job training together with remedial education (but little direct help with parenting); and from infancy up to the age of 6 years the children participated in a structured educational programme with an emphasis on problem-solving and language skills. The families were socially disadvantaged and the mothers had an IQ of 75 or less; 20 were allocated to the

278 ▪

programme and 20 served as untreated controls. Both groups have been followed up to 4th grade level. The WISC IQ results at age 10 showed an 18 point between-group difference (104 vs 86); a significant difference but a smaller one than that when the children were younger. The experimental group children also showed superior scholastic attainments to those of the control group but the differences were less marked than those for IQ, both groups declined steadily through the first 4 years of schooling, the between-group difference progressively lessened, and in absolute terms the experimental groups were performing far below national norms by fourth grade. Within the experimental group there was substantial individual variation in outcome, with the poorest outcomes for those in the most disadvantaged homes. The findings, albeit based on small numbers and with some problems in project design and presentation (Page & Grandon, 1981), show that a prolonged and wide-ranging intervention programme during the preschool years can produce important cognitive gains. However, the follow-up through the first 4 years of schooling has also shown that, after intervention ceased, the benefits diminished markedly with time.

Carolina Abecedarian project. The Abecedarian project was similar to the Milwaukee programme in terms of starting in infancy, providing year-round daily care throughout the preschool years, a focus on language and adaptive social behaviour and a structured approach to teaching (Ramey & Campbell, 1981, 1984; Ramey, MacPhee & Yeates, 1982). Hence, it is most conveniently considered here; however, the project did not include direct work with parents and parental participation was limited and sporadic. Most of the parents were black, all were seriously socially disadvantaged, the mothers had a mean IQ of 84, and three-quarters of the families were female-headed. There was random assignment to experimental and control groups, with outcome data up to 54 months for 49 experimental and 46 control group children and up to 5 years of age for 27 and 23 children, respectively. At 60 months the mean WPPSI IQ (98) for the experimental group was 8 points above that for the controls and far fewer (11 vs 39%) had an IQ of 85 or below—figures comparable to the findings at 48 and 54 months for the total group. It should be noted that the cognitive differences did not begin to appear until about 18 months of age. The experimental group children also differed from controls in adapting better to new situations, in responding more appropriately to task demands, and in making use of language. Fewer of the experimental group mothers were out of work at follow-up and more had obtained further education during the course of the intervention. The experimental programme was accompanied by an attenuation of the correlation between maternal and child IQ scores, but in both groups the home environment and the children's temperamental qualities (those with 'easy' temperaments had higher IQ scores) continued to predict the children's performance. Although the results of the Abecedarian project are more modest than those of the Milwaukee study, the overall pattern of findings is broadly similar. Intervention produced limited but worthwhile cognitive benefits; the effects were not manifest in early infancy, better cognitive performance was associated with better social adaptation, and there were considerable individual differences in response.

Parental programmes. A few programmes have concentrated on work with parents in order to foster the cognitive development of children from low income families. Thus,

279

Journal of Child Psychology and Psychiatry, 1985, vol. 26, pp. 683–704

280 ■

Parent Child Development Centers (PCDC) in the U.S.A. provided a wide-ranging curriculum for mothers, including information on child rearing; teaching on home management and family support combined with preschool education for the children: the families started attending when the children were infants and stopped when they reached 3 years of age (Andrews, Blumenthal, Johnson, Kahn, Fergusson, Lasater, Malone & Wallace, 1982). There was random assignment to experimental and control groups, and multiple methods of outcome evaluation. The results have varied somewhat from centre to centre but all have shown benefits for families receiving the intervention programmes. Mothers in the experimental groups tended to communicate better with their children, were more sensitive to their children's needs, were more emotionally responsive, used more encouragement, and provided more information in their talk with their children. The children showed more social behaviour and more positive interactions with their mothers. The case-control differences on the Stanford–Binet IQ assessments at age 3 years ranged from 4 to 8 points, the experimental group children scoring higher. Preliminary follow-up data 1 year after the end of the programme showed reduced between-group differences.

Tizard and Hewison reading study. The last family intervention project to be discussed was quite different both in its timing (primary school rather than infancy or preschool) and in the minimal nature of the intervention provided. A general population study of children in inner city London schools had shown that those who read to their parents at home had markedly higher reading attainments than those who had not received this kind of help from their parents (Hewison & Tizard, 1980). The finding could not be accounted for in terms of the children's level of intelligence or other aspects of their upbringing. An experimental study was undertaken to assess the effects of parental involvement in the teaching of reading (Tizard, Schofield & Hewison, 1982). Infant school classes were randomly assigned to non-intervention, extra group reading tuition at school, and parental help ('home collaboration') with reading, the books being provided by the school.

At the end of the 2 year intervention period the children in the home collaboration group showed reading skills superior to their controls (a 12 point difference in one school and an 8 point difference in the other), the groups having been comparable prior to the intervention. The extra teacher help groups did not differ in outcome from controls. A follow-up one year after the intervention ended showed that the benefits of parental involvement had markedly diminished in one school (to a 3½ point difference) but had been maintained in the other (11 point difference). Nevertheless, in both schools the parental collaboration resulted in a substantial reduction in the proportion of children reading below age level (79–84% in controls; 46–54% in experimental groups).

There are limitations to the study: randomization was by class rather than by individuals; the effects varied by school; there was not a cross-over, and it was not possible to identify the effective elements of the intervention. Thus, for example, it is not clear whether the benefits stemmed from increased reading experience, from one-to-one reading opportunities, or from effects on esteem or motivation. Nevertheless, the results are impressive in showing that an intervention as simple as getting (often poorly educated) inner city parents to listen to their children read was associated with important gains in reading skills. It is particularly notable that the benefits followed interventions during middle childhood rather than infancy.

Abnormal environments

Institutional rearing. Various early studies in the 1940s and 1950s reported marked intellectual impairment in institution-reared children (see Tizard, 1970). However, other investigations showed cognitive *gains* in children transferred from a poor institution to a better one (e.g. Garvin & Sacks, 1963; Skeels & Dye, 1939), suggesting that the damage did not come from institutional care per se. More recent studies of better quality institutions have confirmed that children reared in them have a level of intelligence that is about average. For example, Tizard and Hodges (1978) found that the 8 year olds in their sample who had been in institutions from infancy had a mean WISC full scale IQ of 99 despite very marked discontinuities in caretaking (some 50–80 parent surrogates), but had gross abnormalities in social behaviour. The mean IQ of 99 was below that (110) in the general population control group but this could be accounted for by the more disadvantaged backgrounds of the institutional children. Similarly, Dixon (1980) found that her sample of 5–8 year olds reared in institutions from infancy had a mean IQ of 108 compared to a mean IQ of 106 in the comparable group of family-fostered children from similarly disadvantaged backgrounds. Again, the institution-reared children differed markedly in behaviour although they did not in measured intelligence.

The lack of effects on general intelligence is striking in view of the marked effects of an institutional upbringing on socio-emotional behaviour (Quinton, Rutter & Liddle, 1984; Rutter, 1981). Nevertheless, although not reflected in IQ scores, there were group differences in classroom behaviour of a kind likely to be relevant for learning. Thus, the institution-reared children in both these studies showed poor task involvement and inattentive overactive behaviour (Roy, 1983). It is not apparent how far these behavioural features in fact impeded either cognitive development or cognitive performance, but clearly the negative potential was there. Other studies have shown that institution-reared children are less likely than controls to continue in education (Quinton & Rutter, unpublished data) and that behavioural disturbance has indirect effects on scholastic attainment as a result of truancy and school drop-out (Maughan, Gray & Rutter, in press).

Family pathology. Numerous studies have shown the increased risk of socio-emotional and behavioural disturbance in the children of parents with some form of chronic psychiatric disorder (Rutter & Quinton, 1984). Less is known about the cognitive sequelae for children reared by mentally ill parents. However, such data as are available show small and inconsistent effects. For example, Winters, Stone, Weintraub and Neale (1981) found that the children of depressed and schizophrenic parents had mean IQ scores about a fifth of a standard deviation below controls. On the other hand, problems in school work are often included among social and behavioural difficulties (Billings & Moos, 1983). Much the same applied to studies of the effects of parental divorce and death. There are no consistent effects on IQ (Rutter, 1981), but often there may be temporary decrements in scholastic performance that persist for at least a year or so (Hetherington, Cox & Cox, 1982; van Eedewegh, Bieri, Parilla & Clayton, 1982).

Journal of Child Psychology and Psychiatry, 1985, vol. 26, pp. 683–704

Several clinical reports have commented on the poor language development of children subjected to physical abuse by parents. However, most studies have failed to control for other family characteristics and it appears that language and cognitive problems are more a function of serious social disadvantage than of abuse *per se* (Elmer, 1977). Moreover, one study showed that verbal abilities were more impaired in children who experienced parental neglect than those who suffered abuse (Allen & Oliver, 1982).

The available data are by no means satisfactory but they are consistent in showing that patterns of upbringing that involve serious discord, discontinuities in parenting, and parental deviance carry a high risk that the children will show socio-emotional problems; however the risk for intellectual impairment is quite slight although that for difficulties in scholastic attainment is rather greater.

Extreme environmental conditions

Lastly, with respect to family influences, there are the children exposed to extreme environmental conditions, being reared in gross social isolation and severe physical confinement. Skuse (1984) had summarized the findings on nine well documented cases and Clarke (1984) has added another. The findings are striking in at least four crucial respects. Firstly, these grossly abnormal patterns of upbringing were associated with severe cognitive deficits at the time the children were discovered at ages ranging from 2½ to 13½ years (Skuse, 1984); all were virtually without spoken language and most showed severe intellectual retardation. Secondly, most of the children showed very substantial cognitive improvement following rescue from their appalling circumstances and seven of the 10 achieved normal levels of intelligence and language; two more gained a normal performance IQ but remained seriously impaired in language. Thirdly, it was usual for improvements in cognitive functioning to be evident within months after removal from the extreme environmental conditions, although it took much longer for normal levels to be achieved. Fourthly, the published reports contain remarkably few systematic data on possible effects on the children's interpersonal relationships.

It may be inferred not only that severe privation led to severe cognitive impairment but also that a complete change of environment led to marked cognitive recovery.

Conclusions on family influences. Although there are major lacunae in the evidence, the findings on family influences point to several reasonably firm conclusions. Firstly, there *are* important effects stemming from the nature of children's experience during their upbringing. Secondly, these effects are most striking during the later preschool years with less impact during the infancy periods; however major environmental changes continue to have major effects on cognitive development throughout the years of childhood. In part, the limited effects seen in infancy probably stem from the difficulties in measuring cognitive performance so early in life but also it appears that early development may show a greater degree of 'canalization', with maturational influences more important at that age than either environmental features or polygenic factors (McCall, 1981). Thirdly, there is no marked critical period for cognitive development. To a very substantial extent the benefits of good experiences in the early years are lost if subsequent experiences are bad; conversely there may be substantial recovery if early bad experiences are followed by good ones in middle childhood. Fourthly, the most striking effects on cognitive development and performance are seen with gross deficits in conditions of rearing: however, as shown both by the ordinal data and the findings on home environment—child IQ correlations there are also smaller effects within the normal range. Fifthly, although it is not possible to specify at all precisely the features of the home environment that provide for optimal cognitive development it is clear that they include: parental responsiveness to children's signals; varied and positive patterns of reciprocal parent–child interaction and communication; and a range of interesting, varied and meaningful experiences and activities with both parents and other people. 'Stimulation' in the sense of sensory bombardment is *not* a useful way of describing the qualities that are necessary. Also, although family discord and disturbance may have some effect on scholastic performance such environments have a much greater adverse effect on socio-emotional and behavioural functioning than on cognition.

■283

SCHOOL INFLUENCES

Variations within the ordinary environment

Studies in both developing and industrialized nations have shown that the experience of schooling is associated with superior cognitive development (see Rutter, 1981). Thus, in countries where schooling is available in only some areas, cognitive skills are greter in those children able to attend school. Forced closure of schools as a result of war or political activities has been followed by IQ decrements of the order of 5 points or so, and continued schooling during later adolescence is associated with a mean IQ gain of some 5–7 points. Traditionally it is usually supposed that IQ predicts scholastic attainment but it is evident also that schooling and improved educational accomplishments may themselves lead to IQ gains.

A further issue concerns the differing importance of school influences according to family circumstances. It has been found that, relatively speaking, pupils from a socially disadvantaged background tend to lose ground in their cognitive performance during the long summer vacation when they are not at school, but this does not occur with those from more favoured families (Heyns, 1978).

In recent years increasing attention has been paid to the extent to which ordinary schools vary in their effects on children's cognitive performance (see Rutter, 1983). These naturalistic studies of school effects have mainly relied on measures of scholastic attainment rather than IQ and it is not known how far variations in the quality of school experiences influence IQ. Nevertheless, the evidence is consistent in showing important school effects on children's educational performance, after taking account of differences between schools in the social and intellectual distributions of the children at the time of school entry. The differences between schools at the extremes of the ranges studied have been marked (with differences in mean levels of attainment of the order of 1 S.D.), indicating that school effects can be very substantial. However, many schools vary little in their effects so that it is not possible to derive any meainingful overall measure of the general strength of school influences.

The qualities of schools associated with good scholastic performance have been studied through the detailed comparison of schools performing better and those performing worse than expected on the basis of their intakes. The findings show a variety of school features to be important. First, there are several that might be considered in terms of their more direct effects on learning. Thus, children's scholastic performance tends to be better in schools with a clear focus on academic goals and a translation of that attitude into practice through the regular setting and marking of homework, a high proportion of time devoted to active teaching, group planning of the curriculum, and checks to ensure that teachers follow the intended practices. Secondly, there are features designed to foster efficient learning through good classroom management—as by lessons beginning and ending on time, clear and unambiguous feedback to pupils on their performance, minimum disciplinary interruptions, and effective classroom teaching techniques. Thirdly, there are school practices that might be thought to operate in terms of aiding high morale, such as adequate but discriminating use of praise and encouragement, good pupils conditions, good models of teacher behaviour; and good care of the school buildings. Fourthly, there are features that serve to set school norms, such as an adequate intellectual balance in the composition of the intake and appropriately high teacher expectations of the pupils. Fifthly, there are actions that might be conceptualized in terms of their effect in fostering pupils' commitment to educational goals; for example, opportunities for most pupils to take responsibility and to participate in the running of their school lives together with out-of-school activities shared between staff and pupils.

It is noteworthy that there are substantial positive correlations between different measures of pupil performance. That is, on the whole, schools with good levels of scholastic attainment also tend to be those with high levels of attendance, generally good behaviour, and a high proportion of pupils staying on at school beyond the period of compulsory schooling (Rutter, Maughan, Mortimer, Ouston & Smith, 1979). Similar associations are seen at an individual level; children who attend poorly tend to do less well in exams, those with disturbed behaviour tend to leave school early without sitting exams. Correlational data of this type cannot delineate mechanisms and processes with any precision. Nevertheless, the strong inference is that much of the cognitive effects stem from influences on self-esteem, patterns of behaviour and task performance, educational motivation, and attitudes to learning. Presumably pedagogic skills are important in determining both how much is taught and how well it is taught. But children's *responses* to that learning environment will be influenced by whether or not they are present (as determined by school attendance and when they leave school), their involvement in the learning task (as determined by features such as attention to instructions and task performance style), their aspirations (as shaped by the expectations of those about them and their own self-concept), and their interest and commitment to learning (as reflected in what they do outside as well as inside school). Whether or not schools serve to foster effective learning in their pupils will be determined by their qualities as a social organization (Minuchin & Shapiro, 1983), as well as by their qualities in relation to the transmission of knowledge as such.

Interventions

Although there have been studies of planned interventions in elementary and in secondary schools, the bulk of research has concerned the effects on IQ and scholastic performance of children experiencing day care (Zigler & Gordon, 1982) or some form of preschool education (Clarke-Stewart & Fein, 1983). As the literature has been extensively reviewed several times, only the key findings will be summarized here.

Preschool education. Numerous studies in the 1960s and early 1970s showed that preschool interventions led to immediate IQ gains but that the benefits did not persist for long after the start of regular schooling. The loss of advantage from the preschool intervention resulted in part from the IQ gains in control groups associated with entry into formal education, and in part from decrements in IQ in the experimental groups. These largely negative findings led to a widespread acceptance that compensatory education was not worthwhile. Undoubtedly, the original expectation that relatively brief educational experiences in the preschool years would lead to lasting beneficial effects on general intelligence was both naive and unwarranted by the empirical evidence available at the time (Clarke & Clarke, 1976). Nevertheless, recent re-evaluations of findings have begun to lead to a readjustment in the initial research appraisal that there were *no* lasting benefits (Berrueta-Clement, Schweinhart, Barnett, Epstein & Weikart, 1984; Lazar & Darlington, 1982; Ramey, Bryant & Suarez, 1984; Schweinhart & Weikart, 1980).

■285

Lazar and Darlington (1982) have reported the findings that resulted from a pooling of the data from 11 of the best designed investigations with appropriate control groups, in which there was a systematic follow-up when the children were aged 9–19 years. It was found that high quality preschool programmes were associated with IQ gains during the first 2 years after the programmes finished, there was a lesser gain for up to 3 or 4 years but no detectable effect at the final follow-up. The findings regarding effects on scholastic achievement were less clearcut but there were significant benefits during the early years of schooling, particularly in maths. In some of the projects the effects on achievement seemed to diminish with time but in the particularly well planned Schweinhart and Weikart (1980) study they increased. In many respects, the most striking lasting benefit of the preschool intervention was the reduced proportion of children who had to repeat a grade or who were placed in special education classes. In addition, the intervention was associated with an increased tendency for the children to report themselves proud of their achievements and for the mothers to be more satisfied with their children's school performance and to have higher aspirations for them. There was evidence from some of the projects that teachers tended to rate the children from the programmes more positively on attitudes to learning and behaviour. It was concluded that early education brought benefits through two routes. First, there were direct effects on cognitive performance (as mediated through the learning of specific skills, improved task orientation, and better persistence). Second, there were benefits through non-cognitive effects on children's self-esteem and self-efficacy and on their attitudes to learning; on parents' hopes and aspirations; and on teachers' expectations of and responses to the children. It was hypothesized that the early education experience may change children from passive to active learners who begin to take the initiative in seeking information, help and interaction with others. When this increased motivation to learn is met by a positive response at home and at school, long-term cognitive gains can result.

The most thorough analysis of the links in the long term of cause and effects

Journal of Child Psychology and Psychiatry, 1985, vol. 26, pp. 683–704

286 ▪

following high quality preschool education is that deriving from the Perry preschool programme (Berrueta-Clement *et al.*, 1984). They have data from five cohorts of low SES 3–4 year old children with IQs in the 60–90 range randomly assigned to an experimental control group. The experimental children received an organized educational programme directed at both intellectual and social development; in addition teachers made a once per week 1½ hour home visit to see each mother and child. Both groups have been followed to age 19 years. IQ differences between the groups did not persist beyond the early years of schooling but other benefits lasted throughout the follow-up period; the experimental group showed improved scholastic achievement, a higher rate of high school graduation, a lower rate of delinquency and a higher rate of employment. A causal path analysis suggested that the initial effect of preschool on intellectual performance generated long term effects through its intermediate direct effects on scholastic achievement and its indirect effects on social maturity and commitment to the educational process. Case studies comparing young people who did and did not respond well to the experimental intervention suggested that long term success was dependent on parental and family support for education, the presence of positive role models (particularly those who demonstrated the value of schooling), a sense of responsibility that extends beyond oneself, and an active goal-oriented approach to life. The findings emphasize the probable operation of transactional indirect effects in the path leading to long-term benefits, the interaction between cognitive and social processes, and the importance of an effective mutually supportive 'mesh' between home and school.

Similar processes were postulated by Pedersen, Faucher and Eaton (1978) in their investigation of the effects on children of one outstanding first grade teacher. The findings showed that the teacher had a major effect on children's academic achievement, work effort and initiative during the following year, but that there were negligible *direct* effects thereafter. On the other hand, her *indirect* effects were substantial because the children had acquired styles of work and behaviour that brought success, which in turn reinforced their efforts. Similarly, their behaviour in class made them more rewarding students for the teachers of later classes who then responded to them in ways that facilitated their continuing success. It cannot be said that these ideas have been rigorously tested but the overall pattern of evidence certainly suggests that preschool education has both cognitive and social effects. The latter may be as important as the former in processes leading to persistence of benefits. However, it is likely that whether or not cognitive gains last will depend not only on whether the children continue in beneficial environments but also on how parents and teachers respond to the initial changes in the children's behaviour and performance. It is probable that the particular patterns of adult–child and of child–child interaction that ensue will contribute to the processes that determine whether the initial gains are built upon or are undermined by subsequent experiences.

Day care and nurseries. The preschool programmes discussed above were explicitly designed to foster the cognitive development of children from a disadvantaged background. It remains to consider other forms of day care in which the main aim is to provide good quality caregiving, as well as the general run of nursery schools and play groups that may be seen as providing an early start to general education rather than any form of compensatory special education (see review by Clarke-Stewart & Fein, 1983; also Zigler & Gordon, 1982).

Although the findings vary somewhat from study to study, it may be concluded that *good quality* day care has no negative effects on intellectual development and it may produce some temporary cognitive enhancement. Whether or not there are cognitive gains seems to depend very largely on the extent to which there are explicit prescribed educational activities together with opportunities for social interaction and exploration of materials. The findings regarding effects of socio-emotional development are both more meagre and less consistent (Rutter, 1981). It seems clear that good quality day care, at least after the age of 2 or 3 years, does not lead to emotional disturbance and may enhance children's social competence. However, again much depends on the quality of care provided, with maladjustment most likely in those who began day care in infancy in centres with little adult–child interaction and conversation (McCartney, Scarr, Phillips, Grajels & Schwarz, 1982).

Sometimes it is assumed that nursery schools have much to offer in terms of their provision of a 'stimulating' language environment that can serve to compensate for an 'unstimulating' disadvanged family environment. The studies by Tizard and her colleagues (Tizard, Carmichael, Hughes & Pinkerton, 1980; Tizard, Hughes, Carmichael & Pinkerton, 1983a, b; Tizard & Hughes, 1984), as well as those of other investigators (see Clarke-Stewart & Fein, 1983), suggest that this may be a misleading assumption. They found that there was more, and more varied, conversational interchange between parents and their children in upper working class homes than the same children experienced at nursery schools. Also, working class children seemed inhibited at school in their language usage. In that it appears that good quality nursery schools *can* aid children's cognitive performance, it may be inferred that the reason they do so is *not* because they provide greater verbal 'stimulation'. Teachers do, however, differ from parents in using language that is more often complex, in asking more questions, and in providing more direct teaching.

It should be emphasized that the Tizard and Hughes (1984) data refer to relatively advantaged working class girls from small two-parent families (thus, they had a mean IQ of 106, which was some 20 points or more above that of the seriously disadvantaged children in most of the preschool intervention programmes) who were studied in relatively stress-free social circumstances (usually with only the mother and one child at home). Accordingly, it cannot be assumed that the conversational interchanges between parents and children would be as rich in socially disadvantaged homes as in the homes studied by Tizard and Hughes. Nevertheless, three findings suggest that the benefits from preschool education do not largely derive from verbal enrichment. First, the data are convincing in demonstrating that the setting of nursery schools does not encourage conversations that explore the development of ideas (because Tizard and Hughes found that the *same* children who appeared verbally inhibited at school were much freer in their use of language at home). Second, preschool education appears to benefit children from average homes as much as those from a very poor background (Clarke-Stewart & Fein, 1983), although the data on this point are quite limited. Thirdly, children in home based day care tend to talk more with their caregivers than do those in special centres, but on the whole the intellectual benefits from the latter are greater (Clarke-Stewart & Fein, 1983). Very tentatively, it may be suggested that language experiences at school and at home may both be beneficial, but for different reasons. Perhaps systematic teaching together with questions and

Journal of Child Psychology and Psychiatry, 1985, vol. 26, pp. 683–704

answer type interchanges benefit cognitive growth through direct learning, whereas the less structured more inductive conversations at home are helpful through encouraging problem solving and sensitivity to other people. Clearly, children's conversations play a part in their language development and in their intellectual development more generally but we remain surprisingly ignorant of just which aspects of those conversations are most likely to promote cognitive growth (Puckering & Rutter, in press).

NATURE OF INFLUENCES AND EFFECTS

288 ■

In conclusion, it is necessary briefly to consider the possible ways in which psycho-social influences may act to facilitate cognitive development and performance. The evidence reviewed in this paper clearly demonstrates the reality of such environmental effects, although it indicates that the effects on IQ are relatively modest within the normal range of environments. The effects on other aspects of cognitive performance are probably rather greater and the effects of markedly disadvantageous circumstances are very substantial with respect to all aspects of cognitive functioning.

The types of environments that have the greatest effect on socio-emotional and behavioural functioning are very different from those with the greatest impact on cognitive development. In particular, discord and discontinuity in relationships seem most important for the former whereas opportunities for active learning seem most influential for the latter. Nevertheless, it is evident that there is overlap. It has been suggested (Rutter, 1985) that what is needed for optimal cognitive development is a combination of active learning experiences that promote cognitive competence together with a social context in which the style of interaction and relationships promotes self-confidence and an active interest in seeking to learn independently of formal instruction. The social context considerations necessarily entail environmental conditions likely to foster social as well as cognitive development. However, the provision of active learning experiences also does so. It is clear that these are *not* most usefully conceptualized in terms of 'stimulation'. Rather they involve the child's active, rather than passive, participation; the provision of varied, interesting and meaningful experiences rather than high level sensory input; direct teaching of specific skills and knowledge; a sensitivity and responsiveness in reacting to children's approaches and questions; and a reciprocity in patterns of interaction. It is obvious that these features bear more than a passing resemblance to the style of authoritative-reciprocal parenting patterns, high in bidirectional communication, thought to be most likely to lead to social responsibility, control of aggression, self-confidence and high self-esteem (see Maccoby & Martin, 1983).

The next question is *how* these influences operate and what changes in the organism they bring about. Traditionally, it would be supposed that the direct cognitive effects operate on some form of cognitive 'structure' that is part of the basic laying down of personality components. However, a consideration of the longitudinal data suggests that this may not be the most helpful way of conceptualizing the process; indeed it may be doubted that there *is* an underlying personality structure laid down in the early years of childhood (Rutter, 1984b). Of course, even very young children have substantial cognitive and interpersonal skills; moreover such skills show some coherence and organization. However, it does not seem that these skills are most helpfully conceptualized in terms of a 'structure' that is either present or absent and which, once present, has a fixity and indestructibility. Perhaps the key data in that connection are the relative impermanence of any effects independent of later environmental circumstances, and the relatively rapid recovery in middle childhood following removal from extremely damaging conditions. Also it may be relevant that both temporary and lasting environmental effects seem to be *least* evident in infancy. For the same reason, it seems dubious whether the main effects are on brain structure and chemistry. It is not that there is any doubt that marked environmental variations *can* lead to structural effects (see Greenough & Schwark, 1984); the scepticism is over this being the main process involved in the continuation of cognitive sequelae following good or bad experiences. In the first place, the physical changes are more evident in the case of either gross sensory deprivation or the restriction of specific sensory inputs (as in vision), rather than in impairments in the *quality* of life experiences as discussed here. Secondly, the modifiability of environmental effects and the relative speed of cognitive changes following radical alterations in life circumstances do not suggest that the processes require any reorganization of brain structure or chemistry.

■289

Perhaps the direct cognitive effects mainly concern the acquisition of knowledge and skills. However, it is most unlikely that these mainly comprise the gaining of information or specific scholastic attainments. It is striking how very limited are the benefits stemming from interventions that are confined to the school environment. Not only may the experience at home provide something not readily available in school but also it seems that the skills involved apply as much to processes of attention, perseverance, task performance and work organization as to particular areas of knowledge. Learning how to learn may be as important as the specifics of what is learned.

In addition to the direct cognitive effects, however, there are equally important non-cognitive effects that influence later cognitive functioning. These include features such as children's concepts of themselves, their aspirations and attitudes to learning, their self-esteem, their commitments to education and their styles of interaction with parents, teachers and others in the environment. The various ways in which environmental effects may lead to continuities and discontinuities in socio-emotional functioning have been considered elsewhere (Rutter, 1986a,b). However, once again it seems that the processes are not best conceptualized in terms of personality structure; on the other hand, it would be equally misleading to view the effects simply in terms of immediate situational effects. Continuities arise because acquired skills and habits open up or close down opportunities; because acquired styles of interaction influence children's responses to new environments; because children's self-concepts influence how they perceive new circumstances and how they respond to new challenges. It may be that this transduction of experiences through incorporation into the child's self system partially explains why experiences in early infancy tend to be less influential (because infants lack some crucial components of self-awareness) and why modest changes in the environment during later childhood have such a minor impact on cognitive development (because the habits, concepts and styles of interaction have had so long to become well established).

Acknowledgement—I am most grateful to Anne Clarke for her detailed and helpful criticisms of an earlier draft of this paper.

Journal of Child Psychology and Psychiatry, 1985, vol. 26, pp. 683-704

REFERENCES

Allen, R. E. & Oliver, J. M. (1982). The effects of child maltreatment on language development. *Child Abuse and Neglect,* **6,** 299-305.

Andrews, S. R., Blumenthal, J. B., Johnson, D. L., Kahn, A. J., Fergusson, C. J., Lasater, T. M., Malone, P. E. & Wallace, D. B. (1982). The skills of mothering: a study of parent child development centers. *Monographs of the Society for Research in Chld Development,* Serial No. 198, **47** (6).

Berrueta-Clement, J. R., Schweinhart, L. J., Barnett, W. S., Epstein, A. S. & Weikart, D. P. (1984). *Changed lives: the effects of the Perry Preschool Program on youths through age 19.* Ypsilanti, Michigan: High Scope Press.

Billings, A. G. & Moos, R. H. (1983). Comparisons of children of depressed and non-depressed parents: a social-environmental perspective. *Journal of Abnormal Child Psychology,* **11,** 463-486.

Birch, H. G. & Gussow, J. D. (1970). *Disadvantaged children: health, nutrition and school failure.* New York: Harcourt, Brace and World.

Bouchard, T. J. & McGue, M. (1981). Familial studies of intelligence: a review. *Science,* **212,** 1055-1059.

Bradley, R. H. & Caldwell, B. M. (1984). The relation of infants' home environment to achievement test performance in first grade: a follow-up study. *Child Development,* **55,** 803-809.

Clarke, A. M. (1982). Developmental discontinuities: an approach to assessing their nature. In L. A. Bond & J. M. Joffe (Eds), *Facilitating infant and early childhood development* (pp. 58-77). Hanover, New Hampshire: University Press of New England.

Clarke, A. M. (1984). Early experience and cognitive development. *Review of Research in Education,* **11,** 125-160.

Clarke, A. M. & Clarke, A. D. B. (1976). *Early experience: myth and evidence.* London: Open Books.

Clarke-Stewart, K. A. & Fein, G. G. (1983). Early childhood programs. In M. M. Haith & J. J. Campos (Eds), *Infancy and developmental psychobiology, Vol. 2. Mussen's handbook of child psychology* (4th edn.), (pp. 917-999). New York: Wiley.

Davie, C. E., Hutt, S. J., Vincent, E. & Mason, M. (1984). *The young child at home.* Windsor, Berks: NFER-Nelson.

Dennis, W. (1973). *Children of the Creche.* New York: Appleton-Century-Crofts.

Douglas, J. W. B. (1964). *The home and the school.* London: MacGibbon and Kee.

Elmer, E. (1977). A follow-up study of traumatized children. *Pediatrics,* **59,** 273-279.

Garber, H. & Heber, F. R. (1977). The Milwaukee project: indications of the effectiveness of early intervention in preventing mental retardation. In P. Mittler (Ed.), *Research to practice in mental retardation—I. Care and intervention.* Baltimore: University Park Press.

Garber, H. & Heber, R. (1982). Modification of predicted cognitive development in high-risk children through early intervention. In M. K. Detterman & R. J. Sternberg (Eds), *How and how much can intelligence be increased?* (pp. 121-137). Norwood, New Jersey: Ablex Publishing Co.

Garvin, J. B. & Sacks, L. S. (1963). Growth potential of preschool-aged-children in institutional care: a positive approach to a negative condition. *American Journal of Orthopsychiatry,* **33,** 399-408.

Gottfried, A. W. (Ed.) (1984). *Home environment and early cognitive development: longitudinal research.* Orlando: Academic Press.

Gray, S. B., Ramsey, B. K. & Klaus, R. A. (1982). *From 3 to 20—the early training project.* Baltimore, Maryland: University Park Press.

Greenough, W. T. & Schwark, H. D. (1984). Age-related aspects of experience: effects upon brain structure. In R. N. Emde & R. J. Harmon (Eds), *Continuities and discontinuities in development* (pp. 69-91). New York: Plenum.

Heber, R., Garber, H., Harrington, S., Hoffman, C. & Falender, C. (1972). Rehabilitation of families at risk for mental retardation, December 1972 Progress Report. Madison: University of Wisconsin.

Hetherington, E. M., Cox, M. & Cox, R. (1982). Effects of divorce on parents and children. In M. E. Lamb (Ed.), *Non-traditional families* (pp. 233-288). Hillsdale, New Jersey: Lawrence Erlbaum.

Hewison, J. & Tizard, J. (1980). Parental involvement and reading attainment. *British Journal of Educational Psychology,* **50,** 209-215.

Heyns, B. (1978). *Summer learning and the effects on schooling.* New York: Academic Press.

Horn, J. M. (1983). The Texas adoption project: adopted children and their intellectual resemblance to biological and adoptive parents. *Child Development,* **54,** 268-275.

290 ■

Jencks, C., Smith, M., Acland, M., Bane, M. J., Cohen, D., Gintis, H., Heyns, B. & Michelson, S. (1973). *Inequality: a reassessment of the effect of family and schooling in America.* London: Allen Lane.

Jensen, A. R. (1973). *Educability and group differences.* London: Methuen.

Kamin, L. J. (1974). *The science and politics of IQ.* Potomac, Maryland: Lawrence Erlbaum.

Klaus, R. & Gray, S. W. (1968). The early training project for disadvantaged children: a report after five years. *Monographs of the Society for Research in Child Development,* Serial No. 120, **33** (4).

Lazar, I. & Darlington, R. (1982). Lasting effects of early education: a report from the consortium for longitudinal studies. *Monographs of the Society for Research in Child Development,* Serial No. 195, **47** (2–3).

Longstreth, L. E. (1981). Revisiting Skeels' final study: a critique. *Developmental Psychology,* **17,** 620–625.

Longstreth, L. E., Davis, B., Carter, L., Flint, D., Owen, J., Rickert, M. & Taylor, E. (1981). Separation of home intellectual environment and maternal IQ as determinants of child IQ. *Developmental Psychology,* **17,** 532–541.

McCall, R. B. (1981). Nature-nurture and the two realms of development: a proposed integration with respect to m ental development. *Child Development,* **52,** 1–12.

McCartney, K., Scarr, S., Phillips, D., Grajek, S. & Schwarz, J. C. (1982). Environmental differences among day care centers and their effects on children's development. In E. F. Zigler & E. W. Gordon (Eds), *Day care: scientific and social policy issues* (pp. 126–151). Boston, Massachusetts: Auburn House.

Maccoby, E. E. & Martin, J. A. M. (1983). Socialization in the context of the family: parent–child interaction. In E. M. Hetherington (Ed.), *Socialization, personality and social development,* Vol. 4. *Mussen's handbook of child psychology* (4th edn), (pp. 1–101). New York: Wiley.

Maughan, B., Gray, G. & Rutter, M. (in press). Reading retardation and antisocial behaviour: a follow-up into employment. *Journal of Child Psychology and Psychiatry.*

Minuchin, P. O. & Shapiro, E. K. (1983). The school as a context for social development. In E. M. Hetherington (Ed.), *Socialization, personality and social development,* Vol. 4. *Mussen's handbook of child psychology* (4th edn), (pp. 197–274). New York: Wiley.

Munsinger, H. (1975). The adopted child's IQ: a critical review. *Psychology Bulletin,* **82,** 623–659.

Page, E. B. & Grandon, G. M. (1981). Massive intervention and child intelligence. The Milwaukee project in critical perspective. *Journal of Special Education,* **15,** 239–256.

Pedersen, E., Faucher, T. A. & Eaton, W. W. (1978). A new perspective on the effects of first grade teachers on children's subsequent adult status. *Harvard Education Review,* **48,** 1–31.

Plomin, R. & DeFries, J. C. (1983). The Colorado adoptive project. *Child Development,* **54,** 276–289.

Puckering, C. & Rutter, M. (in press). Influence of extreme environments on language development. In W. Yule, M. Rutter & M. Bax (Eds), *Language development and disorders.* London: SIMP/Blackwell Scientific, Clinics in Developmental Medicine.

Quinton, D., Rutter, M. & Liddle, C. (1984). Institutional rearing, parental support and marital difficulties. *Psychological Medicine,* **14,** 107–124.

Ramey, C. T. & Campbell, F. A. (1981). Educational intervention for children at risk for mild retardation: a longitudinal analysis. In P. Mittler (Ed.), *Frontiers of knowledge in mental retardation,* Vol. I. *Social, educational and behavioral aspects* (pp. 47–57). Baltimore, Maryland: University Park Press.

Ramey, C. T. & Campbell, F. A. (1984). Preventive education for high risk children: cognitive consequences of the Carolina Abecedarian project. *American Journal of Mental Deficiency,* **88,** 515–524.

Ramey, C. T., Bryant, D. M. & Suarez, T. M. (1984). Preschool compensatory education and the modifiability of intelligence: a critical review. In D. Detterman (Ed.), *Current topics in human intelligence.* Norwood, New Jersey: Ablex Publishing Co.

Ramey, C. T., MacPhee, D. & Yeates, K. (1982). Preventing developmental retardation: a general systems model. In L. Bond & J. Joffe (Eds), *Facilitating infant and early childhood development.* Hanover, New Hampshire: University Press of New England.

Record, R. G., McKeown, T. & Edwards, J. H. (1969). The relation of measured intelligence to birth order and maternal age. *Annals of Human Genetics, London,* **33,** 61–69.

Rowe, D. C. & Plomin, R. (1981). The importance of nonshared (E_1) environmental influences in behavioral development. *Developmental Psychology,* **17,** 517–531.

Roy, P. (1983). Is continuity enough?: substitute care and socialization. Paper presented at the Spring

■ 291

Scientific Meeting, Child and Adolescent Psychiatry Specialist Section, Royal College of Psychiatrists, London, March 1983.

Rutter, M. (1981). *Maternal deprivation reassessed* (2nd edn). Harmondsworth, Middlesex: Penguin Books.

Rutter, M. (1983). School effects on pupil progress: research findings and policy implications. *Child Development*, **54**, 1–29.

Rutter, M. (1984a). Continuities and discontinuities in socio-emotional development: empirical and conceptual perspectives. In R. Emde & R. Harmon (Eds), *Continuities and discontuities in development* (pp. 41–68). New York: Plenum.

Rutter, M. (1984b). Childhood experiences and personality development. *Australian and New Zealand pscyhopathology and development: II. Journal of Psychiatry*, **18**, 314–327.

Rutter, M. (1985b). Family and school influences on behavioural development. *Journal of Child Psychology and Psychiatry*, in press.

Rutter, M. & Madge, N. (1976). *Cycles of disadvantage: a review of research*. London: Heinemann Educational.

Rutter, M., Maughan, B., Mortimore, P., Ouston, J. & Smith, A. (1979). *Fifteen thousand hours: secondary schools and their affects on children*. London: Open Books; Cambridge, MA: Harvard University Press.

Rutter, M. & Quinton, D. (1984). Parental psychiatric disorder: effects on children. *Psychological Medicine*, **14**, 853–880.

Rutter, M., Tizard, J. & Whitmore, K. (Eds) (1970). *Education, health and behaviour*. London: Longmans (reprinted, 1981; Huntington, New York: Krieger).

Scarr, S. (1981). *Race, social class, and individual differences in IQ*. Hillsdale, New Jersey: Lawrence Erlbaum.

Scarr, S. & Kidd, K. K. (1983). Developmental behavior genetics. In M. M. Haith & J. J. Campos (Eds), *Mussen's handbook of child psychology*, Vol. II. *Infancy and developmental psychobiology* (pp. 345–433). New York: Wiley.

Scarr, S. & McCartney, K. (1983). How people make their own environments: a theory of genotype—environment effects. *Child Development*, **54**, 424–435.

Scarr, S. & Weinberg, R. A. (1976). IQ test performance of black children adopted by white families. *American Psychologist*, **31**, 726–739.

Scarr, S. & Weinberg, R. A. (1983). The Minnesota adoptive studies: genetic differences and malleability. *Child Development*, **54**, 260–267.

Schiff, M., Duyme, M., Dumaret, A. & Tomkiewicz, S. (1982). How much *could* we boost scholastic achievement and IQ scores? A direct answer from a French adoption study. *Cognition*, **12**, 165–196.

Schweinhart, L. J. & Weikart, D. P. (1980). *Young children grow up: the effects of the preschool program on youths through age 15*, Monographs of the High/Scope Educational Research Foundation No. 7. Ypsilanti, Michigan: The High/Scope press.

Skeels, H. M. & Dye, H. (1939). A study of the effects of differential stimulation on mentally retarded children. *Proceedings of the American Association for Mental Deficiency*, **44**, 114–136.

Skodak, M. & Skeels, H. M. (1949). A final follow-up study of one hundred adopted children. *Journal of Genetic Psychology*, **50**, 427–439.

Skuse, D. (1984). Extreme deprivation in early childhood—II. Theoretical issues and a comparative review. *Journal of Child Psychology and Psychiatry*, **25**, 543–572.

Snow, M., Jacklin, C. & Maccoby, E. (1981). Birth order differences in peer sociability at 33 months. *Child Development*, **52**, 589–595.

Tizard, J. (1970). The role of social institutions in the causation, prevention and alleviation of mental retardation. In C. Haywood (Ed.), *Social-cultural aspects of mental retardation*. New York: Appleton-Century.

Tizard, B. & Hodges, J. (1978). The effect of early institutional rearing on the development of eight-year-old children. *Journal of Child Psychology and Psychiatry*, **19**, 99–118.

Tizard, B. & Hughes, M. (1984). *Young children learning: talking and thinking at home and at school*. London: Fontana.

Tizard, B., Carmichael, H., Hughes, M. & Pinkerton, G. (1980). Four year olds talking to mothers and teachers. In L. A. Hersov, M. Berger & A. R. Nicol (Eds), *Language and language disorders in childhood*. Book supplement to *Journal of Child Psychology and Psychiatry*, No. 2 (pp. 49–76). New York: Plenum.

292 ▪

Tizard, B., Hughes, M., Carmichael, H. & Pinkerton, G. (1983a). Children's questions and adults' answers. *Journal of Child Psychology and Psychiatry,* **24,** 269–282.

Tizard, B., Hughes, M., Carmichael, H. & Pinkerton, G. (1983b). Language and social class: is verbal deprivation a myth? *Journal of Child Psychology and Psychiatry,* **24,** 533–542.

Tizard, J., Schofield, W. N. & Hewison, J. (1982). Collaboration between teachers and parents in assisting children's reading. *British Journal of Educational Psychology,* **52,** 1–15.

Triseliotis, J. & Russell, J. (1985). *Hard to place: the outcome of late adoptions and residential care.* London: Heinemann Educational.

van Eerdewegh, M. M., Bieri, M. D., Parilla, R. H. & Clayton, P. (1982). The bereaved child. *British Journal of Psychiatry,* **140.** 23–29.

Vernon, P. E. (1970). Intelligence. In W. J. Dockrell (Ed.), *On intelligence.* London: Methuen.

Vernon, P. E. (1979). *Human intelligence: heredity and environment.* San Francisco: Freeman.

Wachs, T. D. & Gruen, G. E. (1982). *Early experience and human development.* New York: Plenum.

Walker, E. & Emory, E. (in press). Commentary: interpretive bias and behavioral genetic research. *Child Development.*

Winters, K. C., Stone, A. A., Weintraub, S. & Neale, J. M. (1981). Cognitive and attentional deficits in children vulnerable to psychopathology. *Journal of Abnormal Child Psychology,* **9,** 435–454.

Yeates, K. O., MacPhee, D., Campbell, F. A. & Ramey, C. T. (1983). Maternal IQ and home environment as determinants of early childhood intellectual competence: a developmental analysis. *Developmental Psychology,* **19,** 731–739.

Zigler, E. F. & Gordon, E. W. (Eds) (1982). *Day care: scientific and social policy issues.* Boston, Massachusetts: Auburn House Publishing Company.

■ 293

Journal of Child Psychology and Psychiatry, 1985, vol. 26, pp. 349–368

FAMILY AND SCHOOL INFLUENCES ON BEHAVIOURAL DEVELOPMENT

Michael Rutter

Department of Child and Adolescent Psychiatry, Institute of Psychiatry, London

294 ■

Abstract—Research findings are reviewed with respect to possible family and school influences on behavioural development, but with special reference to socially disapproved conduct. The hypothesis that statistical associations between environmental variables and children's disorders represent causal connections is considered in terms of the three main alternatives—hereditary influences, the effect of children on their parents, and the operation of some third variable. It is concluded that each has some validity but that nevertheless there are true environmental effects. The mechanisms underlying their operation are discussed with respect to parental criminality, family discord, weak family relationships, ineffective discipline, and peer group influences. Individual differences in response to adversity are discussed in terms of age, sex, temperament, genetic factors, coping processes, patterning of stressors, compensatory good experiences and catalytic factors. The various ways in which environmental effects may persist over time are considered in terms of linkages within the environment as well as within the child. It is concluded that long-term effects are far from independent from intervening circumstances.

Keywords: Behavioural development, individual differences, continuities/discontinuities in development

INTRODUCTION

Numerous studies have shown that children with various kinds of behavioural problems tend to come from homes or schools that are disadvantaged or deviant in some respect (see reviews by Hinde, 1980; Rutter, 1981a, 1982, 1984a; Rutter & Madge, 1976; Rutter & Giller, 1983). As a result it has come to be widely accepted that family difficulties—as reflected in such factors as broken homes, child neglect or marital discord—cause children to have psychiatric disorders. But what evidence is there that family, school and community environments do truly influence children's behaviour? And, insofar as they do, which aspects of the environment matter? Do the effects vary according to the child's age and personal qualities? To what extent do such environmental influences persist and how far are the ill-effects reversible? What mechanisms are involved in the developmental continuities and discontinuities associated with the long-term sequelae of serious adversities in childhood? It is only through answers to questions such as these that the crude statistical associations between family (or school) deviance or disadvantage and child disorder can be translated into any theoretical or practical concepts of how environmental factors may influence the course of psychosocial development. In this selective overview of a

Requests for reprints to: Prof. M. Rutter, Department of Child and Adolescent Psychiatry, Institute of Psychiatry, De Crespigny Park, Denmark Hill, London SE5 8AF, U.K.

Accepted manuscript received 23 *February* 1984

very large topic, therefore, these are the matters to which particular attention is paid. The focus is strictly on behaviour rather than cognition, and within the behavioural domain on extreme variations or deviant outcomes in terms of socially disapproved conduct rather than on variations within the normal range.

ALTERNATIVE EXPLANATIONS

The first question of whether the statistical associations between environmental variables and children's disorders represent causal connections requires an examination of three main alternatives: (a) that the associations represent hereditary rather than environmental influences; (b) that the main effect is from the child to the family rather than a unidirectional parental influence on the children; and (c) that both the family (or school) characteristics and the children's disorders are due to some third variable, such as social disadvantage or physical hazards in the environment.

■295

Genetic transmission

The suggestion that the associations reflect genetic rather than experiential factors constitutes a very real possibility. The question needs to be tackled by means of several different research strategies.

Animal studies. Firstly, environmental effects may be examined directly by means of experiments in which the circumstances of rearing are deliberately altered. For obvious ethical reasons, usually this can be done only in animals. Nevertheless, the findings are clear-cut in showing that marked changes in the environment do indeed have important effects on psychological development (Rutter, 1981a). In these studies we know that the effects were environmental rather than genetic because of the experimental conditions.

Heritability estimates. A second approach is provided by heritability estimates. The findings show that in no case is the genetic determination of psychological attributes so strong that there is no room for environmental effects (McGuffin & Gottesman, 1984; Shields, 1980). Heritability estimates are also useful in showing differences between attributes in the extent of the environmental contribution. For example, it is clear that although genetic factors play some part in juvenile delinquency, environmental factors predominate (Rutter & Giller, 1983). On the other hand, it seems that hereditary influences may be more influential in the case of criminal behaviour that is associated with personality disturbance and that persists from childhood into the adult years.

But, family resemblances also provide another important datum—the extent to which the environmental influences operate within or between families (Rowe & Plomin, 1981). If children in the same family tend to be similar in their characteristics the implication is that they share the most important environmental influences and hence that the crucial factors are likely to be those that affect the family as a whole. This is very much the situation with respect to juvenile delinquency and conduct disorders where it is common for several children in the family to show similar behaviour. The expectation that follows from this observation is that the families of

Journal of Child Psychology and Psychiatry, 1985, vol. 26, pp. 349–368

delinquents are likely to differ markedly from the families of non-delinquents in the overall environments they provide for the children. As we shall see, that is indeed what has been found.

In contrast, if brothers and sisters tend to be dissimilar in their attributes, the implication is that the environmental influences are likely to be ones that impinge differently on each member of the family. That is what seems to be the case with personality features and possibly also emotional disturbance (Loehlin & Nichols, 1976; Scarr, Webber, Weinberg & Wittig, 1981). The suggestion, here, is that it will be factors such as ordinal position, or differential treatment by parents, or stresses specific to the individual, or extra-familial influences that will be most important. But systematic differences between families according to the personality characteristics of the children are not to be expected. In other words, heritability data not only provide some estimate of the overall importance of family influences as determinants of individual differences under the environmental conditions studied, but also provide pointers as to the likelihood that such influences operate in much the same way on all children in the family. The findings suggest that with conduct disturbances to a substantial extent they do, whereas with emotional disturbances and personality features usually they do not.

Rearing in biological and adoptive homes compared. A further variant of the same strategy consists in the comparison of children from similar biological backgrounds according to whether or not they were reared by their biological parents or were adopted in infancy. The findings suggest that when the biological background is seriously deviant or disadvantaged, children who are adopted have a better outcome than those who remain with their biological parents (Bohman & Sigvardsson, 1980; Rutter & Madge, 1976; Rutter & Giller, 1983; Scarr, 1981; Scarr & Weinberg, 1983). Genetic factors still play a part in determining individual differences in behaviour and attainment, but the superior environment of the adoptive homes seemed to result in a general raising of the outcome for the group as a whole. However, it should be added that the evidence regarding the 'protective' effects of adoption is much stronger with respect to intelligence than it is for behaviour. Regrettably, there is a singular paucity of data on the benefits or otherwise of adoption in terms of non-cognitive outcome measures.

Characteristics of adoptive homes. The adoption paradigm, of course, may be used in a second way to examine environmental effects—through the determination of associations between adoptive family characteristics and disorder in the children. Provided selective placement effects can be excluded or controlled for, any such associations must represent environmental influences of one sort or another. This design has been used surprisingly rarely with respect to children's conduct disturbance. There is some evidence of associations between adoptive family characteristics (such as social class, divorce and parental mental disorder) and the children's behaviour and adjustment but the findings are too fragmentary for firm conclusions (Bohman, 1970; Cadoret & Cain, 1980; Mednick, Moffitt, Pollock, Talovic, Gabrielli & Van Dusen, 1983; Raynor, 1980).

Rearing effects after 'controlling' for genetic factors. An alternative strategy is provided by the use of designs that seek to 'control' for possible genetic effects. For example, in our study of children in families with a mentally ill parent we found that marital discord was associated with conduct disturbance in the children even within a subgroup, all of whom had a parent with a life-long personality disorder (Quinton & Rutter, 1984a). Similarly, among institution-reared girls the outcome in adult life was worse for those who experienced disrupted parenting in early childhood even after account had been taken of deviance and disorder in the biological parents (Quinton & Rutter, 1984b). Of course, it was not possible in either study entirely to rule out the possibility that disrupted parenting or marital discord represented some unmeasured genetic variable. On the other hand, this could not apply to Roy's (1983) finding that hyperactivity was more frequent in institution-reared children than in family-fostered children in spite of the fact that the biological backgrounds of the two groups were closely comparable.

■297

Change of environment. Environmental effects may be studied more directly through the consequences of *changes* in the environment. Two rather different examples of this research strategy may be given. Firstly, evidence of the importance of the social group comes from investigations of the effects of a total change in the non-familial environment. For example, West (1982) in his prospective study of London boys found that delinquent activities tended to diminish following a move to somewhere outside London (a change not explicable in terms of the boys' or the families' prior characteristics as measured). These, and other, findings suggest that young people's delinquent activities are influenced by the social group in which they find themselves.

Secondly, it has been found that changes in family circumstances are also associated with effects on the children's behaviour. For example, my colleagues and I (Rutter, 1971) investigated children, all of whom had been separated from their parents as a result of family discord or family problems. Within this group, who had experienced severe early family stress, a change for the better, in terms of a return to harmony or at least a cessation of open discord, was associated with a marked reduction in the risk of conduct disturbance. Similarly, it has been shown by Hetherington, Cox & Cox (1982) and by Wallerstein & Kelly (1980) that whether or not disorders in the children of divorcing parents diminished was a function of whether or not divorce improved family relationships. When the divorce brought harmony, the children's problems tended to improve, but when parental discord and difficulties continued so, too, the children's disorders tended to persist. Other studies (Rutter & Giller, 1983) have given rise to similar findings most of which point to environmental effects associated with changes in the quality of family relationships. However, in some circumstances children's disturbed behaviour acquires self-perpetuating qualities that cause it to persist in spite of alterations in family circumstances (Quinton & Rutter, 1984a; Richman, Stevenson & Graham, 1982).

This design, of course, has even greater power if the effects of changes can be studied in relation to family environments that involve no genetic linkage. Yarrow & Klein (1980) used this strategy with respect to infant behaviour in their study of transfers from foster to adoptive homes but the method has yet to be used to investigate influences on conduct disturbance in older children.

Non-familial environments. The final strategy for disentangling genetic and environmental effects concerns the study of non-familial environments. There is now a substantial literature showing major differences in the behaviour of children according to the characteristics of the institutional environment in which they find themselves.

Journal of Child Psychology and Psychiatry, 1985, vol. 26, pp. 349–368

298∎

Thus, studies of institutions for delinquents, such as probation hostels or correctional schools, have shown large differences between them in rates of absconding and reconviction (Rutter & Giller, 1983). Broadly speaking, the 'successful' institutions were characterized by a combination of firmness, warmth, harmony, high expectations, good discipline and a practical approach to training. Similarly, other studies (Rutter, 1983b) have shown that secondary schools vary greatly in a host of different measures of pupil success. Furthermore, these differences in outcome have been shown to be systematically associated with the qualities of the schools as social organizations.

Obviously, in these institutional studies, there can be no question of genetic transmission in the ordinary sense, in that the staff and pupils have no biological relationship. The consistent association between the characteristics of the institution and the behaviour of the pupils strongly suggests a causal connection that represents an environmental effect. The query here is of a different kind—in which direction does the causal arrow run? Did the institution shape the children's behaviour or, rather, did the qualities of the children make the institution what it was? Of course, that question also arises with the family associations, and we need to consider the various ways in which the problem of how to determine the direction of causation may be tackled.

Child effects on the environment

As with genetic transmission, the first question is whether there is any evidence in favour of the alternative explanation, that is, is there any reason to suppose that children can have effects on how adults behave? This question was first raised in a systematic fashion by Yarrow (1963) with respect to parent–child interaction in foster families, by Thomas, Chess & Birch (1968) in relation to child temperament, and by Bell (1968, 1974) through his reanalysis of the direction of effects in studies of socialization. Since Dell's critique, evidence has accumulated to show that there are important child effects (Bell & Harper, 1977; Belsky & Tolan, 1981; Lerner & Spanier, 1978; Lewis & Rosenblum, 1974; Maccoby & Martin, 1983; Rutter, 1977), although it has to be added that our knowledge on these effects remains rudimentary. Nevertheless, there is no doubt that they exist and the question is whether or not they account for the observed associations between environmental variables and child disorder.

Input differences to schools. That issue may be considered in terms of the research strategies used in studying possible school effects. The question of whether the school affected the children, or, rather, whether the children shaped the functioning of the school may be tackled by determining the timing and patterning of the associations between school characteristics and pupil behaviour or attainments. If the schools influenced the pupils, the correlations should be weak at the time of school entry but strong at the time of school leaving. Conversely, if the pupil characteristics shaped teacher behaviour the reverse should occur, that is the strongest association should be with the intake measures. In our own study (Maughan, Mortimore, Ouston & Rutter, 1980) the former proved to be the case. Thus, for example, the school measures correlated 0.39 with the children's behaviour at intake but 0.92 with that at the end of secondary schooling (both correlations, of course, refer to differences between schools rather than to those between children). The findings on timing and patterning provide strong circumstantial evidence of a causal effect of the school on the child. That is not to say that the reverse does not also occur (almost certainly it does) but it appears there is a true influence on the child stemming from characteristics of the school environment.

Timing and patterning of associations in families. Much the same issues arise with respect to the associations with family variables. Did family discord cause the child to develop behavioural problems or did the presence of a difficult child in the family lead to quarrelling and discord? Did harsh and inconsistent punishment cause the boy to be aggressive or was it that the parents were led to take extreme measures just because the boy's disruptive behaviour failed to respond to more ordinary methods of discipline? Again, there are reasons for supposing that both may occur. For example, Patterson (1982) found that aggressive boys were indeed less responsive than other boys to disciplinary measures; Gardner (1977) showed experimentally that autistic children elicited different patterns of interaction from the adults with whom they were placed. So how may we determine how far and in what circumstances the family factors influence the child rather than vice-versa?

■ 299

Of course, the matter is clear-cut in the case of the many family variables that could not have been caused by the child. Thus, it is obvious that such variables as being the oldest child, having a younger sib born, or being bereaved could not conceivably have resulted from the child's behaviour. In other cases, the fact that the family factors antedated the child's disturbance makes the direction of causation equally clear. This would be so, for example, with many instances of parental criminality or mental disorder and, equally, it would apply in many cases of marital discord. But, often, it is difficult to be at all sure about the timing. For example, prospective longitudinal studies of high-risk populations—such as the West & Farrington (1973, 1977) study of working class London boys—have been able to obtain parental measures before the children became delinquent. But we know that many of the boys showed difficult and troublesome behaviour when they were younger—some years before they appeared in court.

There is no easy way out of this dilemma and often there has to be a reliance on an interpretation of the overall pattern, together with an assessment of which causal process is more likely. Perhaps the situation where this problem arises most obviously concerns the associations between conduct disorder in boys on the one hand and family discord, poor parental supervision and inefficient discipline on the other. A key feature here is that in such families it is usual for several sons to show behavioural disturbance. As already noted, genetic factors do not seem to play a major role in these disorders and hence there is no ready explanation of why so many of the children should show problems if the association with family discord stemmed from the children's behaviour. Rather, it is more plausible that the association stemmed from a general effect of the family on the children resulting from problems in the parents. But this suggestion demands some explanation of why the parents should show such severe difficulties in parenting and in marital relationships. Is it possible to predict these difficulties in advance of the children's birth? Empirical findings show that to some extent it is.

For example, our own study following London children into early adult life (Quinton & Rutter, 1984b; Rutter, Quinton & Liddle, 1983) provides relevant data. It was found that those who experienced severe adversities in their own childhoods were the ones most likely to grow up to show difficulties in many aspects of adult functioning, including marked problems in parenting. People's experiences of rearing when they were young were important determinants of their own qualities as parents when they reached adulthood, as also found by Kruk and Wolkind (1982; Wolkind & Kruk, 1984). Other studies, too, provide limited evidence that characteristics of parents, as assessed prior to the children's birth, predict aspects of parental behaviour (Maccoby & Martin, 1983).

Association with some third variable

300 ▪

The third main alternative to family effects to be considered is that both the parents' behaviour and that of the children are due to some third variable. Thus, one might postulate that the association between parental criminality and delinquency in the sons or that between marital discord and aggressive behaviour in the children are due, not to any causal link between the two, but rather to the fact that both are caused by some other influence such as poverty or poor housing. Of course, this is a possibility that must be borne in mind in any study of hypothesized causal influences, and analyses to investigate the matter were undertaken in all the research considered so far. The results show that it is most unlikely that the family links are an artifact of some broader environmental variable. The associations are remarkably similar in all socio-cultural groups (Robins, 1978; Rutter & Giller, 1983). Of course, that is not to argue that social disadvantage has no effects on behaviour; obviously, it does. Research findings strongly suggest that the styles and qualities of parenting are much influenced by the social context and by the presence of stressors and of emotional support (Belsky, 1981; Belsky, Robins & Gamble, 1984; Bronfenbrenner, 1979; Crnic, Greenberg, Ragozin, Robinson & Basham, 1983; Quinton & Rutter, 1984b). The point being made is the narrower one that the consequences of social disadvantage are not sufficient to explain or account for those family effects that are found in all sectors of society.

Conclusions on environmental effects. We may conclude that the three main types of alternative explanation all have some validity. There are genetic effects, children do influence parents, and family functioning is modified by the broader socio-cultural environment. Nevertheless, these fail to account for all family and school effects. Accordingly, it may be inferred that there is good evidence of environmental influences on behaviour stemming from experiences both within and outside the home. We need to consider now the evidence that might indicate which mechanisms and processes are involved.

MECHANISMS AND PROCESSES

In that connection I shall largely concentrate on those aspect of family functioning found to be associated with conduct disorders and delinquency. Five may be picked out for more detailed consideration (Rutter & Giller, 1983): criminality in the parents, intra-familial discord, weak family relationships, ineffective discipline and peer group influences. These variables cover a wide range and it is necessary to ask which are the crucial dimensions. This is particularly important because the five features overlap greatly. We need to search for means to 'pull apart' variables that ordinarily tend to go together. The procedures may be illustrated by taking just a few specific examples.

Broken homes and family discord

At one time, much emphasis was placed on the supposed importance of broken homes as a cause of delinquency. The notion was that it was the fact of family break-up that was damaging. The idea seemed plausible in that broken homes were indeed statistically associated with delinquency. But what alternative explanations should be considered? One obvious contender is the presence of family discord and quarrelling (Rutter, 1971, 1982). To differentiate the two it is necessary first to split broken homes into those where discord was a prominent feature and those where it was not. Divorce and separation constituted causes that met the first criterion and parental death met the second. Several large-scale studies have data that differentiate these two causes of a broken home; the findings of all of them are agreed in showing that whereas divorce/separation is strongly associated with delinquency, death is only very weakly so. It seems that perhaps discord is more important than break-up *per se*. But if that were so, it should follow that discord in unbroken homes should also lead to delinquency. It has been found that it does. It might also be predicted that temporary separations should predispose to conduct disorders if they arose as a result of discord but not if they occurred for other reasons. Again that has been confirmed. Also, if discord is indeed a causal factor it might be expected that a reduction in discord should be followed by a diminution in the risk of conduct disturbance. Once more, empirical findings show this to be so. We may conclude that the relevant mechanism is likely to involve discordant relationships rather than break-up *per se*.

■301

Weak family relationships

Weak family relationships have also been found to be associated with delinquency. The possible importance of personal relationships is shown by the finding that a good relationship with one parent has an ameliorating effect even in the presence of general family discord (Rutter, 1971; Rutter *et al.,* 1983). However, discord and weak relationships so often accompany one another that it is difficult to separate their effects. When this is the situation, it is necessary to seek special circumstances where this is not the case. Rearing from infancy in a good quality group Home or other institution with multiple changing caretakers provides the nearest approach. Because of the frequent changes in parent-figure and because of the more 'professional' approach to child-rearing, children are less likely to form close bonds and attachments with their caretakers in this setting than if they were brought up in a nuclear family. On the other hand, usually such institutions are not particularly discordant and quarrelsome environments. So the question is what happens to young people reared in that way? Data on that point are limited but they are consistent in showing that conduct disorders are much increased in frequency among children reared from infancy in an institutional setting (Quinton & Rutter, 1984b; Roy, 1983; Rutter *et al.,* 1983; Wolkind, 1974; Yule & Raynes, 1972). Accordingly, it appears that weak family relationships are important in their own right quite apart from their association with discord.

Journal of Child Psychology and Psychiatry, 1985, vol. 26, pp. 349–368

302 ■

Supervision and discipline

But it is necessary also to consider some of the specific influences that shape particular behaviours—the role of adult supervision and discipline. At one time, attention was focused on the use of specific practices, on the severity of discipline, and on matters of consistency (Becker, 1964). But it became clear that these were not the most relevant dimensions and the focus has shifted in recent years (Maccoby & Martin, 1983). It is not yet certain how the findings are best conceptualized, but Patterson (1982) plausibly suggests four dimensions as likely to be most important: (a) the lack of 'house rules' (so that there are no clear expectations of what children may and may not do); (b) lack of parental monitoring of the child's behaviour (so that the parents are not adequately informed about his acts or emotions and hence are not in a good position to respond appropriately); (c) lack of effective contingencies (so that parents nag and shout but do not follow through with any disciplinary plan, and do not respond with an adequate differentiation between praise for prosocial and punishment for antisocial activities); and (d) a lack of techniques for dealing with family crises or problems (so that conflicts lead to tension and dispute but do not result in resolution). The pointers, then, are that we need to focus on an awareness of what children are doing, the process of disciplinary management (including problem-solving methods), and the efficiency of the techniques used.

However, also, the evidence suggests that the socio-emotional context of the discipline (i.e. the pre-existing parent–child relationship and the affective quality of the disciplinary interaction) is at least as important as the particular procedures used. In addition, it appears that key elements in discipline are as likely to be in the parental practices that serve to prevent disruptive behaviour as in any steps taken after the event.

Models of behaviour

So far, most of the dimensions considered have been concerned with one or other aspect of control (either internal or external). But it is clear that control concepts, on their own, provide an inadequate explanation for the specific form or content of children's behaviour (Hirschi, 1969; Elliott, Ageton & Cantor, 1979). In that connection, we need to turn to the role of parental criminality and of peer group influences. Doubtless, they exert their effects through several different means, including those considered already. But, in addition, we need to add the dimension of modelling. Both delinquent peers and criminal parents provide a model of aggression and of antisocial attitudes. Their behaviour constitutes something to be copied and identified with by the children, as well as a setting in which delinquent solutions to problems are regarded as acceptable, or at least to be tolerated. The same applies with delinquent siblings—a possible reason for delinquency being more frequent in boys from large families (Offord, 1982).

To summarize the findings on conduct disorder, it appears that the operative mechanisms probably include emotionally discordant patterns of social interaction, weak family relationships, inefficient supervision and discipline, and deviant models of behaviour. It should be noted that these mechanisms probably apply as much to school influences (Rutter, 1983b) as to family effects.

INDIVIDUAL DIFFERENCES IN RESPONSE TO ADVERSITY

With all these family influences the evidence has been consistent in showing the marked variation in outcomes following even the most extreme adverse experiences. Some children succumb with the development of disorder, but others escape showing resilience in the face of adversity (Garmezy, 1981; Garmezy & Nuechterlein, 1972; Garmezy & Tellegen, 1984; Rutter, 1979; Werner & Smith, 1982). The possible reasons for this individual variation need to be considered.

Age-dependent susceptibilities

The first question that arises with respect to any developmental function is whether or not there are developmentally determined age-specific susceptibilities (Rutter, 1981a, b). Of course, the issue here is not whether adverse effects are generally greater at one age period than another (it would be absurd to assume that all adversities operate in the same way), but rather whether particular environmental influences vary in their effects according to children's social, emotional and intellectual maturity. It seems that some do.

▪303

Thus, the effects of age have been found to be particularly marked in the case of hospital admission, where the age period of greatest risk has proved to be about 6 months to 4 years (Rutter, 1981a).

The effects on selective attachments also seem to be largely restricted to the first few years of life. The pattern of social disinhibition and indiscriminate friendships that is seen in some institution-reared children applies to those admitted in the first 2 years of life and not to those admitted in later childhood (Wolkind, 1974).

Bereavement, in contrast, seems more likely to lead to severe grief reactions in adolescence than in earlier childhood (van Eerdewegh, Bieri, Parrilla & Clayton, 1982; Rutter, 1981b).

Sex differences

The sex of children has been found to influence their response to various family stressors and adversities. In general, it has been found that boys are more vulnerable than girls (Rutter, 1970, 1982). This is most evident with respect to family discord, disharmony and disruption but also it has been observed with other environmental factors.

Temperamental factors

Quite apart from sex and age differences, it is evident that children vary greatly in their temperamental styles, that is in their characteristic mode of behaviour and in the manner in which they respond to differing situations (Plomin, 1983; Porter & Collins, 1982). These temperamental styles have been found to be associated with differences in children's responses to various forms of stress and adversity.

Genetic factors

Genetically determined vulnerabilities may also play a role. Although data on the point are decidedly limited, there is some evidence from studies of fostered or adopted children to suggest that genetic factors associated with delinquency or conduct disturbance may operate, in part, through creating an increased vulnerability to adverse environmental influences (Cloninger, Bohman & Sigvardsson, 1981; Crowe, 1974; Hutchings & Mednick, 1974).

Journal of Child Psychology and Psychiatry, 1985, vol. 26, pp. 349–368

Coping processes

Many such hazards require some reaction or response from the child. Accordingly, it might be thought that the outcome would be influenced by what he does about the stress situation—that is by the coping process (Rutter, 1981b). It is obvious that some coping processes could increase the risk of maladaptation or disorder whereas others could improve adaptation and reduce the risks of a deviant outcome. The notion of effective and ineffective coping is a very plausible one. Unfortunately, we lack good data on what differentiates effective and ineffective mechanisms.

Patterning and multiplicity of stressors

304 ∎

The persistence of ill-effects following stress or adversity depends to a substantial extent on whether or not the environmental hazards continue to impinge on the child. However, there is evidence that the patterning and multiplicity of stressors at any one time is also important (Rutter, 1979, 1981a, b). Thus, the presence of chronic psychosocial adversity makes it more likely that a child will suffer ill-effects from acute stressors. There are interactive effects between psychosocial adversities so that the presence of one potentiates the effect of a second or third (Rutter, 1979, 1983a).

Compensatory good experiences

Another sort of interaction has also been proposed—the balance between pleasant and unpleasant events (Lazarus, Cohen, Folkman, Kanner & Schaefer, 1980). The notion is that the presence of happy experiences, to some extent, can provide a buffer that reduces the impact of unhappy ones. Thus, the shielding influence of a good relationship in the midst of discord and disharmony has been mentioned already. In addition, good experiences at school can, perhaps, do something to compensate for difficulties at home (Quinton & Rutter, 1984b; Rutter, 1979). Success and a sense of self-esteem are important elements in growing up and factors that enhance a person's feelings of their own worth may prove protective. But, again, we lack evidence on the extent to which good experiences can compensate for bad ones.

Catalytic factors

Finally, I need to mention the possibility of 'catalytic' factors. The concept is one of those factors that are largely inert on their own, but, when combined with environmental stresses or hazards, either increase their effect (so-called 'vulnerability' factors), or decrease their impact (so-called 'protective' factors). For example, the presence of a supportive social network and of a cohesive social group are thought to operate in that fashion (Henderson, 1981; Rutter, 1981a, b; Werner & Smith, 1982).

It is clear, then, that any explanation for individual differences in children's response to stress and adversity must include both factors in the child and in his environment, although we do not know their relative importance.

PERSISTENCE OF ENVIRONMENTAL EFFECTS

Up to this point, the effects of family and school influences have been considered without explicit reference to any time frame. Some years ago it was commonly assumed that the effects of serious family adversity or deprivation in early childhood were very long-lasting and very difficult to reverse. However, research findings over the last decade or so have cast increasing doubt on that view (Clarke & Clarke, 1976; Rutter, 1981a) and we need to consider now the extent to which ill-effects persist and, more especially, the factors that determine persistence or non-persistence.

If we are to examine the persistence of effects we must focus attention on that small subgroup of children who experience severe early neglect, deprivation or disadvantage but who then experience a major change of environment followed by a normal pattern of upbringing thereafter.

Apart from single case studies of children rescued in middle childhood from cruel isolated rearing in cupboards and attics (Skuse, 1984), studies of late adoption are about the only examples we have of this phenomenon (Rutter, 1981a). The findings are consistent in showing very substantial recovery in most cases.

It is clear that environmental improvements in middle or late childhood can do much to reverse the ill-effects of early neglect, discord and deprivation. The effects of early bad experiences are not necessarily enduring and to a substantial extent the ill-effects are reversible provided that the environmental change is sufficiently great and that the later environment is sufficiently positive and beneficial. Interestingly, our own data from a follow-up into the mid-1920s of institution-reared girls showed very clearly that this effect extends right into adult life. The findings indicated that a stable harmonious marriage to a non-deviant spouse served to nullify the ill-effects of seriously adverse experiences in childhood (Quinton & Rutter, 1984b). Environmental factors continue to exert their effects well after physical maturity is reached. But just as 'bad' early experiences can be 'neutralized' to a substantial extent by good experiences in later life, so also the converse applies. A good home in the early years does not prevent damage from psychosocial stresses in adolescence. To a substantial extent, whether or not sequelae are enduring is dependent on continuities of experiences and on chain reactions.

However, other considerations must be added before the picture can be regarded as at all complete. There is the possibility that certain experiences have to occur during the early years for social development to proceed normally (Rutter, 1981a). Although the original notion of fixed and absolute 'critical periods' in development has had to be largely abandoned, the concept of 'sensitive periods' during which environmental influences have a particularly marked effect has some validity (Bateson, 1979, 1983). The generally favored candidate for this effect concerns the initial formation of selective attachments. It has been suggested by Bowlby (1969) that these first bonds must develop during the first two years or so if normal social relationships are to be possible later. The evidence to test that hypothesis is quite meagre but the few available data from studies of late-adopted children (Tizard & Hodges, 1978) are interesting and informative. Two main findings require emphasis. Firstly, even children adopted after the age of four years can develop bonds with their adoptive parents. To that extent, either the 'sensitive period' notion is wrong or it extends to a later age than usually supposed. But secondly, in spite of this development of parent–child bonds at age 4 to 6 years, the late-adopted children showed the same social and attentional problems in school as did those who remained in the institution. The implication is that, although attachments can still develop for the first time after infancy, nevertheless, to some extent fully normal social development may be dependent on bonding having taken place at an early age.

The findings are provocative in two respects: first, in their implication of a sensitive period for the optimal development of social relationships; and second, in the implication that the effects may persist into at least middle childhood in spite of a reduced change in family circumstances. Nevertheless, we should be wary about any mechanistic assumptions that the long-term effects of social experiences in the infancy period are independent of later happenings. To begin with, Tizard's data on late adopted children extend only to age 8 years and we do not know whether the findings in later childhood or adolescence would be different. The available evidence from other studies of late adopted children (Triseliotis & Russell, 1984) is inadequate for the resolution of that issue. However, the results of experimental primate studies of total social isolation in infancy may be relevant. On the one hand, the gross social anomalies of these isolation-reared animals persisted into adult life with little evidence of spontaneous recovery (Ruppenthal, Arling, Harlow, Sackett & Suomi, 1976). On the other hand, a variety of experiences in adolescence and adulthood resulted in a surprising degree of recovery of effective social functioning (Novak, 1979). Human data pertinent to this problem are very limited but they point to the same conclusions. Thus, our own study of institution-reared girls showed both: (1) that disrupted parenting in the early years was predictive of adult functioning; and (2) that the quality of marital relationships in adult life hugely modified the effects of these early experiences (Quinton & Rutter, 1984b). A more detailed analysis of the findings was informative in throwing light on the likely mechanisms involved. It was found that disrupted parenting had effects on the children's behaviour but also it was influential in terms of increasing the likelihood of other later adversities. Together these served to influence the circumstances in adolescence in which the choice of marriage partner took place. As a result, girls who suffered poor early social experiences were more likely than other girls to make an unsatisfactory marriage to a deviant man from a similarly disadvantaged background. To a very large extent, the persistent effects of disrupted parenting in infancy were a consequence of that linkage. However, if by good luck the marriage turned out well, the effects of childhood experiences were washed out.

The implication is that we need to re-think our concepts of the ways in which life experiences influence socio-behavioural development. Developmental theories that postulate a 'structure' of personality that is established during the course of the developmental process do not fit the empirical findings. Equally, however, behaviourist theories that conceptualize effects entirely in terms of the here-and-now without the need to invoke developmental considerations are inconsistent with the evidence. Constancy of behaviour over periods of several years is decidedly unusual. Similarly, the effects of early experiences cannot be considered without reference to the effects of later experiences. On the other hand, continuities in development, as well as discontinuities, are very striking. Evidence on the mechanisms that underlie both is very limited but we should consider what little is known on the processes that may be operative (Rutter, 1984b).

DEVELOPMENTAL CONTINUITIES AND DISCONTINUITIES

Selection of environments

As already noted, one important source of continuities is the linkage between different environments. Thus, in our follow-up study into adult life, institutional rearing made it more likely that the women would marry a deviant spouse (Quinton & Rutter, 1984b; Rutter et al., 1983). Similarly, the conditions of upbringing played a part in determining whether the women experienced poor social conditions in adult life, then seriatim social circumstances influenced the women's social functioning. Or, again, institution-reared girls who left the institution to return to discordant families were more likely than other girls to have babies in their 'teens; teenage pregnancy, in turn, was then associated with an increased risk of a poor social outcome. Brown, Harris & Bifulco (1984) have described a closely comparable chain of circumstances in the findings from their latest study of depressed women. The environments change but the experience of one sort of 'bad' environment makes it more likely that the individual will go on to experience other sorts of 'bad' environment.

■ 307

Opportunities

A further mechanism leading to continuities concerns the effects stemming from the opening up or closing down of opportunities. For example, in our study of inner London secondary schools (Rutter, Maughan, Mortimore, Ouston & Smith, 1979), we found powerful effects of the school environment on pupil behaviour and attainments while the children were still at school. We found no direct effects of schooling on the young people's employment one year after school-leaving but there were most important indirect effects as a result of the earlier school influences (Gray, Smith & Rutter, 1980). The school influence on exam qualifications opened up or closed down employment opportunities and in this way produced more lasting chain effects.

Effects on the environment

A third type of linkage over time is provided by the effects of family or school experiences on the environment. For example, Dunn & Kendrick (1982) showed marked behavioural reactions in first born children following the birth of a sibling. This new event introduced an important element of discontinuity but there were linkages with the past and with the future. The mother's previous style of parenting had an effect on how children reacted, but also the arrival of a sibling altered the overall pattern of family interaction. In this way a supposedly 'acute' event had 'chronic' circumstances; as a result the quality of the first born's relationship with his sibling showed a remarkable level of consistency over several years. Perhaps, too, such a changed pattern of family interaction may constitute part of the explanation for the surprisingly lasting effects of recurrent hospital admission (Douglas, 1975; Quinton & Rutter, 1976). Thus, Hinde's experimental studies with rhesus monkeys showed that the long-term effects of brief separation experiences were largely dependent on the extent to which the separation served to disturb and increase tensions in the mother–infant relationship (Hinde & McGinnis, 1977).

Journal of Child Psychology and Psychiatry, 1985, vol. 26, pp. 349–368

Vulnerability, resilience and coping skills

Another mechanism concerns so-called 'sensitization' and 'steeling' effects (Rutter, 1981b). Early events may operate by altering sensitivities to stress or in modifying styles of coping which then protect from, or predispose towards, disorder in later life only in the presence of later stress events (Rutter, 1981b). The suggestion, then, is not that there is any direct persistence of good or ill-effects but rather that patterns of response are established that influence the way the individual reacts to some later stress or adversity. If the pattern is one that increases the harm from later stress it is termed a 'sensitization' effect. Conversely, if it decreases the harm it is spoken of as 'steeling'. The literature contains several examples of both these effects. For example, it seems that the experience of one unpleasant separation may render the individual more likely to be affected adversely by later stressful separations. Conversely, a happy separation experience may prove protective. Similarly, we found that adversities in childhood rendered individuals less resilient in the presence of stresses in adult life (Quinton & Rutter, 1984b; Rutter *et al.*, 1983). There seems little doubt that early events may protect from or predispose towards later disorder through 'sensitization' or 'steeling' effects, but we lack any adequate understanding of how these effects come about, or what determines whether they are protective or damaging.

Habits, attitudes and self-concepts

Alternatively, childhood experiences may have persisting effects as a result of influences on habits, attitudes and self-esteem. Children's self-concepts include feelings of self-esteem, of self-efficacy or ability to control one's destiny, and of ego-resiliency (Harter, 1983). Findings are very limited on the role of these features as mediating mechanisms or modulating influences in children's response to life experiences; nevertheless, several types of findings suggest that they may play a significant role. Thus, it is a commonplace observation that 'problem' parents both fail to plan their lives and also feel unable to control what happens to them (Rutter & Madge, 1976; Tonge, James & Hillam, 1975). We do not know how that feeling of impotency arises but it seems probable that, to a substantial extent, their continuing family difficulties stem from these attitudes and concepts. Thus, for example, we found that institution-reared girls tend to marry on impulse to escape from an unhappy situation, their lack of 'planning' for marriage much increased the likelihood that they would make an unsatisfactory marriage (Quinton & Rutter, 1984b). On the other hand, the girls who experienced good experiences and success of some kind at school (in any aspect of life) were significantly more likely to 'plan' marriage and choose a husband for positive qualities—perhaps because their school success had given them a self-image of people who could control their destinies. Similarly, there is evidence that the taking of a boy to Court for theft, and hence his public 'labelling' as a delinquent, serves to increase the likelihood that he will persist in delinquent activities (Rutter & Giller, 1983). It is probable, too, that some of the school effects on pupils' attainments and behaviour stem from influences on habits, attitudes and self-concepts, as well as from more direct effects on learning (Rutter, 1984b).

'Sleeper' effects

There has been some controversy in the literature on whether or not there are 'sleeper effects' due to 'dormant change' in the organism arising as a result of early life experiences (Clarke & Clarke, 1981, 1982; Seitz, 1981). As already discussed, there is no doubt that there can be delayed effects in the sense of changes in functioning that are causally linked with earlier experiences but yet which do not become manifest in that form until sometime later. However, the concept of 'dormant change' does not seem to be a particularly helpful one in that it does not specify the mechanism involved. Although certainly much has still to be learned regarding the processes involved in long-term effects, it seems probable that usually they are mediated by either some form of immediate effect on the individual (as on habits, attitudes or sensitivities) or some impact on later environment (as with the opening up or closing down of opportunities) or some form of transactional effect involving both.

CONCLUSIONS

These few suggested mechanisms by no means exhaust the possibilities. However, they suffice to make the point that the concept of continuity in development implies meaningful links over the course of time and not a lack of change. The processes involve linkages within the environment as well as within the child. It should be added that even the few available findings point strongly to the poverty of prevailing theories on the nature of psychosocial development and especially on the ways in which it may be influenced by environmental circumstances. We have come to appreciate that there is a crucial difference between risk *indicators* and causal *mechanisms*. As I noted, research findings have served to increase our understanding of the latter. Thus, we have moved from concepts of broken homes, to family discord, to coercive family processes. But still we lack knowledge on exactly how those operate, on which developmental processes are affected, and on the ways in which developmental continuities and discontinuities arise. The findings on family and school influences on behavioural development have done much to clarify the issues but if further progress is to be made it will be necesary to improve both our theoretical concepts and our methods of statistical analysis. If the complex patterns of interaction and of indirect linkage are to be translated into meaningful concepts of developmental processes, it will be crucial to use analytic methods that are designed for the task. These postulated interactions are by no means synonymous with statistical interaction effects in conventional multivariate analyses (see Rutter, 1983a) and we must adapt our methods to ensure that they truly test the concepts in question.

In conclusion, it is apparent that there are important family and school influences on behavioural development. The effects are sizable but they vary markedly across individuals and according to the ecological context; moreover, they are transactional, rather than unidirectional, in nature. The evidence runs counter to the view that early experiences irrevocably change personality development (Rutter, 1981a) and also runs counter to the suggestion that any single process is involved (Sackett, 1982); nevertheless, in some circumstances the indirect effects may be quite long-lasting. Even so, such long-term effects are far from independent from intervening

Journal of Child Psychology and Psychiatry, 1985, vol. 26, pp. 349–368

circumstances. Rather, the continuities stem from a multitude of links over time (Rutter *et al.*, 1983). Because each link is incomplete, subject to marked individual variation and open to modification, recurrent opportunities to break the chain continue right into adult life.

REFERENCES

Bateson, P. (1979). How do sensitive periods arise and what are they for? *Animal Behavior,* **27**, 470–486.

Bateson, P. (1983). The interpretation of sensitive periods. In A. Oliverio & M. Zappella (Eds), *The behavior of human infants* (pp. 57–70). New York: Plenum Press.

Becker, W. C. (1964). Consequences of different kinds of parental discipline. In M. L. Hoffman & L. W. Hoffman (Eds), *Review of child development research*, Vol. 1 (pp. 169–208). New York: Russell Sage Foundation.

Bell, R. W. (1968). A reinterpretation of the direction of effects in studies of socialization. *Psychological Review,* **75**, 81–95.

Bell, R. W. (1974). Contributions of human infants to care-giving and social interaction. In M. Lewis & L. A. Rosenblum (Eds), *The effects of the infant on its caregiver.* New York: Wiley.

Bell, R. W. & Harper, L. V. (Eds) (1977). *Child effects on adults.* Hillsdale, NJ: Erlbaum.

Belsky, J. (1981). Early human experience: a family perspective. *Developmental Psychology,* **17**, 3–23.

Belsky, J. & Tolan, W. (1981). Infants as producers of their own development: an ecological perspective. In R. Lerner & N. Busch-Rossnagel (Eds), *Individuals as producers of their development: a life-span perspective.* New York: Academic Press.

Belsky, J., Robins, J. & Gamble, W. (1984). The determinants of parental competence: toward a contextual theory. In M. Lewis (Ed.), *Beyond the dyad.* New York: Plenum Press.

Bohman, M. (1970). *Adopted children and their families.* Stockholm: Prosprion.

Bohman, M. & Sigvardsson, S. (1980). Negative social heritage. *Adoption and Fostering,* **5**, 25–31.

Bowlby, J. (1969). *Attachment and loss: I. Attachment.* London: Hogarth Press.

Bronfenbrenner, U. (1979). *The ecology of human development: experiments by nature and design.* Cambridge, MA: Harvard University Press.

Brown, G., Harris, T. O. & Bifulco, A. (1984). Long-term effect of early loss of parent. In M. Rutter, C. Izard & P. Read (Eds), *Depression in childhood: developmental perspectives.* New York: Guilford Press (in press).

Cadoret, R. J. & Cain, C. (1980). Sex differences in predictors of antisocial behavior in adoptees. *Archives of General Psychiatry,* **37**, 561–563.

Clarke, A. M. & Clarke, A. D. B. (1976). *Early experience: myth and evidence.* London: Open Books.

Clarke, A. D. B. & Clarke, A. M. (1981). 'Sleeper effects' in development: fact or artifact? *Developmental Review,* **1**, 344–360.

Clarke, A. M. & Clarke, A. D. B. (1982). Intervention and sleeper effects: a reply to Victoria Seitz. *Developmental Review,* **2**, 76–86.

Cloninger, C. R., Bohman, M. & Sigvardsson, S. (1981). Inheritance of alcohol abuse: cross-fostering analysis of adopted men. *Archives of General Psychiatry,* **38**, 861–868.

Crnic, K. A., Greenberg, M. T., Ragozin, A. S., Robinson, N. M. & Basham, R. B. (1983). Effects of stress and social support on mothers and premature and full-term infants. *Child Development,* **54**, 209–217.

Crowe, R. R. (1974). An adoption study of antisocial personality. *Archives of General Psychiatry,* **31**, 785–791.

Douglas, J. W. B. (1975). Early hospital admissions and later disturbances of behaviour and learning. *Developmental Medicine and Child Neurology,* **17**, 456–480.

Dunn, J. & Kendrick, C. (1982). *Siblings: love, envy, and understanding.* Cambridge, MA: Harvard University Press.

Elliott, D. S., Ageton, S. S. & Canter, R. J. (1979). An integrated theoretical perspective on delinquent behavior. *Journal of Research into Crime and Delinquency,* **16**, 3–27.

Gardner, J. (1977). Three aspects of childhood autism: mother–child interactions, autonomic responsivity, and cognitive functioning. PhD Thesis, University of Leicester.

Garmezy, N. (1981). Children under stress: perspectives on antecedents and correlates of vulnerability and resistance to psychopathology. In A. I. Rabin, J. Aronoff, A. M. Barclay & R. A. Zucker (Eds), *Further explorations in personality*. New York: Wiley Interscience.

Garmezy, N. & Nuechterlein, K. (1972). Invulnerable children: the fact and fiction of competence and disadvantage. *American Journal of Orthopsychiatry*, **42**, 328–329 (Abstract).

Garmezy, N. & Tellegen, A. (1984). Studies of stress-resistant children: methods, variables and preliminary findings. In F. Morrison, C. Lord & D. Keating (Eds), *Applied developmental psychology*, Vol. 1, (pp. 231–287). New York: Academic Press.

Gray, G., Smith, A. & Rutter, M. (1980). School attendance and the first year of employment. In L. Hersov & I. Berg (Eds), *Out of school: modern perspectives in truancy and school refusal* (pp. 343–370). Chichester: Wiley.

Harter, S. (1983). Developmental perspectives on the self system. In E. M. Hetherington (Ed.), *Socialization, personality and Social development*, Vol. 4, *Mussen's handbook of child psychology*, Vol. 4 (pp. 275–385). New York: Wiley.

Henderson, S. (1981). Social relationships, adversity and neurosis: an analysis of prospective observations. *British Journal of Psychiatry*, **138**, 391–398.

Hetherington, E. M., Cox, M. & Cox, R. (1982). Effects of divorce on parents and children. In M. Lamb (Ed.), *Nontraditional families* (pp. 233–288). Hillsdale, NJ: Erlbaum.

Hinde, R. A. (1980). Family influences. In M. Rutter (Ed.), *Scientific foundations of developmental psychiatry* (pp. 47–66). London: Heinemann Medical.

Hinde, R. A. & McGinnis, L. (1977). Some factors influencing the effect of temporary mother–infant separation: some experiments with rhesus monkeys. *Psychological Medicine*, **7**, 197–212.

Hirschi, T. (1969). *Causes of delinquency*. Berkeley: University of California Press.

Hutchings, B. & Mednick, S. A. (1974). Registered criminality in the adoptive and biological parents of registered male adoptees. In S. A. Mednick *et al.* (Eds), *Genetics, environment and psychopathology* (pp. 215–227). Amsterdam: North-Holland.

Kruk, S. & Wolkind, S. N. (1982). A longitudinal study of single mothers and their children. In N. Madge (Ed.), *Families at risk* (pp. 119–140). London: Heinemann Educational.

Lazarus, R. S., Cohen, J. B., Folkman, S., Kanner, A. & Schaefer, C. (1980). Psychological stress and adaptation: some unresolved issues. In H. Selye (Ed.), *Guide to stress research*. New York: Van Nostrand Reinhold.

Lerner, R. M. & Spanier, G. B. (Eds) (1978). *Child influence on marital and family interaction: a life span perspective*. New York: Academic Press.

Lewis, M. & Rosenblum, L. A. (Eds) (1974). *The effect of the infant on its caregiver*. New York: Wiley.

Loehlin, J. C. & Nichols, R. C. (1976). *Heredity, environment and personality: a study of 850 sets of twins*. Austin: University of Texas Press.

Maccoby, E. E. & Martin, J. (1983). Socialization in the context of the family: parent–child interaction. In E. M. Hetherington (Ed.), *Socialization, personality and social development*, Vol. 4, *Mussen's handbook of child psychology* (4th edition) (pp. 1–101). New York: Wiley.

Maughan, B., Mortimore, P., Ouston, J. & Rutter, M. (1980). Fifteen thousand hours: a reply to Heath and Clifford. *Oxford Review of Education*, **6**, 289–303.

McGuffin, P. & Gottesman, I. I. (1984). Genetic influences on normal and abnormal development. In M Rutter & L. Hersov (Eds), *Child and adolescent psychiatry: modern approaches* (2nd edition). Oxford: Blackwell Scientific (in press).

Mednick, S. A., Moffitt, T. E., Pollock, V., Talovic, S., Gabrielli, W. F. & Van Dusen, K. T. (1983). The interitance of human deviance. In D. Magnusson & V. Allen (Eds), *Human development: an interactional perspective* (pp. 221–242). New York: Academic Press.

Novak, M. A. (1979). Social recovery of monkeys isolated for the first year of life: II. Long term assessment. *Developmental Psychology*, **15**, 50–61.

Offord, D. R. (1982). Family backgrounds of male and female delinquent. In J. Gunn & D. P. Farrington (Eds), *Abnormal offenders, delinquency, and the criminal justice system* (pp. 129–151). Chichester: Wiley.

Patterson, G. R. (1982). *Coercive family process*. Eugene, Oregon: Castalia Publ. Co.

Plomin, R. (1983). Childhood temperament. In B. B. Lahey & A. E. Kazdin (Eds), *Advances in clinical child psychology*, Vol. 6 (pp. 45–92). New York: Plenum Press.

Porter, R. & Collins, G. M. (Eds) (1982). *Temperamental differences in infants and young children*. Ciba Foundation Symposium 89. London: Pitman Books.

Quinton, D. & Rutter, M. (1976). Early hospital admissions and later disturbances of behaviour: an attempted replication of Douglas' findings. *Developmental Medicine and Child Neurology*, **18**, 447–459.

■311

Quinton, D. & Rutter, M. (1984a). Family pathology and child disorder: a four year prospective study. In A. R. Nicol (Ed.), *Longitudinal studies in child psychology and psychiatry: practical lessons from research experience.* Chichester: Wiley (in press).

Quinton, D. & Rutter, M. (1984b). Parenting behaviour of mothers raised 'in care'. In A. R. Nicol (Ed.), *Longitudinal studies in child psychology and psychiatry: practical lessons from research experience.* Chichester: Wiley (in press).

Raynor, L. (1980). *The adopted child comes of age.* London: Allen & Unwin.

Richman, N., Stevenson, J. & Graham, P. J. (1982). *Preschool to school: a behavioural study.* London: Academic Press.

Robins, L. (1978). Sturdy childhood predictors of adult antisocial behaviour: replications from longitudinal studies. *Psychological Medicine,* **8,** 611–622.

Rowe, D. C. & Plomin, R. (1981). The importance of nonshared (E_1) environmental influences in behavioural development. *Developmental Psychology,* **17,** 517–531.

Roy, P. (1983). Is continuity enough?: Substitute care and socialization. Paper presented at the Spring Scientific Meeting, Child and Adolescent Psychiatry Specialist Section, Royal College of Psychiatrists, London, March.

Ruppenthal, G. C., Arling, G. L., Harlow, H. F., Sackett, G. P. & Suomi, S. J. (1976). A 10-year perspective of motherless–mother monkey behavior. *Journal of Abnormal Psychology,* **85,** 341–349.

Rutter, M. (1970). Sex differences in children's responses to family stress. In E. J. Anthony & C. Koupernik (Eds), *The child in his family* (pp. 165–196). New York: Wiley.

Rutter, M. (1971). Parent–child separation: psychological effects on the children. *Journal of Child Psychology and Psychiatry,* **12,** 233–260.

Rutter, M. (1977). Individual differences. In M. Rutter & L. Hersov (Eds), *Child psychiatry; modern approaches* (pp. 3–21). Oxford: Blackwell Scientific.

Rutter, M. (1979). Protective factors in children's responses to stress and disadvantage. In M. W. Kent & J. E. Rolf (Eds), *Primary prevention of psychopathology,* Vol. 3, *Social competence in children* (pp. 49–74). Hanover, NH: University Press of New England.

Rutter, M. (1981a). *Maternal deprivation reassessed* (2nd edition). Harmondsworth, Middlesex: Penguin.

Rutter, M. (1981b). Stress, coping and development: some issues and some questions. *Journal of Child Psychology and Psychiatry,* **22,** 323–356.

Rutter, M. (1982). Epidemiological–longitudinal approaches to the study of development. In W. A. Collins (Ed.), *The concept of development.* Minnesota Symposia on Child Psychology, Vol. 15 (pp. 105–144). Hillsdale, NJ: Erlbaum.

Rutter, M. (1983a). Statistical and personal interactions: facets and perspectives. In D. Magnusson & V. Allen (Eds), *Human development: an interactional perspective* (pp. 295–319). New York: Academic Press.

Rutter, M. (1983b). School effects on pupil progress: research findings and policy implications. *Child Development,* **54,** 1–29.

Rutter, M. (1984a). Family and school influences: meanings, mechanisms and implications. In A. R. Nicol (Ed.), *Longitudinal studies in child psychology and psychiatry; practical lessons from research experience.* Chichester: Wiley (in press).

Rutter, M. (1984b). Continuities and discontinuities in socio-emotional development: empirical and conceptual perspectives. In R. Emde & R. Harmon (Eds), *Continuities and discontinuities in development.* New York: Plenum Press.

Rutter, M. & Giller, H. (1983). *Juvenile delinquency: trends and perspectives.* Harmondsworth, Middlesex: Penguin.

Rutter, M. & Madge, N. (1976). *Cycles of disadvantage.* London: Heinemann Educational.

Rutter, M., Maughan, B., Mortimore, P., Ouston, J. & Smith, A. (1979). *Fifteen thousand hours: secondary schools and their effects on children.* London: Open Books; Cambridge, MA: Harvard University Press.

Rutter, M., Quinton, D. & Liddle, C. (1983). Parenting in two generations: looking backwards and looking forwards. In N. Madge (Ed.), *Families at risk* (pp. 60–98). London: Heinemann Educational.

Sackett, G. P. (1982). Can single processes explain effects of postnatal influences on primate development. In R. N. Emde & R. J. Harmon (Eds), *The development of attachment and affiliative systems* (pp. 3–12). New York: Plenum Press.

Scarr, S. (Ed.) (1981). *Race, social class and individual differences in IQ.* Hillsdale, NJ: Lawrence Erlbaum.

Scarr, S. & Weinberg, R. A. (1983). The Minnesota adoption studies: genetic differences and malleability. *Child Development,* **54**, 260–267.

Scarr, S., Webber, P. L., Weinberg, R. A. & Wittig, M. A. (1981). Personality resemblance among adolescents and their parents in biologically related and adoptive families. *Journal of Personality and Social Psychology,* **40**, 885–898.

Seitz, V. (1981). Intervention and sleeper effects: a reply to Clarke and Clarke. *Developmental Review,* **1**, 361–373.

Shields, J. (1980). Genetics and mental development. In M. Rutter (Ed.), *Scientific foundations of developmental psychiatry* (pp. 8–24). London: Heinemann Medical.

Skuse, D. (1984). Extreme deprivation in early childhood: II. Therapeutic issues and a comparative review. *Journal of Child Psychology and Psychiatry,* **25**, 543–572.

Thomas, A., Chess, S. & Birch, H. G. (1968). *Temperament and behavior disorders in children.* New York: University Press.

Tizard, B. & Hodges, J. (1978). The effect of early institutional rearing on the development of eight-year-old children. *Journal of Child Psychology and Psychiatry,* **19**, 99–118.

Tonge, W. L., James, D. S. & Hillam, S. M. (1975). *Families without hope: a controlled study of 33 problem families.* British Journal of Psychiatry Special Publication No. 11.

Triseliotis, J. & Russell, J. (1984). *Hard to place: the outcome of adoption and residential care of children.* London: Heinemann Educational.

van Eerdewegh, M. M., Bieri, M. D., Parrilla, R. H. & Clayton, P. J. (1982). The bereaved child. *British Journal of Psychiatry,* **140**, 23–29.

Wallerstein, J. S. & Kelly, J. B. (1980). *Surviving the break up: how children and parents cope with divorce.* New York: Basic Books.

Werner, E. E. & Smith, R. S. (1982). *Vulnerable, but invincible: a longitudinal study of resilient children and youth.* New York: McGraw-Hill.

West, D. J. (1982). *Delinquency: its roots, careers and prospects.* London: Heinemann Educational.

West, D. J. & Farrington, D. P. (1973). *Who becomes delinquent?* London: Heinemann Educational.

West, D. J. & Farrington, D. P. (1977). *The delinquent way of life.* London: Heinemann Educational.

Wolkind, S. (1974). The components of "affectionless psychopathy" in institutionalized children. *Journal of Child Psychology and Psychiatry,* **15**, 215–220.

Wolkind, S. N. & Kruk, S. (1984). From child to parent: early separation and the adoption to motherhood. In A. R. Nicol (Ed.), *Longitudinal studies in child psychology and psychiatry: practical lessons from research experience.* Chichester: Wiley (in press).

Yarrow, L. J. (1963). Dimensions of maternal care. *Merrill-Palmer Quarterly of Behavior and Development,* **9**, 101–114.

Yarrow, L. J. & Klein, R. P. (1980). Environmental discontinuity associated with transition from foster to adoptive homes. *International Journal of Behavioral Development,* **3**, 311–322.

Yule, W. & Raynes, N. V. (1972). Behavioural characteristics of children in residential care in relation to indices of separation. *Journal of Child Psychology and Psychiatry,* **13**, 149–258.

■313

Proceedings of the Royal Society of Medicine, 1973, vol. 66, pp. 1221–1225

314■

Meeting 8 May 1973

Why are London Children so Disturbed? [Abridged]

Professor Michael Rutter
(*Institute of Psychiatry, De Crespigny Park, Denmark Hill, London SE5 8AF*)

In many respects the Isle of Wight is reasonably representative of England as a whole (Rutter *et al.* 1970) and our findings on the prevalence of child psychiatric disorder could safely be generalized to other areas of small towns. However, it would be unwise to assume that the situation would be the same in the major cities with their very different life circumstances. Accordingly, the present study was designed to determine if there were differences in the rates of child psychiatric disorder between an inner London borough and the Isle of Wight; and, if differences were found, to examine reasons for the differences in order to elucidate possible causal or precipitating factors which might suggest what remedies were required.

Methods
Children aged 10 years were selected as the population for study. The London borough was one for which extensive information was already available from other studies (Wing & Hailey 1972) and which, in most respects, was reasonably typical of the inner London area.

The strategy of investigation followed was based on the earlier Isle of Wight surveys (Rutter *et al.* 1970). A two-stage procedure was used to identify children with psychiatric disorder. First, the total population was studied using a revised version of our teacher's questionnaire (Rutter 1967) as the screening instrument. On this basis, children were selected for further study, either if they formed part of a randomly selected control group or if they had deviant scores on the teacher's questionnaire. In the second stage this group of children was studied intensively by means of a standardized parental interview of demonstrated reliability (Graham & Rutter 1968) and an individual diagnosis was made for each child.

As the teacher's questionnaire was the sole screening instrument, the prevalence figures for both areas were underestimates of true prevalence. However, as the object of the study was to estimate the relative difference between the two areas in rates of disorder, this did not matter for our purposes, so long as the underestimate was similar in each case (a point which we checked).

Whereas the Isle of Wight population at the time of study included almost no children whose parents were immigrant, the London population included a substantial minority of such children. Accordingly, in order to provide comparable groups of children from both areas, the children from immigrant families were excluded from this comparison.

Prevalence
The rate of deviance (as assessed from the teacher's questionnaire) in London (ILB) children was nearly double that in Isle of Wight (IOW) boys and girls (Fig 1). Overall, the deviance rate in London was 19.1% compared to 10.6% on the Isle of Wight (*P*<0.001). Both 'neurotic' or emotional type deviance and 'conduct' type deviance were considerably more frequent in the London 10-year-olds (*P*<0.001) (Fig 2). The findings for individual items on the questionnaire

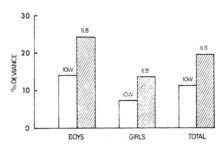

Fig 1 *Deviance on teacher questionnaire in IOW and ILB*

showed that deviance of almost all types was much more frequent in London. A series of checks showed that deviant scores had the same meaning and that the questionnaire was an equally valid screening instrument in the two areas, confirming that there was a true area difference in rates of deviant behaviour (Rutter, Cox, Tupling, Berger & Yule 1973). Nevertheless, deviance is not the same as psychiatric disorder which includes considerations of developmental course and of impaired function and requires individual diagnosis.

In London nearly 12% of boys showed psychiatric disorder compared with 6% on the Isle of Wight (Fig 3). About 5% of ILB girls showed psychiatric disorder – a rate double that on the Isle of Wight. Overall, the London rate was just over 8% compared with 4% on the Island. It may

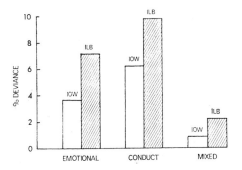

Fig 2 *Type of deviance in IOW and ILB*

be concluded that 10-year-old children living in inner London not only show more behavioural deviance than do IOW children of the same age, but also they exhibit more psychiatric disorder. It was again necessary to search for possible biasing factors which might account for the differences in prevalence; none was found (Rutter, Cox, Tupling, Berger & Yule 1973).

A parallel study (Berger, Yule & Rutter 1973, in preparation) showed that specific reading retardation was also twice as frequent in ILB children as in IOW children.

Reasons for Differences
The next question is why the rate of psychiatric disorder should be so much higher in London. For this purpose we followed a strategy which utilized a two-stage approach: (1) To identify the factors associated with psychiatric disorder *within* the inner London borough and *within* the Isle of Wight. (2) To determine if there were differences *between* the London borough and the Isle of Wight with respect to those same adverse influences associated with disorder *within* the two populations.

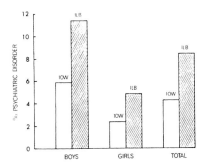

Fig 3 *Prevalence of psychiatric disorder in IOW and ILB (after teacher questionnaire screening only)*

(1) The parental interview was used to assess family interaction, relationships and style of life (Brown & Rutter 1966, Rutter & Brown 1966). Systematic and standardized techniques of known reliability were used to evaluate both attitudes or feelings and events or activities in the home. A much shorter interview was carried out with fathers, and both parents completed a health questionnaire. The two local authorities kindly provided information on school characteristics. This paper outlines only the main trends; more detailed findings are given elsewhere (Rutter, Yule, Quinton, Rowlands, Yule & Berger 1973).

In both areas severe marital discord was considerably commoner in the families of children with psychiatric disorder (Fig 4), meaning that unhappy, disruptive, quarrelsome homes are associated with psychiatric disorder in the children. Probably for the same reason, a 'broken home' (that is a home in which the child is not living with his two natural parents) was also associated with psychiatric disorder in London. It was not in the Isle of Wight to the same extent but this is explicable in terms of the very different circum-

■ 315

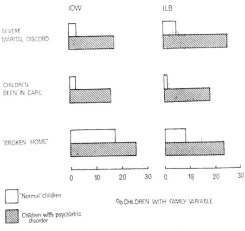

Fig 4 *Family disturbance and child psychiatric disorder in IOW and ILB*

Proceedings of the Royal Society of Medicine, 1973, vol. 66, pp. 1221–1225

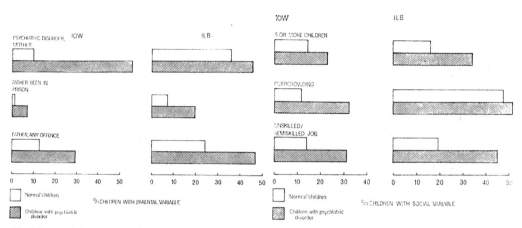

316■

Fig 5 *Parental deviance and child psychiatric disorder in IOW and ILB*

Fig 6 *Social circumstances and child psychiatric disorder in IOW and ILB*

stances associated with broken homes in the two areas. The proportion of children admitted 'into care' and placed in children's homes or with foster families is another index of family disturbance. Children admitted to short-term, as well as long-term care, frequently come from and return to disturbed families (Schaffer & Schaffer 1968, Wolkind & Rutter 1973). Among the normal children in both areas only about 2% had been admitted into care for as long as one continuous week, but among those with psychiatric disorder the proportion was 16–19%. It may be concluded from these findings that, as in other studies (Rutter 1971), family discord and disturbance is strongly associated with psychiatric disorder in the children.

Psychiatric disorder in the mother, as assessed from a systematic interview with her, was strongly associated with psychiatric problems in the IOW children (Fig 5). Half the mothers of children with psychiatric disorder had some form of psychiatric disorder themselves, compared to a rate of only 10% in the mothers of normal children. Most of the disorders in the mothers consisted of mild, chronic or recurrent depressive or neurotic conditions. The same association of disorder between mother and child was not found in London largely because of the very high rate of disorder in the mothers of the normal children. In both populations the mean score on a health questionnaire which tapped neurotic and psychosomatic symptoms of mothers of children with psychiatric disorder was significantly above that of the mothers of normal children.

Few of the fathers in both normal groups had been in prison and the rate in the fathers of the children with disorder was three times as high (difference short of significance). Considering any proven offences against the law, again the rate was twice as high in the fathers of children with

psychiatric disorder. Thus, as found in previous studies (Rutter 1966), parental illness and deviance of various sorts were associated with child psychiatric disorder.

In both London and the Isle of Wight large family size was associated with problems in the children (Fig 6). The cut-off point which differentiated the groups of normal and disordered children was different in the two cases and, although in Fig 6 the association appears stronger in London, in fact it was generally stronger in the Isle of Wight. This is illustrated by the findings on overcrowding where the difference is stronger on the Isle of Wight. In both populations there was an association between child psychiatric disorder and father's job, disorder being commoner when the father held a semi- or un-skilled job; this association was more marked in London. In short, there was a tendency for various sorts of social disadvantage or low social status to be associated with disorder in the children.

So far, school characteristics have only been analysed for the inner London borough, and Fig 7 presents the findings in terms of deviance on the teacher's questionnaire. Several school attributes were strongly associated with deviance in the children. Deviance ran at a high rate in schools with a high turnover of teachers or children, with a high proportion of children entitled to free meals, or with a large proportion of 'non-indigenous' children – that is children with immigrant parents. Of course, particularly with these last two variables, the findings might reflect selective factors in the children admitted to the schools rather than anything about the schools themselves. In order to reduce the possible effect of selective intake, the findings in Fig 7 are given after exclusion of all free-meals children and all non-indigenous children. The findings are just as strong after exclusion of these children and the

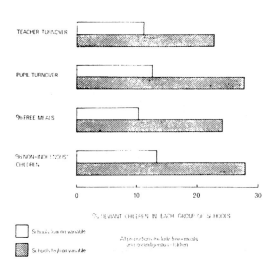

Fig 7 *School characteristics and child deviance (ILB)*

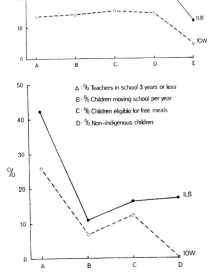

Fig 8 *Above: family/social characteristics in IOW and ILB. Below: school characteristics in IOW and ILB. IOW/ILB differences can be gauged from the difference in height between the curves; the shape of the curves is of no significance and the graphic method of presentation does not imply continuity between points*

results suggest that, however it may be caused, something in the school itself plays some part in the association with deviance in the children.

These findings have been solely concerned with the factors associated with deviance in the children *within* the two areas. It was found that in both populations child psychiatric disorder was associated with family disturbance, parental deviance, social disadvantage and features of the schools.

(2) The next stage of the investigation was to determine, with respect to these same variables, whether there was any difference *between* the two populations. For this purpose, the two randomly chosen control groups were compared.

The average marriage rating for the London families was somewhat 'worse' than for the Isle of Wight families and more children were admitted into short-term care. The official Home Office figures (1970) were used for the number of children currently in long-term care in the two areas. The rate of children in care for the borough of which our area now forms part was 12.5 per 1000, nearly three times the rate for the Isle of Wight (Fig 8).

Twice as many London fathers had been convicted of some offence and seven times as many had been to prison. Psychiatric disorder in the mothers was over twice as common in London and the health questionnaire score of both parents was also higher in the metropolis.

There was a tendency for semi- and un-skilled jobs to be commoner among London fathers (difference short of significance). Overcrowding,

however, was nearly four times as frequent, and large families (4 or more children) were nearly three times as common in London. In short, the family, parental and social circumstances associated with child psychiatric disorder were much more a feature of London than of the Isle of Wight.

All the features associated with deviance were commoner in the inner London borough than in the Isle of Wight (Fig 8). Thus, 43% of the London teachers had been with the authority for three years or less compared with 26% on the Isle of Wight. In London there was an 11% pupil turnover as against 7% on the Island. The proportion of free-meals children was higher and there was an average of 18% non-indigenous children compared with 0% on the Isle of Wight.

Discussion
The conclusions of this two-area study of child psychiatric disorder are, therefore, reasonably clear-cut. It was possible to identify four sets of

Proceedings of the Royal Society of Medicine, 1973, vol. 66, pp. 1221–1225

318▪

variables which were associated with child disorder *within* the two communities, and in almost all cases these same factors also differentiated *between* the two communities. In so far as these factors may be regarded as contributing to causal influences (and there is evidence from other studies that they do), it may be concluded that the high prevalence of psychiatric disorder in London 10-year-olds is due in part to the fact that a relatively high proportion of London families are discordant and disrupted, that families are often large and living in overcrowded homes which they do not own, and that the schools are more often characterized by a high rate of turnover in staff and pupils. These findings provide important clues as to aspects of family life, social circumstances and school conditions which require attention if the rate of child psychiatric disorder is to be reduced. Nevertheless, it is important to recognize that we know relatively little about the mechanisms involved. Many of the factors are interrelated and our preliminary analyses have so far done little to separate the effects of each variable.

Our findings on primary school differences, which are in keeping with other studies of secondary schools (Power *et al.* 1972; Gath *et al.* 1972), are important in suggesting that some schools may be more successful than others in reducing the rates of problems in their children. But what is it about the school which makes the difference? Is it the way the teachers respond to the children or does the answer lie in the nature of peer-group pressures? Is it a question of group 'morale', of quality of teaching, of attitudes to attainment or of the type of contact between school and home? What help needs to be given to schools to enable them to do their job better? We do not know but we need to find out.

Similar issues arise in the disentangling of the psychological and social processes underlying the associations between family and social circumstances and disorder in the children. There is a great need to separate out the different mechanisms involved in the various types of privation, deprivation and distortion of family life and relationships (Rutter 1972).

Finally, it is necessary to add that our conclusion, that the area differences in child psychiatric disorder are partially explicable in terms of area differences in family and school characteristics, only pushes the questions back one stage further. Why is psychiatric disorder commoner in the mothers of London children than in the mothers of Isle of Wight children? Why are there higher rates of criminality and discord? The answer does not lie in terms of deviant and disturbed families drifting to London, because the rate of disorder is just as high in children born and bred in London of parents born and bred in London as in migrants from other parts of Britain. So far we have not been able to determine whether it is due to selective out-migration, but we are examining that possibility in a separate four-year longitudinal study. Nor does it appear to be due to higher rates of biological damage during the birth process in London. Perinatal mortality rates were closely similar in the two populations at the time of the children's birth (Registrar-General 1962). Genetic data are lacking but it seems unlikely that the answer lies there in view of the high rate of population turnover in London. By a process of exclusion it seems that it must be something about life in an inner London borough which predisposes to deviance, discord or disorder. We hope to take the problem further by other analyses of our data but it is clear that further work will be required to answer the questions about what it is about life in London which leads to these problems. The answer to that question should have far-reaching implications for social policy as well as service provision.

Acknowledgments: This study was undertaken in collaboration with many colleagues. I am particularly indebted to Mrs B Yule, Mr M Berger, Mr W Yule, Dr A Cox, Mr D Quinton, Miss O Rowlands and Miss C Tupling. The project is supported by grants from the Foundation for Child Development and the Social Science Research Council.

REFERENCES

Brown G W & Rutter M (1966) *Human Relations* 19, 241–263
Gath D, Cooper B & Gattoni F E G
(1972) *Psychological Medicine* 2, 185
Graham P & Rutter M
(1968) *British Journal of Psychiatry* 114, 581
Home Office
(1970) Children in Care in England and Wales. HMSO, London
Power M J, Benn R T & Morris J N
(1972) *British Journal of Criminology* 12, 111
Registrar-General (1962) Statistical Review of England and Wales for the Year 1960. Part I, Tables, Medical. HMSO, London
Rutter M
(1966) Children of Sick Parents. Oxford University Press, London
(1967) *Journal of Child Psychology and Psychiatry* 8, 1
(1971) *Journal of Child Psychology and Psychiatry* 12, 233
(1972) Maternal Deprivation Reassessed.
Penguin, Harmondsworth
Rutter M & Brown G W (1966) *Social Psychiatry* 1, 38–53
Rutter M, Cox A, Tupling C, Berger M & Yule W
(1973) Submitted for publication
Rutter M, Tizard J & Whitmore K *eds* (1970) Education, Health and Behaviour. Longmans, Green, London
Rutter M, Yule B, Quinton D, Rowlands O, Yule W & Berger M
(1973) Submitted for publication
Schaffer H R & Schaffer E B (1968) Child Care and the Family.
Occasional Papers on Social Administration No. 25. Bell, London
Wing J K & Hailey A M *eds* (1972) Evaluating a Community Psychiatric Service: The Camberwell Register 1964–71. Oxford University Press, London
Wolkind S & Rutter M
(1973) *Journal of Child Psychology and Psychiatry* 14, 97

Part VI
Principal scientific publications

1958 Papers and book chapters
A report of two cases of the juvenile form of amaurotic familial idiocy (cerebromacular degeneration) (Jefferson, M. & Rutter, M.). *Journal of Neurology, Neurosurgery and Psychiatry*, **21**, 31–37.

1963 Papers and book chapters
Genetic and environmental factors in the development of primary reaction patterns (Rutter, M., Korn, S. & Birch, H.G.). *British Journal of Social and Clinical Psychology*, **2**, 161–173.
Interaction of temperament and environment in the production of behavioural disturbances in children (Chess, S., Thomas, A., Rutter, M. & Birch, H.G.). *American Journal of Psychiatry*, **120**, 142–147.
Psychosocial factors in the short-term prognosis of physical disease. I. Peptic ulcer (Rutter, M.). *Journal of Psychosomatic Research*, **7**, 45–60.
Some current research issues in American child psychiatry (Rutter, M.). *Millbank Memorial Fund Quarterly*, **41**, 339–370.
The psychiatrist and the general hospital (Kenyon, F.E. & Rutter, M.). *Comprehensive Psychiatry*, **4**, 80–89.

1964 Papers and book chapters
Intelligence and childhood psychiatric disorder (Rutter, M.). *British Journal of Social and Clinical Psychology*, **3**, 120–129.
Temperamental characteristics in infancy and the later development of behavioural disorders (Rutter, M., Birch, H.G., Thomas, A. & Chess, S.). *British Journal of Psychiatry*, **110**, 651–661.

1965 Papers and book chapters
Classification and categorization in child psychiatry (Rutter, M.). *Journal of Child Psychology and Psychiatry*, **6**, 71–83.
Medical aspects of the education of psychotic (autistic) children (Rutter, M.). In *Some Approaches to Teaching Autistic Children* (ed. P.T.B. Weston), London: Pergamon.
Speech disorders in a series of autistic children (Rutter, M.). In *Children with Communication Problems* (ed. A.W. Franklin), pp. 39–47. London: Pitman.
The influence of organic and emotional factors on the origins, nature and outcome of childhood psychosis (Rutter, M.). *Developmental Medicine and Child Neurology*, **7**, 518–528.

1966 Books and monographs
Children of Sick Parents: An Environmental and Psychiatric Study (Institute of Psychiatry Maudsley Monographs No.16) (Rutter, M.). London: Oxford University Press.

1966 Papers and book chapters
Behavioural and cognitive characteristics of a series of psychotic children (Rutter, M.). In *Early Childhood Autism: Clinical, Educational and Social Aspects* (ed. J.K. Wing), pp. 51–81. London: Pergamon.
Cerebral involvement in Duchenne-type muscular dystrophy (Rutter, M.). *Developmental Medicine and Child Neurology*, **8**, 85–86.
Interrelations between the choreiform syndrome, reading disability and psychiatric disorder in children of 8–11 years (Rutter, M., Graham, P. & Birch, H.G.). *Developmental Medicine and Child Neurology*, **8**, 149–159.
Prognosis: psychotic children in adolescence and early adult life (Rutter, M.). In *Early Childhood Autism: Clinical, Educational and Social Aspects* (ed. J.K. Wing), pp. 83–100. London: Pergamon.

Psychiatric disorder in 10 and 11 year old children (Rutter, M. & Graham, P.). *Proceedings of the Royal Society of Medicine*, **59**, 328–387.

The measurement of family activities and relationships (Brown, G.W. & Rutter, M.). *Human Relations*, **19**, 241–263.

The reliability and validity of measures of family life and relationships in families containing a psychiatric patient (Rutter, M. & Brown, G.W.). *Social Psychiatry*, **1**, 38–53.

1967   Papers and book chapters

A children's behaviour questionnaire for completion by teachers: preliminary findings (Rutter, M.). *Journal of Child Psychology and Psychiatry*, **8**, 1–11.

A five to fifteen year follow-up study of infantile psychosis. Part I. Description of sample (Rutter, M. & Lockyer, L.). *British Journal of Psychiatry*, **113**, 1169–1182.

A five to fifteen year follow-up study of infantile psychosis. Part II. Social and behavioural outcome (Rutter, M., Greenfield, D. & Lockyer, L.). *British Journal of Psychiatry*, **113**, 1183–1199.

Childhood asthma: a psychosomatic disorder? Some epidemiological considerations (Graham, P., Rutter, M., Yule, W. & Pless, I.B.). *British Journal of Preventive and Social Medicine*, **21**, 78–85.

Prognosis of infantile neurosis and psychosis (Rutter, M.). In *Proceedings of the IV World Congress of Psychiatry, Madrid, 1966 (Excerpta Medica International Congress)*, Series No.150.

Psychotic disorders in early childhood (Rutter, M.). In *Recent Developments in Schizophrenia: A Symposium (British Journal of Psychiatry Special Publication no. 1)* (eds A. Coppen & A. Walk), pp. 133–158. Ashford: Royal Medico-Psychological Association.

1968   Papers and book chapters

Child psychiatry (Rutter, M.). In *Studies in Psychiatry* (eds M. Shepherd & D. Davies). London: Oxford University Press.

Concepts of autism: a review of research (Rutter, M.). *Journal of Child Psychology and Psychiatry*, **9**, 1–25.

Educational aspects of childhood maladjustment: some epidemiological findings (Yule, W. & Rutter, M.). *British Journal of Educational Psychology*, **39**, 1–14.

Lésion cérébrale organique hyperkinesie et retard mental (Rutter, M.). *La Psychiatrie de L'Enfant*, **11**, 475–492.

Organic brain dysfunction and child psychiatric disorders (Graham, P. & Rutter, M.). *British Medical Journal*, **3**, 695–700.

The reliability and validity of the psychiatric assessment of the child. I. Interview with the child (Rutter, M. & Graham, P.). *British Journal of Psychiatry*, **114**, 563–579.

The reliability and validity of the psychiatric assessment of the child. II. Interview with the parent (Graham, P. & Rutter, M.). *British Journal of Psychiatry*, **114**, 581–592.

1969   Papers and book chapters

A five- to fifteen-year follow-up study of infantile psychosis. III. Psychological aspects (Lockyer, L. & Rutter, M.). *British Journal of Psychiatry*, **115**, 865–882.

A tri-axial classification of mental disorders in childhood: An International Study (Rutter, M., Lebovici, S., Eisenberg, L., Snezsnevskij, A.V., Sadoun, R., Brooke, E. & Lin, T-Y.). *Journal of Child Psychology and Psychiatry*, **10**, 41–61.

The concept of dyslexia (Rutter, M.). In *Planning for Better Learning* (eds P.H. Wolff & R. MacKeith). London: Heinemann/SIMP.

1970   Books and monographs

A Neuropsychiatric Study in Childhood (Clinics in Developmental Medicine 35/36) (Rutter, M., Graham, P. & Yule, W.). London: Heinemann/SIMP.

Education, Health and Behaviour (eds M. Rutter, J. Tizard & K. Whitmore). London: Longman. Reprinted, 1981, Melbourne, FL: Krieger.

1970   Papers and book chapters

A five to fifteen year follow-up study of infantile psychosis. IV. Patterns of cognitive ability (Lockyer, L. & Rutter, M.). *British Journal of Social and Clinical Psychology*, **9**, 152–163.

Autistic children: infancy to adulthood (Rutter, M.). *Seminars in Psychiatry*, **2**, 435–450.

Psychological development: predictions from infancy (Rutter, M.). *Journal of Child Psychology and Psychiatry*, **11**, 49–62.

Psychosocial disorders in childhood and their outcome in adult life (Rutter, M.). *Journal of the Royal College of Physicians, London*, **4**, 211–218.

Sex differences in children's response to family stress (Rutter, M.). In *The Child in his Family: Children at Psychiatric Risk, Vol.3* (eds E.J. Anthony & C. Koupernik), pp. 165–196. New York, NY: John Wiley & Sons.

1971   Books and monographs

Infantile Autism: Concepts, Characteristics and Treatment (ed. M. Rutter). Edinburgh & London: Churchill Livingstone. Translation: Japanese, 1978, Tokyo: Bunkodo Blue Books.

1971   Papers and book chapters

A developmental and behavioral approach to the treatment of pre-school autistic children (Rutter, M. & Sussenwein, F.). *Journal of Autism and Childhood Schizophrenia*, **1**, 376–396.

Causes of infantile autism: some considerations from recent research (Rutter, M. & Bartak, L.). *Journal of Autism and Childhood Schizophrenia*, **1**, 20–32.

Normal psychosexual development (Rutter, M.). *Journal of Child Psychology and Psychiatry*, **11**, 259–283.

Parent–child separation: psychological effects on the children (Rutter, M.). *Journal of Child Psychology and Psychiatry*, **12**, 233–260.

Psychiatry (Rutter, M.). In *Mental Retardation: An Annual Review III* (ed. J. Wortis), pp. 186–221. New York, NY: Grune & Stratton.

The description and classification of infantile autism (Rutter, M.). In *Infantile Autism* (ed. D.W. Churchill), pp. 8–28. Springfield, IL: Chas C. Thomas.

1972 Books and monographs

Maternal Deprivation Reassessed (Rutter, M.). Harmondsworth: Penguin Books. 2nd edn 1981. Translations: Italian, 1974, Bologna: Societa Editrice Il Milano; Swedish, 1975, Lund: Aldus Bokforlaget (Bonnier Group); Portuguese, 1978, Sao Paulo: Editoria des Humanismo, Ciencia e Tecnologia; German, 1978, Deutsch Ugend Institut/Juventa Verlag; Dutch, 1979, Utrecht: Het Spectrum; Japanese, 1979, Tokyo: Seishin Shobo; French, 1983, Centre Technique National d'Etudes et de Recherches; Spanish, 1990, Ediciones Morata; reprinted 1976 as *The Qualities of Mothering*, New York, NY: Jason Aronson.

The Child with Delayed Speech (*Clinics in Developmental Medicine 43*) (eds M. Rutter & J.A.M. Martin). London & Philadelphia: Heinemann/SIMP & Lippincott.

1972 Papers and book chapters

Childhood schizophrenia reconsidered (Rutter, M.). *Journal of Autism and Childhood Schizophrenia*, **2**, 315–317.

Classification of mental retardation: issues arising in the fifth WHO seminar on psychiatric diagnosis, classification, and statistics (Tarjan, M.D., Tizard, J., Rutter, M., Becab, M., Brooke, E.M., De La Cruz, F., Lin, T-Y., Montenegro, H., Strotzka, H. & Sartorius, N.). *American Journal of Psychiatry*, **128** (suppl. 11), 34–45.

Maternal deprivation reconsidered (Rutter, M.). *Journal of Psychosomatic Research*, **16**, 241–250.

Psychiatric disorder and intellectual impairment in childhood (Rutter, M.). *British Journal of Hospital Medicine*, **8**, 137–140.

Relationships between child and adult psychiatric disorders (Rutter, M.). *Acta Psychiatrica Scandinavica*, **48**, 3–21.

■321

1973 Papers and book chapters

A home-based approach to the treatment of autistic children (Howlin, P., Marchant, R., Rutter, M. & Berger, M.). *Journal of Autism and Childhood Schizophrenia*, **3**, 308–336.

Analyzing mothers' speech to young autistic children: a methodological study (Howlin, P., Cantwell, D., Marchant, R., Berger, M. & Rutter, M.). *Journal of Abnormal Child Psychology*, **1**, 317–339.

Children who have been 'in care': an epidemiological study (Rutter, M. & Wolkind, S.). *Journal of Child Psychology and Psychiatry*, **14**, 97–105.

Enuresis and behavioural deviance: some epidemiological considerations (Rutter, M., Yule, W. & Graham, P.). In *Bladder Control and Enuresis* (*Clinics in Developmental Medicine 48/49*) (eds I. Kolvin, R.C. MacKeith & S.R. Meadow). London: Heinemann/SIMP.

Indications for research: III (Rutter, M.). In *Bladder Control and Enuresis* (*Clinics in Developmental Medicine 48/49*) (eds I. Kolvin, R.C. MacKeith & S.R. Meadow). London: Heinemann/SIMP

Preliminary communication. An evaluation of the proposal for a multi-axial classification of child psychiatric disorders (Rutter, M., Shaffer, D. & Shepherd, M.). *Psychological Medicine*, **3**, 244–250.

Psychiatric disorders in the young adolescent: a follow-up study (Graham, P. & Rutter, M.). *Proceedings of the Royal Society of Medicine*, **66**, 1226–1229.

Special educational treatment of autistic children: a comparative study. I. Design of study and characteristics of units (Bartak, L. & Rutter, M.). *Journal of Child Psychology and Psychiatry*, **14**, 161–179.

Special educational treatment of autistic children: a comparative study. II. Follow-up findings and implications for services (Rutter, M. & Bartak, L.). *Journal of Child Psychology and Psychiatry*, **14**, 241–270.

Specific reading retardation (Rutter, M. & Yule, W.). In *The Review of Special Education* (eds L. Mann & D. Sabatino). Philadelphia, PA: Buttonwood Farms.

Temperamental characteristics as predictors of behavior disorders in children (Graham, P., Rutter, M. & George, S.). *American Journal of Orthopsychiatry*, **43**, 328–339.

The assessment and treatment of pre-school autistic children (Rutter, M.). *Early Child Development and Care*, **3**, 13–29.

Why are London children so disturbed? (Rutter, M.). *Proceedings of the Royal Society of Medicine*, **66**, 1221–1225.

1974 Papers and book chapters

Children of West Indian immigrants. I. Rates of behavioural deviance and of psychiatric disorder (Rutter, M., Yule, W., Berger, M., Yule, B., Morton, J. & Bagley, C.). *Journal of Child Psychology and Psychiatry*, **15**, 241–262.

Dimensions of parenthood: some myths and some suggestions (Rutter, M.). In *The Family in Society: Dimensions of parenthood. Report of Seminar held at All-Souls College, Oxford, 10–13 April, 1973* (Department of State and Official Bodies). London: HMSO.

Emotional disorder and educational under-achievement (Rutter, M.). *Archives of Disease in Childhood*, **49**, 249–256.

Epidemiological strategies and psychiatric concepts in research on the vulnerable child (Rutter, M.). In *The Child in His Family: Children at Psychiatric Risk, Vol.3* (eds E. Anthony & C. Koupernik), pp. 167–179. New York, NY: John Wiley & Sons.

Graded change in the treatment of the behaviour of autistic children (Yule, W., Berger, M., Rutter, M. & Yule, B.). *Journal of Child Psychology and Psychiatry*, **15**, 221–227.

Over- and under-achievement in reading: distribution in the general population (Yule, M., Rutter, M., Berger, M. & Thompson, J.). *British Journal of Educational Psychology*, **44**, 1–12.

The development of infantile autism (Rutter, M.). *Psychological Medicine*, **4**, 147–163.

1975 Books and monographs

A Guide to a Multi-Axial Classification Scheme for Psychiatric Disorders in Childhood and Adolescence (Rutter, M., Shaffer, D. & Sturge, C.). London: Institute of Psychiatry.

A Multi-Axial Classification of Child Psychiatric Disorders (Rutter, M., Shaffer, D. & Shepherd, M.). Geneva: World Health Organization.

Helping Troubled Children (Rutter, M.). Harmondsworth: Penguin Books. Reprinted 1976 , New York, NY: Plenum). Translations: German, 1981, Munchen: Ernst Reinhardt Verlag; Japanese, 1983, Tokyo: Rugaru Sha; Russian, 1988, Moscow: Progres Publishers.

1975 Papers and book chapters

A comparative study of infantile autism and specific developmental receptive language disorder. I. The children (Bartak, L., Rutter, M. & Cox, A.). *British Journal of Psychiatry*, **126**, 127–145.

A comparative study of infantile autism and specific developmental receptive language disorder. II. Parental charactieristics (Cox, A., Rutter, M., Newman, S. & Bartak, L.). *British Journal of Psychiatry*, **126**, 146–159.

Attainment and adjustment in two geographical areas. I. The prevalence of psychiatric disorder (Rutter, M., Cox, A., Tupling, C., Berger, M. & Yule,W.). *British Journal of Psychiatry*, **126**, 493–509.

Attainment and adjustment in two geographical areas. II. The prevalence of specific reading retardation (Berger, M., Yule, W. & Rutter, M.). *British Journal of Psychiatry*, **126**, 510–519.

Attainment and adjustment in two geographical areas. III. Some factors accounting for area differences (Rutter, M., Yule, B., Quinton, D., Rowlands, O., Yule, W. & Berger, M.). *British Journal of Psychiatry*, **126**, 520–533.

Language and cognition in autistic and 'dysphasic' children (Bartak, L. & Rutter, M.). In *Language, Cognitive Deficits and Retardation* (ed. N. O'Connor), pp. 193–202. London: Butterworth.

Psychiatric outcome of localized head injury in children (Shaffer, D., Chadwick, O. & Rutter, M.). In *Outcome of Severe Damage to the Central Nervous System (Ciba Foundation Symposium 34)* (eds R. Porter & S. FitzSimons), pp. 191–213. Amsterdam: Elsevier/Excerpta Medica/North Holland.

Psychological disorders in crippled children: a comparative study of children with and without brain damage (Seidel, U.P., Chadwick, O.F.D. & Rutter, M.). *Developmental Medicine and Child Neurology*, **17**, 563–573.

The birth of human developmental psychology (Rutter, M.). In *Child Alive: New Insights into the Development of Young Children* (ed. R. Lewin), pp. 12–22. London: Temple Smith.

The children of West Indian immigrants. II. Intellectual performance and reading attainment (Yule, W., Berger, M., Rutter, M. & Yule, B.). *Journal of Child Psychology and Psychiatry*, **16**, 1–17.

The children of West Indian immigrants. III. Some circumstances and family patterns (Rutter, M., Yule, B., Morton, J. & Bagley, C.). *Journal of Child Psychology and Psychiatry*, **16**, 105–123.

The concept of specific reading retardation (Rutter, M. & Yule, W.). *Journal of Child Psychology and Psychiatry*, **16**, 181–197.

The measurement of staff–child interaction in three units for autistic children (Bartak, L. & Rutter, M.). In *Varieties of Residential Experience* (eds J. Tizard, I. Sinclair & R.V.G Clarke) London: Routledge & Kegan Paul.

1976 Books and monographs

Cycles of Disadvantage: A Review of Research (Rutter, M. & Madge, N.). London: Heinemann Educational.

1976 Papers and book chapters

Adolescent turmoil: fact or fiction? (Rutter, M., Graham, P., Chadwick, O.F.D. & Yule, W.). *Journal of Child Psychology and Psychiatry*, **17**, 35–56.

An evaluation of an interview assessment of marriage (Quinton, D., Rutter, M. & Rowlands, O.). *Psychological Medicine*, **6**, 557–586.

Differences between mentally retarded and normally intelligent autistic children (Bartak, L. & Rutter, M.). *Journal of Autism and Childhood Schizophrenia*, **6**, 109–120.

Early hospital admissions and later disturbances of behaviour: an attempted replication of Douglas' findings (Quinton, D. & Rutter, M.). *Developmental Medicine and Child Neurology*, **18**, 447–459.

Language and autism (Baker, L., Cantwell, P., Rutter, M. & Bartak, L.). In *Autism: Diagnosis, Current Research and Management* (ed. E. Ritvo), pp. 12–149. Holliswood, NY: Spectrum Publications.

Research report: Institute of Psychiatry Department of Child and Adolescent Psychiatry (Rutter, M.). *Psychological Medicine*, **6**, 505–516.

Research report: Isle of Wight studies, 1964–1974 (Rutter, M.). *Psychological Medicine*, **6**, 313–332.

The epidemiology and social implications of specific reading retardation (Yule, W. & Rutter, M.). In *The Neuropsychology of Learning Disorders* (eds R.M. Knights & D.J. Bakker). Baltimore, MD: University Park.

1977 Books and monographs

Child Psychiatry: Modern Approaches (eds Rutter, M. & Hersov, L.). Oxford & Baltimore, MD: Blackwell Scientific & University Park Press. 2nd and subsequent edns published as *Child and Adolescent Psychiatry: Modern Approaches*. 2nd edn 1985 (eds Rutter, M., Taylor, E. & Hersov, L.); 3rd edn 1994 (eds Rutter, M., Taylor, E. & Hersov, L.). Translations: Italian, 1980, Bologna: Zanichelli; Japanese, 1982, Kyoto: Rugaru Sha Press.

322 ■

1977 Papers and book chapters

A comparative study of infantile autism and specific developmental receptive language disorders. III. Discriminant function analysis. (Bartak, L., Rutter, M. & Cox, A.). *Journal of Autism and Childhood Schizophrenia*, **7**, 383–396.

Bias resulting from missing information: some epidemiological findings (Cox, A., Rutter, M., Yule, B. & Quinton, D.). *British Journal of Preventive and Social Medicine*, **31**, 131–136.

Brain damage syndromes in childhood: concepts and findings (Rutter, M.). *Journal of Child Psychology and Psychiatry*, **18**, 1–21.

Cognitive characteristics of parents of autistic children (Lennox, C., Callias, M. & Rutter, M.). *Journal of Autism and Childhood Schizophrenia*, **7**, 243–261.

Compliance and resistance in autistic children (Clark, P. & Rutter, M.). *Journal of Autism and Childhood Schizophrenia*, **7**, 33–48.

Families of autistic and dysphasic children. II. Mothers' speech to the children (Cantwell, D.P., Baker, L. & Rutter, M.). *Journal of Autism and Childhood Schizophrenia*, **7**, 313–327.

Genetic influences and infantile autism (Folstein, S. & Rutter, M.). *Nature*, **265**, 726–728.

Infantile autism: a genetic study of 21 twin pairs (Folstein, S. & Rutter, M.). *Journal of Child Psychology and Psychiatry*, **18**, 297–321.

Prospective studies to investigate behavioral change (Rutter, M.). In *The Origins and Course of Psychopathology* (eds J.S. Strauss, H.M. Babigian & M. Roff). New York, NY: Plenum.

Psychiatric disorder: ecological factors and concepts of causation (Rutter, M. & Quinton, D.). In *Ecological Factors in Human Development* (ed. H. McGurk). Amsterdam: North-Holland.

Surveys to answer questions: some methodological considerations (Rutter, M.). In *Epidemiological Approaches in Child Psychiatry* (ed. P.J. Graham), pp. 1–30. London: Academic Press.

The analysis of language level and language function: a methodological study (Cantwell, D., Howlin, P. & Rutter, M.). *British Journal of Disorders of Communication*, **12**, 119–135.

1978 Books and monographs

Autism: A Reappraisal of Concepts and Treatment (eds Rutter, M. & Schopler, E.). New York, NY: Plenum. Translation: Japanese, 1982, Tokyo: Reimei Shobo.

1978 Papers and book chapters

A comparative study of infantile autism and specific developmental receptive language disorder. IV. Analysis of syntax and language function (Rutter, M.). *Journal of Child Psychology and Psychiatry*, **19**, 351–362.

Communication deviance and diagnostic differences (Rutter, M.). In *The Nature of Schizophrenia: New Approaches to Research and Treatment* (eds L.C. Wynne, R.L. Cromwell & S. Matthysee), pp. 512–516. New York, NY: John Wiley & Sons.

Diagnosis and definition of childhood autism (Rutter, M.). *Journal of Autism and Childhood Schizophrenia*, **8**, 139–169.

Diagnostic validity in child psychiatry (Rutter, M.). *Advances in Biological Psychiatry*, **2**, 2–22.

Early sources of security and competence (Rutter, M.). In *Human Growth and Development* (eds J.S. Bruner & A. Garton). London: Oxford University Press.

Family, area and school influences in the genesis of conduct disorders (Rutter, M.). In *Aggression and Antisocial Behaviour in Childhood and Adolescence* (*Journal of Child Psychology and Psychiatry Book Series No. I*) (eds L. Hersov, M. Berger & D. Shaffer). Oxford: Pergamon.

Hyperkinetic disorder in psychiatric clinic attenders (Sandberg, S. Rutter, M. & Taylor, E.). *Developmental Medicine and Child Neurology*, **20**, 279–299.

Prevalence and types of dyslexia (Rutter, M.). In *Dyslexia: An Appraisal of Current Knowledge* (eds A.L. Benton & D. Pearl), pp. 3–28. New York, NY: Oxford University Press.

Research and prevention of psychosocial disorder in childhood (Rutter, M.). In *Social Care Research* (eds J. Barnes & N. Connolly). London: Bedford Square Press.

1979 Books and monographs

Changing Youth in a Changing Society: Patterns of Adolescent Development and Disorder (Rutter, M.). London: Nuffield Provincial Hospitals Trust. Reprinted 1980, Cambridge, MA: Harvard University Press.

Fifteen Thousand Hours: Secondary Schools and their Effects on Children (Rutter, M., Maughan, B., Mortimore, P., Ouston, J. & Smith, A.). London & Cambridge, MA: Open Books & Harvard University Press. Reprinted 1994, London: Paul Chapman.

1979 Papers and book chapters

Autism: psychopathological mechanisms and therapeutic approaches (Rutter, M.). In *Cognitive Growth and Development: Essays in Memory of Herbert G. Birch* (ed. M. Bortner), pp. 273–299. New York, NY: Brunner/Mazel.

Families of autistic and dysphasic children. I. Family life and interaction patterns (Cantwell, D.P., Baker, L. & Rutter, M.). *Archives of General Psychiatry*, **36**, 682–687.

Invulnerability, or why some children are not damaged by stress (Rutter, M.). In *New Directions in Children's Mental Health* (ed. S.J. Shamsie), pp. 53–75. New York, NY: Spectrum.

Language, cognition and autism (Rutter, M.). In *Congenital and Acquired Cognitive Disorders* (ed. R. Katzman), pp. 247–264. New York, NY: Raven Press.

Maternal deprivation 1972–1978: new findings, new concepts, new approaches (Rutter, M.). *Child Development*, **50**, 283–305.

Protective factors in children's responses to stress and disadvantage (Rutter, M.). In *Primary Prevention of Psychopathology: Vol.3: Social Competence in Children* (eds M.W. Kent & J.E. Rolf), pp. 49–74. Hanover, NH: University Press of New England.

■323

Psychosocial issues in planning for the future (Rutter, M.). In *The Child in the World of Tomorrow* (ed. S. Doxiadis), pp. 125–131. Oxford: Pergamon.

Separation experiences: a new look at an old topic (Rutter, M.). *Journal of Pediatrics*, **95**, 147–154.

Task difficulty and task performance in autistic children (Clark. P. & Rutter, M.). *Journal of Child Psychology and Psychiatry*, **20**, 271–285.

1980 Books and monographs

Scientific Foundations of Developmental Psychiatry (ed. Rutter, M.). London & Baltimore, MD: Heinemann Medical & University Park Press. Translation: Spanish, 1985, Barcelona: Salvat Editores.

1980 Papers and book chapters

A prospective study of children with head injuries. I. Design and methods (Rutter, M. & Chadwick, O.). *Psychological Medicine*, **10**, 633–645.

DSM–III: a step forward or back in terms of the classification of child psychiatric disorders? (Rutter, M. & Shaffer, D.). *Journal of the American Academy of Child Psychiatry*, **19**, 371–394.

Head injury and later reading disability (Shaffer, D., Bijur, P., Chadwick, O. & Rutter, M.). *Journal of the American Academy of Child Psychiatry*, **19**, 592–610.

Language training with autistic children: how does it work and what does it achieve? (Rutter, M.). In *Language and Language Disorders in Childhood* (eds L.A. Hersov, M. Berger & A.R. Nicol), pp. 147–172. Oxford: Pergamon.

Neurobehavioural associations and syndromes of 'minimal brain dysfunction' (Rutter, M. & Chadwick, O.). In *Clinical Neuroepidemiology* (ed. F.C. Rose), pp. 330–338. Tunbridge Wells: Pitman Medical.

Raised lead levels and impaired cognitive/behavioural functioning: a review of the evidence (Rutter, M). *Developmental Medicine and Child Neurology Supplement*, **42**, 1–36.

School attendance and the first years of employment (Gray, G., Smith, A. & Rutter, M.). In *Out of School: Modern Perspectives in Truancy and School Refusal* (eds L. Hersov & I. Berg), pp. 343–370. Chichester: John Wiley & Sons.

School influences on pupil progress: research strategies and tactics (Rutter, M., Maughan, B., Mortimore, P., Ouston, J. & Smith, A.). *Journal of Child Psychology and Psychiatry*, **21**, 366–369.

Secondary school practice and pupil success (Rutter, M.). In *Education for the Inner City* (ed. M. Marland). London: Heinemann Educational.

The long-term effects of early experience (Rutter, M.). *Developmental Medicine and Child Neurology*, **22**, 800–815.

1981 Papers and book chapters

A prospective study of children with head injuries. II. Cognitive sequelae (Chadwick, O., Rutter, M., Brown, G., Shaffer, D. & Traub, M.). *Psychological Medicine*, **11**, 49–61.

A prospective study of children with head injuries. III. Psychiatric sequelae (Brown, G., Chadwick, O., Shaffer, D., Rutter, M. & Traub, M.). *Psychological Medicine*, **11**, 63–78.

A prospective study of children with head injuries: IV. Specific cognitive deficits (Chadwick, O., Rutter, M., Shaffer, D. & Shrout, P.E.). *Journal of Clinical Neuropsychology*, **3**, 101–120.

Autistic children's responses to structure and to interpersonal demands (Clark, P. & Rutter, M.). *Journal of Autism and Developmental Disorders*, **11**, 201–217.

Epidemiological/longitudinal strategies and causal research in child psychiatry (Rutter, M.). *Journal of the American Academy of Child Psychiatry*, **20**, 513–544.

Intellectual performance and reading skills after localised head injury in childhood (Chadwick, O., Rutter, M., Thompson, J. & Shaffer, D.). *Journal of Child Psychology and Psychiatry*, **22**, 117–139.

Isle of Wight and Inner London studies (Rutter, M.). In *Prospective Longitudinal Research: An Empirical Basis for Primary Prevention of Psychosocial Disorders* (eds S.A. Mednick & A.E. Baert), pp. 122–130. Oxford: Oxford University Press.

Longitudinal studies: a psychiatric perspective (Rutter, M.). In *Prospective Longitudinal Research: An Empirical Basis for Primary Prevention of Psychosocial Disorders* (eds S.A. Mednick & A.E. Baert), pp. 326–335. Oxford: Oxford University Press.

Longitudinal studies of autistic children (Rutter, M.). In *Prospective Longitudinal Research: An Empirical Basis for Primary Prevention of Psychosocial Disorders* (eds S.A. Mednick & A.E. Baert), pp. 267–269. Oxford: Oxford University Press.

Longitudinal studies of institutional children and children of mentally ill parents (Rutter, M. & Quinton, D.). In *Prospective Longitudinal Research: An Empirical Basis for Primary Prevention of Psychosocial Disorders* (eds S.A. Mednick & A.E. Baert), pp. 297–304. Oxford: Oxford University Press.

Psychiatric interviewing techniques: I. Methods and measures (Rutter, M. & Cox, A.). *British Journal of Psychiatry*, **138**, 273–282.

Psychiatric interviewing techniques: II. Naturalistic study: eliciting factual information (Cox, A., Hopkinson, K. & Rutter, M.). *British Journal of Psychiatry*, **138**, 283–291.

Psychiatric interviewing techniques: III. Naturalistic study: eliciting feelings (Hopkinson, K., Cox, A. & Rutter, M.). *British Journal of Psychiatry*, **138**, 406–415.

Psychiatric interviewing techniques: IV. Experimental study: four contrasting styles (Rutter, M., Cox, A., Egert, S., Holbrook, D. & Everitt, B.). *British Journal of Psychiatry*, **138**, 456–465.

Psychiatric interviewing techniques: V. Experimental study: eliciting factual information (Cox, A., Rutter, M. & Holbrook, D.). *British Journal of Psychiatry*, **139**, 29–37.

Psychiatric interviewing techniques: VI. Experimental study: eliciting feelings (Cox, A., Holbrook, D. & Rutter, M.). *British Journal of Psychiatry*, **139**, 144–152.

Psychiatric sequelae and cognitive recovery after severe head injury in childhood (Chadwick, O., Brown, G., Shaffer, D. & Rutter, M.). In *Prospective Longitudinal Research: An Empirical Basis for*

Primary Prevention of Psychosocial Disorders (eds S.A. Mednick & A.E. Baert), pp. 270–274. Oxford: Oxford University Press.

Psychological sequelae of brain damage in children (Rutter, M.). *American Journal of Psychiatry*, **138**, 1533–1544.

Social/emotional consequences of day care for pre-school children (Rutter, M.). *American Journal of Orthopsychiatry*, **51**, 4–28.

Stress, coping and development: some issues and some questions (Rutter, M.). *Journal of Child Psychology and Psychiatry*, **22**, 323–356.

The characteristics of situationally and pervasively hyperactive children: implications for syndrome definition (Schachar, R., Rutter, M. & Smith, A.). *Journal of Child Psychology and Psychiatry*, **22**, 375–392.

The city and the child (Rutter, M.). *American Journal of Orthopsychiatry*, **51**, 610–625.

1982 Papers and book chapters

Concepts of autism: a review of research (Rutter, M.). In *New Directions in Childhood Psychopathology, Vol. 2, Deviations in Development* (eds S.I. Harrison & J.F. McDermott, Jr.), pp. 979–1017. New York, NY: International Universities Press.

Developmental neuropsychiatry: concepts, issues and problems (Rutter, M.). *Journal of Clinical Neuropsychology*, **4**, 91–115.

Epidemiological-longitudinal approaches to the study of development (Rutter, M.). In *The Concept of Development. (Minnesota Symposia on Child Psychology, Vol. 15)* (ed. W.A. Collins), pp. 105–144. Hillsdale, NJ: Lawrence Erlbaum.

Mother and pre-school child interaction: a sequential approach (Mrazek, D.A., Dowdney, L., Rutter, M. & Quinton, D.). *Journal of the American Academy of Child Psychiatry*, **21**, 453–464.

Prevention of children's psychosocial disorders: myth and substance (Rutter, M.). *Pediatrics*, **70**, 883–894.

Psychological therapies: issues and prospects (Rutter, M.). *Psychological Medicine*, **12**, 723–740.

Surveys to answer questions: some methodological considerations (Rutter, M.). *Acta Psychiatrica Scandinavica*, **65** (suppl. 296), 64–76.

Syndromes attributed to "minimal brain dysfunction" in childhood (Rutter, M.). *American Journal of Psychiatry*, **139**, 21–33.

Temperament: concepts, issues and problems (Rutter, M.). In *Temperamental Differences in Infants and Young Children* (eds R. Porter & G. Collins), pp. 1–16. London: Pitman Books.

Towards the resolution of conflicting findings (Boulin, D., Freeman, B.J., Geller, E., Ritvoe, E.R., Rutter, M. & Yuwiler, A.). *Journal of Autism and Developmental Disorders*, **12**, 97–98.

1983 Books and monographs

A Measure of our Values: Goals and Dilemmas in the Upbringing of Children (Rutter, M.). London: Friends' Home Service Committee.

Developmental Neuropsychiatry (ed. Rutter, M.). New York, NY: Guilford Press.

Juvenile Delinquency: Trends and Perspectives (Rutter, M. & Giller, H.). Harmondsworth: Penguin Books.

Lead versus Health: Sources and Effects of Low Level Lead Exposure (eds M. Rutter & R. Russell Jones). Chichester: John Wiley & Sons.

Stress, Coping and Development (eds N. Garmezy & M. Rutter). New York, NY: McGraw-Hill. Reprinted 1988, Baltimore, MD: Johns Hopkins University Press.

1983 Papers and book chapters

Children in lesbian and single parent households (Golombok, S., Spencer, A. & Rutter, M.). *Journal of Child Psychology and Psychiatry*, **24**, 551–572.

Cognitive deficits in the pathogenesis of autism (Rutter, M.). *Journal of Child Psychology and Psychiatry*, **24**, 513–531.

Developmental psychopathology (Rutter, M. & Garmezy, N.). In *Socialization, Personality, and Social Development, Vol. 4, Mussen's Handbook of Child Psychology (4th edn)* (ed. E.M. Hetherington), pp. 775–911. New York, NY: John Wiley & Sons.

Epidemiological-longitudinal approaches to the study of development (Rutter, M.). In *Epidemiological Approaches in Child Psychiatry. II. (International Symposium, Mannheim, 1981)* (eds M.H. Schmidt & H. Remschmidt). Stuttgart: Thieme Verlag.

Hyperactivity and minimal brain dysfunction: epidemiological perspectives on questions of cause and classification (Rutter, M., Chadwick, O. & Schachar, R.). In *The Child at Psychiatric Risk* (ed. R.E. Tarter), pp. 80–107. New York, NY: Oxford University Press.

Parenting in two generations: looking backwards and looking forwards (Rutter, M., Quinton, D. & Liddle, L.). In *Families at Risk* (ed. N. Madge), pp. 60–98. London: Heinemann Educational.

School effects on pupil progress: research findings and policy implications (Rutter, M.). *Child Development*, **54**, 1–29.

Statistical and personal interactions: facets and perspectives (Rutter, M.). In *Human Development: An Interactional Perspective* (eds D. Magnusson & V. Allen), pp. 295–319. New York, NY: Academic Press.

The family, the child and the school (Rutter, M.). In *Middle Childhood: Developmental Variation and Dysfunction Between Six and Fourteen Years* (eds M.D. Levine & P. Satz). New York, NY: Academic Press.

1984 Papers and book chapters

"Project future": the way forward for child psychiatry (Rutter, M.). *Journal of the American Academy of Child Psychiatry*, **23**, 577–581.

■325

Continuities and discontinuities in socio-emotional development: empirical and conceptual perspectives (Rutter, M.). In *Continuities and Discontinuities in Development* (eds R. Emde & R. Harmon), pp. 41–68. New York, NY: Plenum.

Institutional rearing, parenting difficulties, and marital support (Quinton, D., Rutter, M. & Liddle, C.). *Psychological Medicine*, **14**, 107–124.

Long-term follow-up of women institutionalized in childhood – factors promoting good functioning in adult life (Rutter, M. & Quinton, D.). *British Journal of Developmental Psychology*, **18**, 225–234.

Observation of parent and child interaction with two-to-three year olds (Dowdney, L, Mrazek, D., Quinton, D. & Rutter, M.). *Journal of Child Psychology and Psychiatry*, **25**, 379–407.

Parental psychiatric disorder: effects on children (Rutter, M. & Quinton, D.). *Psychological Medicine*, **14**, 853–880.

Parents with children in care. I. Current circumstances and parenting skills (Quinton, D. & Rutter, M.). *Journal of Child Psychology and Psychiatry*, **25**, 211–229.

Parents with children in care. II. Intergenerational continuities (Quinton, D. & Rutter, M.). *Journal of Child Psychology and Psychiatry*, **25**, 231–250.

Psychopathology and development. I. Childhood antecedents of adult psychiatric disorder (Rutter, M.). *Australian and New Zealand Journal of Psychiatry*, **18**, 225–234.

Psychopathology and development. II. Childhood experiences and personality development (Rutter, M.). *Australian and New Zealand Journal of Psychiatry*, **18**, 314–327.

The domain of developmental psychopathology (Sroufe, A. & Rutter, M.). *Child Development*, **58**, 17–29.

1985 Papers and book chapters

Aggression and the family (Rutter, M.). *Acta Paedopsychiatrica*, **6**, 11–25.

Black pupils' progress in secondary school. I. Reading attainment between 10 and 14 (Maughan, B., Dunn, G. & Rutter, M.). *British Journal of Developmental Psychology*, **3**, 113–121.

Education: improving practice through increasing understanding (Maughan, B. & Rutter, M.). In *Children, Youth, and Families: The Action-Research Relationship* (ed. R.N. Rapoport), pp. 26–49. Cambridge: Cambridge University Press.

Effects of lead on children's behaviour and cognitive performance: a critical review (Yule, W. & Rutter, M.). In *Dietary and Environmental Lead: Human Health Effects* (ed. K.R. Mahaffey). Amsterdam: Elsevier.

Epidemiology of child psychiatric disorder: methodological issues and some substantive findings (Rutter, M. & Sandberg, S.). *Child Psychiatry and Human Development*, **15**, 209–233.

Family and school influences on behavioural development (Rutter, M.). *Journal of Child Psychology and Psychiatry*, **26**, 349–368.

Family and school influences on cognitive development (Rutter, M.). *Journal of Child Psychology and Psychiatry*, **26**, 683–704

Infantile autisms (Rutter, M.). In *The Clinical Guide to Child Psychiatry* (eds D. Shaffer, A. Erhardt & L. Greenhill), pp. 48–78. New York, NY: Free Press.

Parenting qualities, concepts, measures and origins (Dowdney, L., Skuse, D., Rutter, M. & Mrazek, D.). In *Recent Research in Developmental Psychopathology (Journal of Child Psychology and Psychiatry Monograph Supplement No. 4)* (ed. J. Stevenson), pp. 19–42. Oxford: Pergamon.

Reading retardation and anti-social behaviour: a follow-up into employment (Maughan, B., Gray, G. & Rutter, M.). *Journal of Child Psychology and Psychiatry*, **26**, 741–758.

Resilience in the face of adversity. Protective factors and resistance to psychiatric disorder (Rutter, M.). *British Journal of Psychiatry*, **147**, 598–611

The nature and qualities of parenting provided by women raised in institutions (Dowdney, L., Skuse, D., Rutter, M., Quinton. D. & Mrazek, D.). *Journal of Child Psychology and Psychiatry*, **26**, 599–625.

The treatment of autistic children (Rutter, M.). *Journal of Child Psychology and Psychiatry*, **26**, 193–214.

1986 Books and monographs

Depression in Young People: Developmental and Clinical Perspectives (eds M. Rutter, C. Izard & P. Read). New York, NY: Guilford Press.

1986 Papers and book chapters

Agreement between teachers' ratings and observations of hyperactivity, inattentiveness and defiance (Schachar, R., Sandberg, S. & Rutter, M.). *Journal of Abnormal Child Psychology*, **14**, 331–345.

Black pupils' progress in secondary school. II. Examination attainments (Maughan, B. & Rutter, M.). *British Journal of Developmental Psychology*, **4**, 19–29.

Child psychiatry: looking 30 years ahead (Rutter, M.). *Journal of Child Psychology and Psychiatry*, **27**, 803–840.

Child psychiatry: the interface between clinical and developmental research (Rutter, M.). *Psychological Medicine*, **16**, 151–169.

Conduct disorder and hyperactivity. II. A cluster analytic approach to the identification of a behavioural syndrome (Taylor, E., Everitt, B., Thorley, G., Schachar, R., Rutter, M. & Wieselberg, M.). *British Journal of Psychiatry*, **149**, 768–777.

Family and school influences on cognitive development (Rutter, M.). In *Social Relationships and Cognitive Development* (eds R.A. Hinde, A.N. Perret-Clermon & J. Stevenson-Hinde). London: Oxford University Press.

Meyerian psychobiology, personality development and the role of life experiences (Rutter, M.). *American Journal of Psychiatry*, **143**, 1077–1087.

Social child psychiatry: the next 25 years (Rutter, M.). In *Psychiatry and Its Related Disciplines: The Next 25 Years* (eds R. Rosenberg, F. Schulsinger & E. Stromgren). Copenhagen: WPA/Schutz-Gralisk A/S.

326

The study of school effectiveness (Rutter, M.). In *Kwaliteit van Onderwigs in Het Geding* (eds J.C. van der Wolf & J.J Hox), pp. 32–43. Lisse: Swets and Zeitlingen.

1987 Books and monographs

Language Development and Disorders (Clinics in Developmental Medicine 101/102) (eds Yule, W. & Rutter, M.). London: MacKeith Press/Blackwell Scientific.

Treatment of Autistic Children (Howlin, P. & Rutter, M. with Berger, M., Hemsley, R., Hersov, L. & Yule, W.). Chichester: John Wiley & Sons. Translation: Japanese, 1996, Kyoto: Rugara Sha.

1987 Papers and book chapters

Autism and pervasive developmental disorders: concepts and diagnostic issues (Rutter, M. & Schopler, E.). *Journal of Autism and Developmental Disorders*, **17**, 159–186.

Autism: familial aggregation and genetic implications (Folstein, S. & Rutter, M.). In *Neurobiological Issues in Autism* (eds E. Schopler & G. Mesibov), pp. 83–105. New York, NY: Plenum.

Changes in family function and relationships in children who respond to methylphenidate (Schachar, R., Taylor, E., Wieselberg, M., Thorley, G. & Rutter, M.). *Journal of the American Academy of Child and Adolescent Psychiatry*, **26**, 728–732.

Continuities and discontinuities from infancy (Rutter, M.). In *Handbook of Infant Development* (2nd edn) (ed. J. Osofsky), pp. 1256–1296. New York, NY: John Wiley & Sons.

Developmental language disorders: some thoughts on causes and correlates (Rutter, M.) In *Proceedings of the First International Symposium on Specific Speech and Language Disorders in Children*. Brentford: Association for All Speech Impaired Children.

Parental mental disorder as a psychiatric risk factor (Rutter, M.). In *American Psychiatric Association Annual Review, Vol. 6* (eds R.E. Hales & A.J. Frances), pp. 647–663. Washington, DC: American Psychiatric Association.

Parental mental illness as a risk factor for psychiatric disorders in childhood (Rutter, M. & Quinton, D.). In *Psychopathology: An International Perspective* (eds D. Magnusson & A. Ohman), pp. 199–219. New York, NY: Academic Press.

Psychosocial resilience and protective mechanisms (Rutter, M.). *American Journal of Orthopsychiatry*, **57**, 316–331.

Pupil progress in selective and non-selective schools (Maughan, B. & Rutter, M.). *Schools Organization*, **7**, 50–68.

Temperament, personality and personality disorder (Rutter, M.). *British Journal of Psychiatry*, **150**, 443–458.

The role of cognition in child development and disorder (Rutter, M.). *British Journal of Medical Psychology*, **60**, 1–16.

Which boys respond to stimulant medication? A controlled trial of methylphenidate in boys with disruptive behaviour (Taylor, E., Schachar, R., Thorley, G., Everitt, B. & Rutter, M.). *Psychological Medicine*, **17**, 121–143.

■327

1988 Books and monographs

Assessment and Diagnosis in Child Psychopathology (eds M. Rutter, A.H. Tuma & I.S. Lann). London & New York, NY: Fulton & Guilford Press.

Parenting Breakdown: The Making and Breaking of Intergenerational Links (Quinton, D. & Rutter, M.). Aldershot: Avebury.

Studies of Psychosocial Risk: The Power of Longitudinal Data (ed. M. Rutter). Cambridge: Cambridge University Press.

1988 Papers and book chapters

Autism and pervasive developmental disorders: concepts and diagnostic issues (Rutter, M. & Schopler, E.). In *Diagnosis and Assessment in Autism* (eds E. Schopler & G. Mesibov), pp. 15–36. New York, NY: Plenum.

Autism: biological concepts and treatment prospects (Rutter, M.). In *A Challenge to Child Psychiatry* (eds R. Takagi & L. Wing), pp. 31–54. Tokyo: Iwasaki Gakujutsu Shuppensha.

Autism: familial aggregation and genetic implications (Folstein, S. & Rutter, M.). *Journal of Autism and Developmental Disorders*, **18**, 3–30.

Biological basis of autism: implications for intervention (Rutter, M.). In *Preventive and Curative Intervention in Mental Retardation* (eds F.J. Menolascino & J.A. Stark), pp. 265–294. Baltimore: Brookes Publishing.

Cerebral blood flow and metabolism of oxygen and glucose in young autistic adults (Le Couteur, A., Trygstad, O., Evered, C., Gillberg, C. & Rutter, M.). *Psychological Medicine*, **18**, 823–831.

Child health and the environment (Golding, J., Hull, D. & Rutter, M.). In *Child Health in a Changing Society* (ed. J.O. Forfar), pp. 122–154. Oxford: Oxford University Press.

Childhood depression: epidemiology, etiological models, and treatment implications (Rutter, M.). *Integrative Psychiatry*, **6**, 1–21.

Diagnosis and description of autism: current concepts and approaches (Rutter, M.). In *Autismus Hente und Morgen* (International Association of Autism – Europe) (eds H. Blohm, W. Judt and E. Pohl-Wenzel). Hamburg: Bundesverband.

Diagnosis and subclassification of autism: concepts and instrument development (Rutter, M., Le Couteur, A., Lord, C., Macdonald, H., Rios, P. & Folstein, S.). In *Diagnosis and Assessment in Autism* (eds E. Schopler & G. Mesibov), pp. 239–259. New York, NY: Plenum.

Epidemiological approaches to developmental psychopathology (Rutter, M.). *Archives of General Psychiatry*, **45**, 486–495.

Functions and consequences of relationships: some psychopathological considerations (Rutter, M.). In *Relations within Families: Mutual Influences* (eds R.A. Hinde & J. Stevenson-Hinde), pp. 332–353. Oxford: Clarendon Press.

Infantile autism and urinary excretion of peptides and protein-associated peptide complexes (Le Couteur, A., Trygstad, O., Evered, C., Gillberg, C. & Rutter, M.). *Journal of Autism and Developmental Disorders*, **18**, 181–190.

Psychiatric interviewing techniques. A second experimental study: eliciting feelings (Cox, A., Rutter, M. & Holbrook, D.). *British Journal of Psychiatry*, **152**, 64–72.

Psychosocial risk trajectories and beneficial turning points (Rutter, M.). In *Early Influences Shaping the Individual* (ed. S. Doxiadis), pp. 229–239. New York, NY: Plenum.

Review symposium: the comprehensive experiment: a comparison of the selective and non-selective school organisation (Rutter, M.). *British Journal of Sociology of Education*, **9**, 107–112.

Selective subcortical abnormalities in autism (Jacobson, R., Le Couteur, A., Howlin, P. & Rutter, M.).*Psychological Medicine*, **18**, 39–48.

The assessment of lifetime psychopathology: a comparison of two interviewing styles (Harrington, R., Hill, J., Rutter, M., Joh, K., Fudge, H., Zoccolillo, M. & Weissman, M.). *Psychological Medicine*, **18**, 487–493.

1989 Papers and book chapters

Adult personality functioning assessment (APFA). An investigator-based standardised interview (Hill, J., Harrington, R., Fudge, H., Rutter, M. & Pickles, A.). *British Journal of Psychiatry*, **155**, 24–35.

Age as an ambiguous variable in developmental research: some methodological considerations from developmental psychopathology (Rutter, M.). *International Journal of Behavioral Development*, **12**, 1–34.

Annotation: child psychiatric disorders in ICD–10. (Rutter, M.). *Journal of Child Psychology and Psychiatry*, **30**, 499–513.

Approche psycho-educative pour le traitement des autistes (Rutter, M.). In *Autisme et Troubles du Développement Global de l'Enfant* (eds G. LeLord, J.P. Muh, M. Petit & D. Savage), pp. 172–188. Paris: Expansion Scientifique Française.

Attention deficit disorder/hyperkinetic syndrome: conceptual and research issues regarding diagnosis and classification (Rutter, M.). In *Attention Deficit Disorder: Clinical and Basic Research* (eds. T. Sagvolden and T. Archer), pp. 1–24. Hillsdale, NJ: Lawrence Erlbaum.

Autism diagnostic interview: a standardized investigator-based instrument (Le Couteur, A., Rutter, M., Lord, C., Rios, P., Robertson, S., Holdgrafer, M. & McLennan, J.). *Journal of Autism and Developmental Disorders*, **19**, 363–387.

Autism Diagnostic Observation Schedule: a standardized observation of communicative and social behavior (Lord, C., Rutter, M. & Goode, S.). *Journal of Autism and Developmental Disorders*, **19**, 185–212.

Infantile autism and developmental receptive dysphasia: a comparative follow-up into middle childhood (Cantwell, D.P., Baker, L., Rutter, M. & Mawhood, L.). *Journal of Autism and Developmental Disorders*, **19**, 19–31.

Intergenerational continuities and discontinuities in serious parenting difficulties (Rutter, M.). In *Child Maltreatment* (eds D. Cicchetti & V. Carlson), pp. 317–348. New York, NY: Cambridge University Press.

Isle of Wight revisited: twenty-five years of child psychiatric epidemiology (Rutter, M.). *Journal of the American Academy of Child and Adolescent Psychiatry*, **28**, 633–653.

Mothers' speech to autistic children: a preliminary causal analysis (Howlin, P. & Rutter, M.). *Journal of Child Psychology and Psychiatry*, **30**, 819–843.

Pathways from childhood to adult life (Rutter, M.). *Journal of Child Psychology and Psychiatry*, **30**, 23–51.

Psychiatric disorder in parents as a risk factor in children (Rutter, M.). In *Prevention of Psychiatric Disorders in Child and Adolescent: The Project of the American Academy of Child and Adolescent Psychiatry (OSAP Prevention Monograph 2)* (eds D. Shaffer, I. Philips, N. Enver, M. Silverman & V.Q. Anthony), pp. 157–189. Rockville, MD: Office for Substance Abuse Prevention, US Department of Health and Human Services.

Recognition and expression of emotional cues by autistic and normal adults (Macdonald, H., Rutter, M., Howlin, P., Rios, P., Le Couteur, A., Evered, C. & Folstein, S.). *Journal of Child Psychology and Psychiatry*, **30**, 865–877.

Temperament: conceptual issues and clinical implications (Rutter, M.). In *Temperament in Childhood* (eds G.A. Kohnstamm, J.E. Bates & M.K Rothbart), pp. 463–479. Chichester: John Wiley & Sons.

1990 Books and monographs

Straight and Devious Pathways from Childhood to Adulthood (eds L. Robins & M. Rutter). New York, NY: Cambridge University Press.

1990 Papers and book chapters

Adult outcome of childhood and adolescent depression. I. Psychiatric status (Harrington, R., Fudge, H., Rutter, M., Pickles, A. & Hill, J.). *Archives of General Psychiatry*, **47**, 465–473.

Changing patterns of psychiatric disorder over adolescence (Rutter, M.). In *Adolescence and Puberty* (eds J. Bancroft & J.M. Reinisch), pp. 124–145. New York, NY: Oxford University Press.

Classification of abnormal psychosocial situations: preliminary report of a revision of a WHO scheme (van Goor-Lambo, G., Orley, J., Poutska, F. & Rutter, M.). *Journal of Child Psychology and Psychiatry*, **31**, 229–241.

Commentary: some focus and process considerations regarding effects of parental depression on children (Rutter, M.). *Developmental Psychology*, **26**, 60–67.

Genetic factors in child psychiatric disorders: I. A review of research strategies (Rutter, M., Bolton, P., Harrington, R., Le Couteur, A., Macdonald, H. & Simonoff, A.). *Journal of Child Psychology and Psychiatry*, **31**, 3–37.

Genetic factors in child psychiatric disorders: II. Empirical findings (Rutter, M., Macdonald, H., Le Couteur, A., Harrington, R., Bolton, P. & Bailey, A.). *Journal of Child Psychology and Psychiatry*, **31**, 39–83.

Genetic influences in autism (Bolton, P. & Rutter, M.). *International Review of Psychiatry*, **2**, 65–78.

Improving the quality of psychiatric data: classification, cause and course (Rutter, M. & Pickles, A.). In *Data Quality in Longitudinal Research* (eds D. Magnusson & L.R. Bergman), pp. 32–57. Cambridge: Cambridge University Press.

Interface between research and clinical practice in child psychiatry: some personal reflections. Discussion paper (Rutter, M.). *Journal of the Royal Society of Medicine*, **83**, 444–447.

Psychosocial resilience and protective mechanisms (Rutter, M.). In *Risk and Protective Factors in the Development of Psychopathology* (eds J. Rolf, A. Masten, D. Cicchetti, K. Nuechterlein & S. Weintraub), pp. 181–214. New York, NY: Cambridge University Press.

1991 *Books and monographs*

Biological Risk Factors for Psychosocial Disorders (eds M. Rutter & P. Casaer). Cambridge: Cambridge University Press.

1991 *Papers and book chapters*

A fresh look at 'maternal deprivation' (Rutter, M.). In *The Development and Integration of Behaviour* (ed. P. Bateson), pp. 331–374. Cambridge: Cambridge University Press.

Adult outcomes of childhood and adolescent depression. II. Links with antisocial disorder (Harrington, R., Fudge, H., Rutter, M., Pickles, A. & Hill, J.). *Journal of the American Academy of Child and Adolescent Psychiatry*, **30**, 434–439.

Age changes in depressive disorders: some developmental considerations (Rutter, M.). In *The Development of Emotion and Dysregulation* (eds J. Garber & K. Dodge), pp. 273–300. Cambridge: Cambridge University Press.

Autism (Bailey, A.J. & Rutter, M.). *Science Progress*, **75**, 389–402.

Autism as a genetic disorder (Rutter, M.). In *The New Genetics of Mental Illness* (eds P. McGuffin & R. Murray), pp. 225–244. Oxford: Heinemann Medical.

Autism: pathways from syndrome definition to pathogenesis (Rutter, M.). *Comprehensive Mental Health Care*, **1**, 5–26.

Can schools change? I. Outcomes at six London secondary schools (Maughan, B., Pickles, A., Rutter, M. & Ouston, J.). *School Effectiveness and School Improvement*, **1**, 188–210.

Can schools change? II. Practice at six London secondary schools (Ouston, J., Maughan, B. & Rutter, M.). *School Effectiveness and School Improvement*, **2**, 3–13.

Childhood experiences and adult psychosocial functioning (Rutter, M.). In *The Childhood Environment and Adult Disease (Ciba Foundation Symposium No. 156)* (eds G.R. Bock & J. Whelan), pp. 189–200. Chichester: John Wiley & Sons.

Comorbidity in child psychopathology: concepts, issues and research strategies (Caron, C. & Rutter, M.). *Journal of Child Psychology and Psychiatry*, **32**, 1063–1080.

Growing up as a twin: twin–singleton differences in psychological development (Rutter, M. & Redshaw, J.). *Journal of Child Psychology and Psychiatry*, **32**, 885–896.

Nature, nurture, and psychopathology: a new look at an old topic (Rutter, M.). *Development and Psychopathology*, **3**, 125–136.

Person–environment interactions; concepts, mechanisms and implications for data analysis (Rutter, M. & Pickles, A.). In *Conceptualization and Measurement of Organism–Environment Interaction* (eds T.D. Wachs & R. Plomin), pp. 105–141. Washington, DC: American Psychological Association.

Quantitative genetics and developmental psychopathology (Plomin, R., Remde, R. & Rutter, M.). In *Internalizing and Externalizing Expressions of Dysfunction: Rochester Symposium on Developmental Psychopathology, Vol.2* (eds D. Cicchetti & S.L.Toth), pp. 155–202. Hillsdale, NJ: Lawrence Erlbaum.

Reliability and validity of a psychosocial axis in patients with child psychiatric disorder (Shaffer, D., Gould, M.S., Rutter, M. & Sturge, C.). *Journal of the American Academy of Child and Adolescent Psychiatry*, **30**, 109–115.

Statistical and conceptual models of "turning points" in developmental processes (Pickles, A. & Rutter, M.). In *Problems and Methods in Longitudinal Research: Stability and Change* (eds D. Magnusson, L.R. Bergman, G. Rudinger & B. Törestad), pp. 133–165. Cambridge: Cambridge University Press.

1992 *Papers and book chapters*

Adolescence as a transition period: continuities and discontinuities in conduct disorder (Rutter, M.). *Journal of Adolescent Health*, **13**, 451–460.

Classification of pervasive developmental disorders: some concepts and practical considerations (Rutter, M. & Schopler, E.). *Journal of Autism and Developmental Disorders*, **22**, 459–482.

Effects of age and pubertal status on depression in a large clinical sample (Angold, A. & Rutter, M.). *Development & Psychopathology*, **4**, 5–28.

Fragile X in families multiplex for autism and related phenotypes: prevalence and criteria for cytogenetic diagnosis (Bolton, P., Pickles, A., Butler, L., Summers, D., Webb, T., Lord, C., Le Couteur, A., Bailey, A. & Rutter, M.). *Psychiatric Genetics*, **2**, 277–300.

Language delay and social development (Rutter, M., Mawhood, L. & Howlin, P.). In *Specific Speech and Language Disorders in Children* (eds P. Fletcher & D. Hall), pp. 63–78. London: Whurr Publishers.

Psychosocial stressors: concepts, causes and effects (Rutter, M. & Sandberg, S.). *European Child and Adolescent Psychiatry*, **1**, 3–13.

Research report: the Medical Research Council Unit in Child Psychiatry (Taylor, E. & Rutter, M.). *Psychological Medicine*, **22**, 805–813.

■329

Season of birth: issues, approaches and findings for autism (Bolton, P., Pickles, A., Harrington, R., Macdonald, H. & Rutter, M.). *Journal of Child Psychology and Psychiatry*, **3**, 509–531.

The outcome of conduct disorder: implications for defining adult personality disorder and conduct disorder (Zoccolillo, M., Pickles, A., Quinton, D. & Rutter, M.). *Psychological Medicine*, **22**, 971–986.

The role of eye-contact in goal-detection: evidence from normal infants and children with autism or mental handicap (Phillips, W., Baron-Cohen, S. & Rutter, M.). *Development and Psychopathology*, **4**, 375–383.

1993   Books and monographs

Developing Minds: Challenge and Continuity across the Lifespan (Rutter, M. & Rutter, M.). Harmondsworth & New York: Penguin Books & Basic Books.

1993   Papers and book chapters

An overview of paediatric neuropsychiatry (Rutter, M.). In *The Brain and Behaviour: Organic Influences on the Behaviour of Children* (eds F. Besag & R. Williams), *Educational and Child Psychology* (suppl.), **10**, pp. 4–11.

Analyzing twin resemblance in multisymptom data: genetic applications of a latent class model for symptoms of conduct disorder in juvenile boys (Eaves, L.J., Silberg, J.L. Hewitt, J.K, Rutter, M., Meyer, J.M., Neale, M.C. & Pickles, A.). *Behavior Genetics*, **23**, 5–19.

Assessment of psychosocial experiences in childhood: methodological issues and some illustrative findings (Sandberg, S., Rutter, M., Giles, S., Owen, A., Champion, L., Nicholls, J. & Prior, V.). *Journal of Child Psychology and Psychiatry*, **34**, 879–897.

Autism: syndrome definition and possible genetic mechanisms (Rutter, M., Bailey, A., Bolton, P. & Le Couteur, A.). In *Nature, Nurture, and Psychology* (eds R. Plomin & G.E. McClearn), pp. 269–284. Washington, DC: APA Books.

Cause and course of psychopathology: some lessons from longitudinal data (Rutter, M.). *Paediatric and Perinatal Epidemiology*, **7**, 105–120.

Child and adult depression: a test of continuities with data from a family study (Harrington, R.C., Fudge, H., Rutter, M.L., Bredenkamp, D., Groothues, C. & Pridham, J). *British Journal of Psychiatry*, **162**, 627–633.

Developmental psychopathology as a research perspective (Rutter, M.). In *Longitudinal Research on Individual Development: Present Status and Future Perspectives* (eds D. Magnusson & P. Casaer), pp. 127–152. Cambridge: Cambridge University Press.

Genes, personality, and psychopathology: a latent class analysis of liability to symptoms of attention-deficit hyperactivity disorder in twins (Eaves, L., Silberg, J., Hewitt, J.K., Meyer, J., Rutter, M., Simonoff, E., Neale, M. & Pickles, A.). In *Nature, Nurture, and Psychology* (eds R. Plomin & G.E. McClearn), pp. 285–303. Washington, DC: APA Books.

How informative are twin studies of child psychopathology? (Rutter, M., Simonoff, E. & Silberg, J.). In *Twins as a Tool of Behavioral Genetics* (eds T.J. Bouchard Jr. & P. Propping), pp. 179–194. Chichester: John Wiley & Sons.

Partners, peers, and pathways: assortative pairing and continuities in conduct disorder (Quinton, D., Pickles, A., Maughan, B. & Rutter, M.). *Development and Psychopathology*, **5**, 763–783.

Prevalence of the fragile X anomaly amongst autistic twins and singletons (Bailey, A., Bolton, P., Butler, L., Le Couteur, A., Murphy, M., Scott, S., Webb, T. & Rutter, M.). *Journal of Child Psychology and Psychiatry*, **34**, 675–688.

Resilience: some conceptual considerations (Rutter, M.). *Journal of Adolescent Health*, **14**, 626–631. Translation: French, 1994, Mécanismes protecteurs. In *Préadolescence: Théorie, Recherche et Clinique* (eds M. Bolognini, B. Plancherel, R. Nùñez & W. Bettschart). Paris: ESF Editeur.

Thinking and relationships: mind and brain (Rutter, M. & Bailey, A.). In *Understanding Other Minds: Perspectives from Autism* (eds S. Baron-Cohen, H. Tager-Flusberg & D. Cohen), pp. 481–504. Oxford: Oxford University Press.

Using the ADI-R to diagnose autism in preschool children (Lord, C., Storoschuk, S., Rutter, M. & Pickles, A.). *Infant Mental Health*, **14**, 234–252.

Whither behavior genetics? A developmental psychopathology perspective (Rutter, M., Silberg, J. & Simonoff, E.). In *Nature, Nurture, and Psychology* (eds R. Plomin & G.E. McClearn), pp. 433–456. Washington, DC: APA Books.

1994   Books and monographs

Development through Life: A Handbook for Clinicians (eds M. Rutter & D. Hay). Oxford: Blackwell Scientific.

Stress, Risk and Resilience in Children and Adolescents: Processes, Mechanisms and Interventions (eds R.J. Haggerty, L.R. Sherrod, N. Garmezy & M. Rutter). New York, NY: Cambridge University Press.

1994   Papers and book chapters

A case control family history study of autism (Bolton, P., Macdonald, H., Pickles, A., Rios, P., Goode, S., Crowson, M., Bailey, A. & Rutter, M.). *Journal of Child Psychology and Psychiatry*, **35**, 877–900.

A simple method for censored age-of-onset data subject to recall bias: mothers' reports of age of puberty in male twins (Pickles, A., Neale, M., Simonoff, E., Rutter, M., Hewitt, J., Meyer, J., Crouchley, R., Silberg, J. & Eaves, L.). *Behavior Genetics*, **24**, 457–468.

Abnormal psychosocial situations: preliminary results of a WHO and a German multicenter study (van Goor-Lambo, G., Orley, J., Poutska, F. & Rutter, M.). *European Child and Adolescent Psychiatry*, **3**, 229–241.

Adult outcome of conduct disorders in childhood: implications for concepts and definitions of patterns of psychopathology (Rutter, M., Harrington, R., Quinton, D. & Pickles, A.). In *Adolescent Problem Behaviors: Issues and Research* (eds R. Ketterlinus & M. Lamb), pp. 57–80. Hillsdale, NJ: Lawrence Erlbaum.

Adult outcomes of childhood and adolescent depression. III. Links with suicidal behaviours (Harrington, R., Bredenkamp, D., Groothues, C., Rutter, M., Fudge, H. & Pickles, A.). *Journal of Child Psychology and Psychiatry*, **35**, 1309–1319.

Autism and known medical conditions: myth and substance (Rutter, M., Bailey, A., Bolton, P. & Le Couteur, A.). *Journal of Child Psychology and Psychiatry*, **35**, 311–322.

Autism diagnostic interview revised: a revised version of a diagnostic interview for caregivers of individuals with possible pervasive developmental disorders (Lord, C., Rutter, M. & Le Couteur, A.). *Journal of Autism and Developmental Disorders*, **24**, 659–685.

Beyond longitudinal data: causes, consequences, changes and continuity (Rutter, M.). *Journal of Consulting and Clinical Psychology*, **62**, 928–940.

Concepts of causation, tests of causal mechanisms and implications for intervention (Rutter, M.). In *Youth Unemployment and Society* (eds A.C. Petersen & J.T. Mortimer), pp. 147–171. New York, NY: Cambridge University Press.

Family discord and conduct disorder: cause, consequence or correlate? (Rutter, M.). *Journal of Family Psychology*, **8**, 170–186.

Field trial for autistic disorder in DSM-IV (Volkmar, F., Klin, A., Siegel, B., Szatmari, P., Lord, C., Campbell, M., Freeman, B.J., Cicchetti, D. & Rutter, M.). *American Journal of Psychiatry*, **151**, 1361–1367.

La résilience: quelques considérations théoretiques (Rutter, M.). In *Préadolescence: Théorie, Recherche et Clinique* (eds M. Bolognini, B. Plancherel, R. Nùñez & W. Bettschart), pp. 147–158. Paris: ESF Editeur.

Poor readers in secondary schools (Maughan, B., Hagell, A., Rutter, M. & Yule, W.). *Reading and Writing: An Interdisciplinary Journal*, **6**, 125–150.

Psychiatric genetics: research challenges and pathways forward (Rutter, M.). *American Journal of Medical Genetics (Neuropsychiatric Genetics)*, **54**, 185–198.

Stress research: accomplishments and tasks ahead (Rutter, M.). In *Stress, Risk, and Resilience in Children and Adolescent* (eds R.J. Haggerty, L.R. Sherrod, N. Garmezy & M. Rutter), pp. 354–385. New York, NY: Cambridge University Press.

Survival models for developmental genetic data: age of onset of puberty and antisocial behavior in twins (Pickles, A., Crouchley, R., Simonoff, E., Eaves, L., Meyer, J., Rutter, M., Hewitt, J. & Silberg, J.). *Genetic Epidemiology*, **11**, 155–170.

Temperament: changing concepts and implications (Rutter, M.). In *Prevention and Early Intervention: Individual Differences as Risk Factors for the Mental Health of Children* (eds W.B. Carey & S.C. McDevitt), pp. 23–24. New York, NY: Brunner/Mazel.

The application of structural equation modeling to maternal ratings of twins' behavioral and emotional problems (Silberg, J., Erickson, M., Meyer, J., Eaves, L., Rutter, M. & Hewitt, J.). *Journal of Consulting and Clinical Psychology*, **62**, 510–521.

1995 Books and monographs

Psychosocial Disorders in Young People: Time Trends and their Causes (eds M. Rutter & D. Smith, D.). Chichester: John Wiley & Sons.

Psychosocial Disturbances in Young People: Challenges for Prevention (ed. M. Rutter). Cambridge: Cambridge University Press.

1995 Papers and book chapters

A 15–20 year follow-up of adult psychiatric patients. Psychiatric disorder and social functioning (Quinton, D., Gulliver, L. & Rutter, M.). *British Journal of Psychiatry*, **167**, 315–323.

Autism as a strongly genetic disorder: evidence from a British twin study (Bailey, A., Le Couteur, A., Gottesman, I., Bolton, P., Simonoff, E., Yuzda, E. & Rutter, M.). *Psychological Medicine*, **25**, 63–77.

Autism, mental retardation, multiple exostoses and short stature in a female with 46,X,t(X;8)(p22.13;q22.1) (Bolton, P., Powell, J., Rutter, M., Buckle, V., Yates, J.R.W., Ishikawa-Brush, Y. & Monaco, A.P.). *Psychiatric Genetics*, **5**, 51–55.

Behavioural problems in childhood and stressors in early adult life: a twenty year follow-up of London school children (Champion, L.A., Goodall, G. & Rutter, M.). *Psychological Medicine*, **25**, 231–246.

Childhood disintegrative disorder: results of the DSM-IV autism field trial (Volkmar, F. & Rutter, M.). *Journal of the American Academy of Child and Adolescent Psychiatry*, **34**, 1092–1095.

Clinical implications of attachment concepts: retrospect and prospect (Rutter, M.). *Journal of Child Psychology and Psychiatry*, **36**, 549–571.

Latent class analysis of recurrence risk for complex phenotypes with selection and measurement error: a twin and family history study of autism (Pickles, A., Bolton, P., Macdonald, H., Bailey, A., Le Couteur, A., Sim, L. & Rutter, M.). *American Journal of Human Genetics*, **57**, 717–726.

Multiple raters of disruptive child behavior: using a genetic strategy to examine shared views and bias (Simonoff, E., Pickles, A., Hewitt, J., Silberg, J., Rutter, M., Loeber, R., Meyer, J., Nerale, M. & Eaves, L.). *Behavior Genetics*, **25**, 311–326.

Psychosocial adversity: risk, resilience and recovery (Rutter, M.). *Southern African Journal of Child and Adolescent Psychiatry*, **7**, 75–88.

Relationship between mental disorders in childhood and adulthood (Rutter, M.). *Acta Psychiatrica Scandinavica*, **91**, 73–85.

The adult personality functioning assessment (APFA): factors influencing agreement between subject and informant (Hills, J., Fudge, H., Harrington, R., Pickles, A. & Rutter, M.). *Psychological Medicine*, **25**, 263–275.

The child and adolescent psychiatric assessment (CAPA) (Angold, A., Prendergast, M., Cox, A., Harrington, R., Simonoff, E. & Rutter, M.). *Psychological Medicine*, **25**, 739–753.

The Pre-Linguistic Autism Diagnostic Observation Schedule (PL-ADOS) (Di Lavore, P.C., Lord, C. & Rutter, M.). *Journal of Autism and Developmental Disorders*, **25**, 355–379.

To what extent can children with autism understand desire? (Phillips, W., Baron-Cohen, S. & Rutter, M.).*Development & Psychopathology*, **7**, 151–169.

Understanding individual differences in environmental risk exposure (Rutter, M., Champion, L., Quinton, D., Maughan, B. & Pickles, A.). In *Examining Lives in Context: Perspectives on the Ecology of Human Development* (eds P. Moen, G.H. Elder Jr. & K. Lüscher), pp. 61–93. Washington, DC: American Psychological Association.

1996   Papers and book chapters

A broader phenotype of autism: the clinical spectrum in twins (Le Couteur, A., Bailey, A.J., Goode, S., Pickles, A., Robertson, S., Gottesman, I. & Rutter, M.). *Journal of Child Psychology and Psychiatry*, **37**, 785–801.

An update on the status of the Rutter parents' and teachers' scales (Elander, J. & Rutter, M.). *Child Psychology and Psychiatry Review*, **1**, 31–35.

Autism research: prospects and priorities (Rutter, M.). *Journal of Autism and Developmental Disorders* (special issue), **26**, 257–275.

Autism: towards an integration of clinical, genetic, neuropsychological and neurobiological perspectives (Bailey, A., Phillips, W. & Rutter, M.). *Journal of Child Psychology and Psychiatry Annual Review*, **37**, 89–126.

Commentary: risk mechanisms in development: some conceptual and methodological considerations (O'Connor, T. & Rutter, M.). *Developmental Psychology* (special issue), **32**, 787–795.

Concepts of antisocial behaviour, of cause and of genetic influences (Rutter, M.); Concluding Remarks (Rutter, M.). In *Genetics of Criminal and Antisocial Behaviour (Ciba Symposium No. 194.)* (eds G. Bock & J. Goode), pp. 1–15 & pp. 26–271. Chichester: John Wiley & Sons.

Developmental pathways in depression: multiple meanings, antecedents, and endpoints (Harrington, R., Rutter, M. & Fombonne, E.). *Development and Psychopathology*, **8**, 601–616.

Developmental psychopathology as an organizing research construct (Rutter, M.). In *The Lifespan Development of Individuals: Behavioral, Neurobiological and Psychosocial Perspectives* (ed. D. Magnusson), pp. 394–413. Cambridge & New York, NY: Cambridge University Press.

Developmental psychopathology: concepts and prospects (Rutter, M.). In *Frontiers of Developmental Psychopathology* (eds M.F. Lenzenweger & J. Haugaard), pp. 209–237. New York, NY: Oxford University Press.

Family trends and children's futures (Rutter, M.). In *The Child in the World of Tomorrow: The Next Generation* (eds S. Nakou & S. Pantelakis). Oxford: Pergamon.

Genetic and environmental influences on the covariation between hyperactivity and conduct disturbance in juvenile twins (Silberg, J., Rutter, M., Meyer, J., Maes, H., Hewitt, J., Simonoff, E., Pickles, A., Loeber, R. & Eaves, L.). *Journal of Child Psychology and Psychiatry*, **37**, 803–816.

Genetic influences on mild mental retardation: concepts, findings and research implications (Rutter, M., Shonkoff, E. & Plomin, R.). *Journal of Biosocial Science* (special issue), **28**, 509–526.

Head circumference and pervasive developmental disorder (Woodhouse, W., Bailey, A., Rutter, M., Bolton, P., Baird, G. & Le Couteur, A.). *Journal of Child Psychology and Psychiatry*, **37**, 785–801.

Heterogeneity among juvenile antisocial behaviours: findings from the VTSABD (Silberg, J., Meyer, J., Pickles, A., Simonoff, E., Eaves, L., Hewitt, J., Maes, H. & Rutter, M.). In *Genetics of Criminal and Antisocial Behaviour (Ciba Symposium No. 194.)* (eds G. Bock & J. Goode), pp. 76–86. Chichester: John Wiley & Sons.

Mental retardation: genetic findings, clinical implications and research agenda (Simonoff, E., Bolton, P. & Rutter, M.). *Journal of Child Psychology and Psychiatry*, **37**, 259–280.

Precision, reliability and accuracy in the dating of symptom onsets in child and adolescent psychopathology (Angold, A., Erkanli, A., Costello, E.J. & Rutter, M.). *Journal of Child Psychology and Psychiatry*, **37**, 657–664.

Reading problems and antisocial behaviour: developmental trends in comorbidity (Maughan, B., Pickles, A., Hagell, A., Rutter, M. & Yule, W.). *Journal of Child Psychology and Psychiatry*, **37**, 405–418.

Specificity of brain–behavioural relationships revisited: from epileptic personality to behavioural phenotypes (Rutter, M. & Yule, W.). In *Children, Research and Policy* (eds B. Bernstein & J. Brannen), pp. 29–46. London: Taylor & Francis.

The genetics of children's oral reading performance (Reynolds, C.A., Hewitt, J.K., Erickson, M.T., Silberg, J.L., Rutter, M., Simonoff, E., Meyer, J. & Eaves, L.J.). *Journal of Child Psychology and Psychiatry*, **37**, 425–434.

Transitions and turning points in developmental psychopathology: as applied to the age span between childhood and mid-adulthood (Rutter, M.). *International Journal of Behavioral Development*, **19**, 603–626.

Use and development of the Rutter parents' and teachers' scales (Elander, J. & Rutter, M.). *International Journal of Methods in Psychiatric Research*, **6**, 63–78.

1997   Books and monographs

Behavioral Genetics (3rd edn) (Plomin, R., DeFries, J.C., McClearn, G.E. & Rutter, M.). New York, NY: W.H. Freeman.

1997   Papers and book chapters

A family study of autism: cognitive patterns and levels in parents and siblings (Fombonne, E., Bolton, P., Prior, J., Jordan H. & Rutter, M.). *Journal of Child Psychology and Psychiatry*, **38**, 667–683.

Afterword: maternal depression and infant development: cause and consequence; sensitivity and specificity (Rutter, M.). In *Postpartum Depression and Child Development* (eds L. Murray & P.J. Cooper), pp. 295–315. New York, NY: Guilford Press.

Antisocial behavior: developmental psychopathology perspectives (Rutter, M.). In *Handbook of Antisocial Behavior* (eds D. Stoff, J. Breiling & J.D. Maser), pp. 115–124. New York, NY: John Wiley & Sons.

Autism and other behavioral disorders (Simonoff, E. & Rutter, M.). In *Emery and Rimoin's Principles and Practice of Medical Genetics (3rd edn)* (eds D.L. Rimoin, J.M. Connor & R.E. Pyeritz), pp. 1791–1806. New York, NY: Churchill Livingstone International.

Commentary: child psychiatric disorder: measures, causal mechanisms, and interventions (Rutter, M.). *Archives of General Psychiatry*, **54**, 785–789.

Comorbidity: concepts, claims and choices (Rutter, M.). *Criminal Behaviour and Mental Health*, **7**, 265–286.

Genetic and environmental influences on child reports of manifest anxiety and symptoms of separation anxiety and overanxious disorders: a community-based twin study (Topolski, T.D., Hewitt, J.K., Eaves, L.J., Silberg, J.L. Meyer, J.M., Rutter, M., Pickles, A. & Simonoff, E.). *Behavior Genetics*, **27**, 15–28.

Genetic influences and autism (Rutter, M., Bailey, A., Simonoff, E. & Pickles, A.). In *Handbook of Autism and Pervasive Developmental Disorders (2nd edn)* (eds D.J. Cohen & F.R. Volkmar), pp. 370–387. New York, NY: John Wiley & Sons.

Genetics and developmental psychopathology: 1. Phenotypic assessment in the Virginia twin study of adolescent behavioral development (Hewitt, J.K., Silberg, J.L., Rutter, M., Simonoff, E., Meyer, J.M., Maes, H., Pickles, A., Neale, M.C, Loeber, R., Erickson, M.T., Kendler, K.S., Heath, A.C., Truett, K.R., Reynolds, C.A. & Eaves, L.J.). *Journal of Child Psychology and Psychiatry*, **38**, 943–963.

Genetics and developmental psychopathology: 2. The main effects of genes and environment on behavioral problems in the Virginia twin study of adolescent behavioral development (Eaves, L.J., Silberg, J.L., Meyer, J.M., Maes, H.H., Simonoff, E., Pickles, A., Rutter, M., Neale, M.C., Reynolds, C.A., Erickson, M.T., Heath, A.C., Loeber, R., Truett, K.R. & Hewitt, J.K.). *Journal of Child Psychology and Psychiatry*, **38**, 965–980.

Heterogeneity of antisocial behavior: causes, continuities and consequences (Rutter, M., Maughan, B., Meyer, J., Pickles, A., Silberg, J., Simonoff, E. & Taylor, E.). In *Nebraska Symposium on Motivation: Vol. 44: Motivation and Delinquency* (eds R. Dienstbier & D.W. Osgood), pp. 45–118. Lincoln, NE: University of Nebraska Press.

Implications of genetic research for child psychiatry (Rutter, M.). *Canadian Journal of Psychiatry*, **42**, 569–576.

Integrating nature and nurture: implications of person–environment correlations and interactions for developmental psychopathology (Rutter, M., Dunn, J., Plomin, R., Simonoff, E., Pickles, A., Maughan, B., Ormel, J., Meyer, J. & Eaves, L.). *Development and Psychopathology* (special issue), **9**, 335–366.

Molecular and cytogenetic investigations of the fragile X region including the FRAX A and FRAX E CGG trinucleotide repeat sequences in familes multiplex for autism and related phenotypes (Gurling, H.M.D., Bolton., P.F., Vincent, J., Melmer, G. & Rutter, M.). *Human Heredity*, **47**, 254–262.

Nature–nurture integration: the example of antisocial behavior (Rutter, M.). *American Psychologist*, **52**, 390–398.

Obstetric complications in autism: consequence or causes of the condition? (Bolton, P., Murphy, M., Macdonald, H., Whitlock, B., Pickles, A. & Rutter, M.). *Journal of the American Academy of Child and Adolescent Psychiatry*, **36**, 272–281.

Opportunities for psychiatry from genetic findings (Rutter, M. & Plomin, R.). *British Journal of Psychiatry*, **171**, 209–219.

Psychiatric disorders in the relatives of depressed probands. I. Comparison of prepubertal, adolescent and early adult onset cases (Harrington, R., Rutter, M., Weissman, M., Fudge, H., Groothues, C., Bredenkamp, D., Pickles, A., Rende, R. & Wickramaratne, P.). *Journal of Affective Disorders*, **42**, 9–22.

Psychiatric disorders in the relatives of depressed probands. II. Familial loading for comorbid non-depressive disorders based upon proband age of onset (Rende, R., Weissman, M., Rutter, M., Harrington, R., Pickles, A. & Wickramaratne, P.). *Journal of Affective Disorders*, **42**, 23–28.

Psychosocial adversities in childhood and adult psychopathology (Rutter, M. & Maughan, B.). *Journal of Personality Disorders*, **11**, 4–18.

Retrospective reporting of childhood adversity: issues in assessing long-term recall (Maughan, B. & Rutter, M.). *Journal of Personality Disorders*, **11**, 19–33.

The Virginia twin study of adolescent behavioral development: influences of age, sex, and impairment in rates of disorder (Simonoff, E., Pickles, A., Meyer, J., Silberg, J.L., Maes, H.H., Loeber, R., Rutter, M., Hewitt, J.K. & Eaves, L.J.). *Archives of General Psychiatry*, **54**, 801–808.

1998 *Books and monographs*

Antisocial Behaviour by Young People (Rutter, M., Giller, H. & Hagell, A.). Cambridge: Cambridge University Press.

1998 *Papers and book chapters*

A clinicopathological study of autism (Bailey, A., Luthert, P., Dean, A., Harding, B., Janota, I., Montgomery, M., Rutter, M. & Lantos, P.). *Brain*, **121**, 889–905.

A comparative study of Greek children in long-term residential group care: I. Social, emotional and behavioural effects (Vorria, P., Rutter, M., Pickles, A., Wolkind, S. & Hobsbaum, A.). *Journal of Child Psychology and Psychiatry*, **39**, 225–236.

A comparative study of Greek children in long-term residential group care: II. Possible mediating mechanisms (Vorria, P., Rutter, M., Pickles, A., Wolkind, S. & Hobsbaum, A.). *Journal of Child Psychology and Psychiatry*, **39**, 237–245.

■333

A full genome screen for autism with evidence for linkage to a region on chromosome 7q (International Molecular Genetic Study of Autism Consortium) (Rutter, M.). *Human Molecular Genetics*, **7**, 517–578.

Assortative mating for major psychiatric diagnoses in two population-based samples (Maes, H.H.M., Neale, M.C., Kendler, K.S., Hewitt, J.K., Silberg, J.L., Foley, D.L., Meyer, J.M., Rutter, M., Simonoff, E., Pickles, A. & Eaves, L.J.). *Psychological Medicine*, **28**, 1389–1401.

Autism, affective and other psychiatric disorders: patterns of familial aggregation (Bolton, P.F., Pickles, A., Murphy, M. & Rutter, M.). *Psychological Medicine*, **28**, 385–395.

Child development, molecular genetics, and what to do with genes once they are found (Plomin, R. & Rutter, M.). *Child Development*, **69**, 1223–1242.

Continuities and discontinuities in antisocial behavior from childhood to adult life (Maughan, B. & Rutter, M.). In *Advances in Clinical Child Psychology, Vol. 20* (eds T.H. Ollendick & R.J. Prinz), pp. 1–47. New York, NY: Plenum Press.

Developmental catch-up, and deficit, following adoption after severe global early privation (Rutter, M. and the English & Romanian Adoptees Study Team). *Journal of Child Psychology and Psychiatry*, **39**, 465–476.

Diagnosing autism: analyses of data from the autism diagnostic interview (Volkmar, R., Klin, A., Siegel, B., Szatmari, P., Lord, C., Campbell, M., Freeman, B.J., Cicchetti, D.V. & Rutter, M.). In *DSM–IV Source Book. Vol. 4* (eds T.A. Widiger & A.J. Frances), pp. 607–624. Washington, DC: American Psychiatric Association.

Genetic influences on childhood hyperactivity: contrast effects imply parental rating bias, not sibling interaction (Simonoff, E., Pickles, A., Silberg, J., Rutter, M. & Eaves, L.). *Psychological Medicine*, **28**, 825–837.

Genetic perspectives in mental retardation (Simonoff, E., Bolton, P. & Rutter, M.). In *Handbook of Mental Retardation and Development* (eds J. Burack, R. Hodapp & E. Zigler), pp. 41–79. New York, NY: Cambridge University Press.

Genotype–environment correlations in late childhood and early adolescence: antisocial behavioral problems and coercive parenting (O'Connor, T.G., Deater-Deckard, K., Fulker, D., Rutter, M. & Plomin, R.). *Developmental Psychology*, **34**, 970–981.

Independence of childhood life events and chronic adversities: a comparison of two patient groups and controls (Sandberg, S., McGuinness, D., Hillary, C. & Rutter. M.). *Journal of American Academy of Child and Adolescent Psychiatry*, **37**, 728–735.

Individual differences and levels of antisocial behavior (Rutter, M.). In *Biosocial Bases of Violence* (eds A. Raine, D. Farrington, P. Brennan & S.A. Mednick). New York, NY: Plenum.

Intergenerational continuities and discontinuities: some research considerations (Rutter, M.) In Commentary, Special Section, (eds L.A. Serbin & D. M.Stack). *Developmental Psychology*, **34**, 1269–1273.

Practitioner review: routes from research to clinical practice in child psychiatry: retrospect and prospect (Rutter, M.). *Journal of Child Psychology and Psychiatry*, **39**, 805–816.

Retrospective recall recalled (Rutter, M., Maughan, B., Pickles, A. & Simonoff, E.) In *The Individual in Developmental Research: Essays in Honor of Marian Radke Yarrow* (eds R.B. Cairns & P.C. Rodkin), pp. 219–243. Thousand Oaks, CA: Sage.

The validity of parent-based assessment of the cognitive abilities of two-year-olds (Saudino, K.J., Dale, P.S., Oliver, B., Petrill, S.A., Richardson, V., Rutter, M., Simonoff, E., Stevenson, J. & Plomin, R.). *British Journal of Developmental Psychology*, **16**, 349–363.

Understanding intention in normal development and in autism (Phillips, W., Baron-Cohen, S. & Rutter, M.). *British Journal of Developmental Psychology*, **16**, 337–348.

1999 *Papers and book chapters*

Attachment disturbances and disorders in children exposed to early severe deprivation (O'Connor, T., Bredenkamp, D. & Rutter, M. with the ERA study team). *Infant Mental Health Journal*, **20**, 10–29.

Autism screening questionnaire: diagnostic validity (Berument, S.K., Rutter, M., Lord, C., Pickles, A. & Bailey, A.). *British Journal of Psychiatry*, **175**, 444–451.

Autism: two-way interplay between research and clinical work (Emanuel Miller Memorial Lecture 1998) (Rutter, M.). *Journal of Child Psychology and Psychiatry*, **40**, 169–188.

Effects of qualities of early institutional care on cognitive attainment (Castle, J., Groothues, C., Bredenkamp, D., Beckett, C., O'Connor, T., Rutter, M. & the ERA study team). *American Journal of Orthopsychiatry*, **69**, 424–437.

Genes and behaviour: health potential and ethical concerns (Rutter, M.). In *Inventing Heaven – Quakers Confront the Challenge of Genetic Engineering* (eds C. Skidmore & A. Carroll), pp. 66–88. Reading: Sowle Press.

Genetic and environmental influences on ratings of manifest anxiety by parents and children (Topolski, T.D., Hewitt, J.K., Eaves, L., Meyer, J.M., Silberg, J.L., Simonoff, E. & Rutter, M.). *Journal of Anxiety Disorders*, **13**, 371–397.

Genetics and child psychiatry: I. Advances in quantitative and molecular genetics (Rutter, M., Silberg, J., O'Connor, T. & Simonoff, E.). *Journal of Child Psychology and Psychiatry*, **40**, 3–18.

Genetics and child psychiatry: II. Empirical research findings (Rutter, M., Silberg, J., O'Connor, T. & Simonoff, E.). *Journal of Child Psychology and Psychiatry*, **40**, 19–55.

Implications of attachment theory for child care policies (Rutter, M. & O'Connor, T). In *Handbook of Attachment* (eds J. Cassidy & P. Shaver), pp. 823–844. New York, NY: Guilford Press.

Preventing anti-social behaviour in young people: the contribution of early intervention (Rutter, M.). In *Transforming Children's Lives: The Importance of Early Intervention* (ed. R. Bayley), pp. 21–25. London: Family Policy Studies Centre.

Psychosocial adversity and child psychopathology (Rutter, M.). *British Journal of Psychiatry*, **174**, 480–493.

Quasi-autistic patterns following severe early global privation (Rutter, M., Anderson-Wood, L., Beckett, C., Bredenkamp, D., Castle, J., Groothues, C., Kreppner, J., Keaveney, L., Lord, C & O'Connor, T). *Journal of Child Psychology and Psychiatry*, **40**, 537–549.

Resilience concepts and findings: implications for family therapy (Rutter, M.). *Journal of Family Therapy*, **21**, 119–144.

Social context: meanings, measures and mechanisms (Rutter, M.). *European Review*, **7**, 139–149.

The influence of genetic factors and life stress on adolescent female depression (Silberg, J., Pickles, A., Rutter, M., Hewitt, J., Simonoff, E., Maes, H., Carbonneau. R., Murelle, L., Foley. D & Eaves, L.). *Archives of General Psychiatry*, **56**, 225–232.

Tobacco, alcohol and drug use in 8–16 year old twins (Maes, H.H., Woodard, C.E., Murrelle, L., Meyer, J.M., Silberg, J.L., Hewitt, J.K., Rutter, M., Simonoff, E., Pickles, A., Carbonneau, R., Neale, M.C., Eaves, L.J.). *Journal of Studies on Alcohol*, **60**, 293–305.

2000 Papers and book chapters

Attachment disorder behavior following early severe deprivation: extension and longitudinal follow-up (O'Connnor, T., Rutter, M. & the ERA Study Team) *Journal of the American Academy of Child and Adolescent Psychiatry*, **39**, 703–712.

Autism and developmental receptive language disorder – a comparative follow-up in early adult life: I. Cognitive and language outcomes (Mawhood, L., Howlin, P. & Rutter, M.). *Journal of Child Psychology and Psychiatry*, **41**, 547–559.

Autism and developmental receptive language disorder – a comparative follow-up in early adult life: II. Social, behavioural and psychiatric outcomes (Howlin, P., Mawhood, L. & Rutter, M.). *Journal of Child Psychology and Psychiatry*, **41**, 561–578.

Children in substitute care: some conceptual considerations and research implications (Rutter, M.). *Children and Youth Services Review*, **27**, 685–703.

Complementary approaches to the assessment of personality disorder: the Personality Assessment Schedule and Adult Personality Functioning Assessment compared (Hill, J., Fudge, H., Harrington, R., Pickles, A. & Rutter, M.). *British Journal of Psychiatry*, **176**, 434–438.

Developmental catch-up, and deficit, following adoption after severe global early privation (Rutter, M. and the English & Romanian Adoptees Study Team). In *The Nature-Nurture Debate: The Essential Readings* (eds S.J. Ceci & W.M. Williams). Oxford: Blackwell.

Developmental psychology: concepts and challenges (Rutter, M. & Sroufe, A.). *Development and Psychopathology*, **12**, 265–296.

Explanations for apparent late onset criminality in a high risk sample of children followed up in adult life (Elander, J., Rutter, M., Simonoff, E. & Pickles, A.). *British Journal of Criminology*, **40**, 497–509.

Familial aggregation for conduct disorder symptomatology: the role of genes, marital discord and family adaptability (Meyer, J.M., Rutter, M., Silberg, J.L., Maes, H.H., Simonoff, E., Shillady, L.L., Pickles, A., Hewitt, J.K. & Eaves, L.J.). *Psychological Medicine*, **30**, 759–774.

Genetic studies of autism: from the 1970s into the millennium (Rutter, M.). *Journal of Abnormal Child Psychology*, **28**, 3–14.

Institutional care: risk from family background or pattern of rearing? (Roy, P., Rutter, M. & Pickles, A.). *Journal of Child Psychology and Psychiatry*, **41**, 139–149.

Introduction (Rutter, M.); Closing remarks (Rutter, M.). In *The Nature of Intelligence: Novartis Symposium 233* (eds G. Bock, J. Goode & K. Webb), pp. 1–5 & pp. 281–287. Chichester: John Wiley & Sons.

Longitudinal study of adolescent and adult conviction rates among children referred to psychiatric services for behavioural or emotional problems (Elander, J., Simonoff, E., Pickles, A., Holmshaw, J. & Rutter, M.). *Criminal Behaviour and Mental Health*, **10**, 40–59.

Negative life events and family negativity: accomplishments and challenges (Rutter, M.). In *Where Inner and Outer Worlds Meet: Psychosocial Research in the Tradition of George W. Brown* (ed. T. Harris), pp. 123–149. London: Routledge.

Personality traits of the relatives of autistic probands (Murphy, M., Bolton, P.F., Pickles, A., Fombonne, E., Piven, J. & Rutter, M.) *Psychological Medicine*, **30**, 1411–1424.

Psychosocial influences: critiques, findings and research needs (Rutter, M.). *Development and Psychopathology*, **12**, 375–405.

Recovery and deficit following profound early deprivation (Rutter, M., O'Connor, T., Beckett, C., Castle, J., Croft, C., Dunn, J., Groothues, C. & Kreppner, J.). In *Inter-Country Adoption: Developments, Trends and Perspectives* (ed. P. Selman), pp. 107–125. London: British Association for Adoption and Fostering.

Research into practice: future prospects (Rutter, M.). In *Speech and Language Impairment in Children: Causes, Characteristics, Intervention and Outcome* (eds D.V.M. Bishop & L.B. Leonard), pp. 273–290. Hove: Psychology Press.

Resilience reconsidered: conceptual considerations and empirical findings (Rutter, M.). In *Handbook of Early Childhood Intervention* (eds J. Schonkof & S. Meisels), pp. 651–682. Cambridge: Cambridge University Press.

The ADOS–G (Autism Diagnostic Observation Schedule – Generic): a standard measure of social and communication deficits associated with the spectrum of autism (Lord, C., Risi, S., Lambrecht, L., Cook, E.H., Leventhal, B.L., DiLavore, P., Pickles, A. & Rutter, M.). *Journal of Autism and Developmental Disorders*, **30**, 205–223.

The Awkward Moments test: a naturalistic measure of social understanding in autism (Heavey, L., Phillips, W., Baron-Cohen, S. & Rutter, M.). *Journal of Autism and Developmental Disorders*, **30**, 225–236.

The effects of global severe privation on cognitive competence: extension and longitudinal follow-up (O'Connor, T., Rutter, M., Beckett, C., Keaveney, L., Kreppner, J., and the ERA study team). *Child Development*, **71**, 376–390.

Variable expression of the autism broader phenotype: findings from extended pedigrees (Pickles, A., Starr, E., Kazak, S., Bolton, P., Papanikolau, K., Bailey, A.J., Goodman, R. & Rutter, M.). *Journal of Child Psychology and Psychiatry*, **41**, 491–502.

2001 Books and monographs

Guidelines for Researchers and for Research Ethics Committees on Psychiatric Research Involving Human Participants (Rutter, M.). Council Report CR82. London: Gaskell.

2001 Papers and book chapters

Antisocial children grown up (Maughan, B. & Rutter, M.). In *Conduct Disorders in Childhood and Adolescence* (eds J. Hill & B. Maughan), pp. 507–552. Cambridge: Cambridge University Press.

Comparison of multiple measures of ADHD symptomatology: a multivariate genetic analysis (Nadder, T.S., Silberg, J.L., Maes, H.H., Rutter, M. & Eaves, L.). *Journal of Child Psychology and Psychiatry*, **42**, 475–486.

Conduct disorder: future directions. An afterword (Rutter, M.). In *Conduct Disorders in Childhood and Adolescence* (eds J. Hill & B. Maughan), pp. 553–572. Cambridge: Cambridge University Press.

Development and current functioning in adolescents with Asperger syndrome: a comparative study (Gilchrist, A.C., Green, J.M., Cox, A.D., Burton, D., Rutter, M. & LeCouteur, A.). *Journal of Child Psychology and Psychiatry*, **42**, 227–240.

Do high threat life events really provoke the onset of psychiatric disorder in children? (Sandberg, S., Rutter, M., Pickles, A, McGuinness, D. & Angold, A.). *Journal of Child Psychology and Psychiatry*, **42**, 523–532.

Prevalence and developmental course of "secret language" (Thorpe, K., Greenwood, R., Eivers, A. & Rutter, M.). *International Journal of Language and Communication Disorders*, **36**, 43–62.

Psychosocial adversity: risk, resilience and recovery (Rutter, M.). In *The Context of Youth Violence: Resilience, Risk and Protection* (eds J. Richman & M.W. Fraser), pp. 13–41. Westport, CT: Praeger.

In press Books and monographs

Sorting Out Sex Differences in Antisocial Behavior: Findings from the First Two Decades of the Dunedin Longitudinal Study (Moffitt, T., Caspi, A., Rutter, M. & Silva, P.). Cambridge: Cambridge University Press.

In press Papers and book chapters

A family genetic study of autism associated with profound mental retardation (Starr, E., Berument, S.K., Pickles, A., Tomlins, M., Bailey, A., Papanikolau, E. & Rutter, M.). *Journal of Autism and Developmental Disorders*.

Autism and other behavioral disorders (Simonoff, E. & Rutter, M.). In *Emery and Rimoin's Principles and Practice of Medical Genetics, 4th Edn* (ed. D.L. Rimoin). London: Churchill Livingstone.

Child psychiatric symptoms and psychosocial impairment: relationship and prognostic significance (Pickles, A., Rowe, R., Simonoff, E. & Rutter, M.). *British Journal of Psychiatry*.

Child psychiatry in the era following sequencing the genome (Rutter, M.). In *Attention, Genes and ADHD* (eds F. Levy & D. Hay). Hove: Brunner-Routledge.

Family influences on behavior and development: challenges for the future (Rutter, M.). In *Retrospect and Prospect in the Psychological Study of Families* (eds J. McHale & W. Grolnick Hillsdale). Hillsdale, NJ: Lawrence Erlbaum.

Genetic and environmental causes of variation in interview assessments of disruptive behavior in adolescent twins (Eaves, L., Maes, H., Rutter, M. & Silberg, J.L.). *Behavior Genetics*.

Genetic moderation of environmental risk for depression and anxiety in adolescent girls (Silberg, J., Rutter, M., Neale, M. & Eaves, L.). *British Journal of Psychiatry*.

Specificity and heterogeneity in children's responses to profound privation (Rutter, M., Kreppner, J., O'Connor, T. & ERA Study Team). *British Journal of Psychiatry*.

Testing hypotheses on specific environmental risk mechanisms for psychopathology (Rutter, M., Pickles, A., Murray, R. & Eaves, L.). *Psychological Bulletin*.

The development of a brief screening measure of emotional disturbance in children (Parker, G., Yiming, C., Tan, S. & Rutter, M.). *Journal of Child Psychology and Psychiatry*.

The emergence of developmental psychopathology (Rutter, M.). In *Psychology in Britain: Historical Essays and Personal Reflections* (eds G.C. Bunn, A.D. Lovie & G.D. Richards), pp. 422–432. London: British Pyschological Society.

Twins as a natural experiment to study the causes of language delay: report to the Mental Health Foundation (Rutter, M., Thorpe, K., Golding, J., Greenwood, R. & North, K). London: Mental Health Foundation.

Index

Compiled by Linda English